# Prescription for Healthy Weight Loss & Optimum Health

**A Lifelong Winning Strategy**

- **A New Way of Eating & Physical Activity Habits for Long-Term Weight & Body Fat Reduction**
- **Antioxidants & Anti-inflammatory Foods**
- **30 Day Meal Plan & Recipes—Good Taste & Simplicity**
- **Efficient Weight Loss of 8-10 lbs/month or More**
- **Healthy Fast Food Choices**
- **Control Diabetes, Cholesterol, Syndrome X**
- **Effective Control of Craving & Overeating**

Optimal Health to you, Karen.

**Bill C. Johnson, MD, PhD**
**and Daniel Chong-Jimenez, B.S.**

Billy C. Johnson MD. Ph.D

Llumina Press

This book is intended as a source of information only, not as a medical manual. The information presented in this book is designed to help you make informed decisions about your health and quality of life. The book is not considered a substitute for the advice of a qualified medical professional that must always be consulted before beginning any health program, such as diet and exercise. It is not intended as a substitute for any treatment prescribed by your physician. Always consult with your medical provider for advice and help regarding any recommendation in this book.

In writing this book, all efforts have been made to ensure that the information contained in this book is accurate as of the date published. The author and publisher expressly disclaim responsibility for any adverse effects that may come about from the use of the information given in this book.

Mention of specific organizations, companies, or institutions in this book does not imply endorsement by the author and publisher, nor does mention of specific organization, companies, or institution imply an endorsement by them.

Some of the names of contributors and participants in this book have been changed to protect their privacy and identity.



FIRST EDITION

Johnson, Billy C.
The Prescription for Healthy Weight Loss and Optimum Health/ by Billy C. Johnson and Daniel Chong-Jimenez – 1st ed.



ISBN: 1-59526-391-8 PB
1-59526-392-6 E-Book

Printed in the United States of America by Llumina Press

Library of Congress Control Number: 2006924706

*Dedicated to my friends, teachers, and family who have diligently helped to mold and shape my life – mentally and spiritually:*

*Professor James F. Preston, Ph.D., My Doctorate Research Adviser, Department of Cell & Molecular Biology, University of Florida, Gainesville, FL.*

*The late Eduard Friedrich, MD. Chairman, Department of Obstetrics & Gynecology, University of Florida Medical School, Gainesville, FL.*

*Professor Linda Morgan, MD. Director of Gynecology Oncology, University of Florida Medical School, Gainesville, FL.*

*Professor Leon Tancer, MD. Former Chairman, Department of Obstetrics & Gynecology, Maimonides Medical Center, Brooklyn, NY.*

*Professor Norma Perez Veridiano, MD, JP. Chairman, Department of Obstetrics & Gynecology, Brookdale Medical Center, Brooklyn, NY.*

*Professor Nick Khulpateea, MD. Director, Gynecology & Oncology, Coney Island Medical Center, Brooklyn, NY.*

*Professor Sushma Nakra, MD. Department of Obstetrics & Gynecology, Coney Island Medical Center, Brooklyn, NY.*

*The late Rev. Edwin King – a great mentor and teacher.*

*My late brother, Francis BobRay, Plainfield, NJ – the most gentle, kind, and compassionate person that I have ever known. His invaluable guidance and insight greatly contributed to my growth as a person.*

*My beloved mother, Mary K. Johnson, who made all things possible. She taught me to be humble, caring, and to be loving even of those undeserving. Most of all, she taught me to believe in myself.*

# CONTENTS

# ACKNOWLEDGEMENTS

I would like to thank the host of people from all walks of life whose knowledge, dedication, and discipline contributed to the development of the UDP Weight Loss and Wellness Program. When I began my research five years ago, I underestimated the amount of work and sacrifice it would take to complete the project. My curiosity and research began with a personal quest to find better and benign ways to control my diabetes and cholesterol. My findings were simple but profound and powerful: we as physicians can all be more successful in preventing and combating diseases if we teach our patients to take care of their own health, rather than prescribing health for them.

I wanted to prove this point. Those who helped me through the years are so many that it's impossible to mention all of them by name. It could not have been done without them.

No work would be complete without sincere appreciation for the researchers that unselfishly dedicate their life to the pursuit of knowledge that would benefit humanity.

In this regards, my greatest respect and admiration goes to Dr. Simopoulos. Her research and writings got me interested in the role of Omega-3 fatty acids and their impact on our mental and physical health.

My thanks go to Chef Dan and to all the people who contributed their recipes and support. The makeover and use of these recipes allowed the individualization of the UDP program into an effective one that offers more than just recipes and boring meal plans.

My sincere thanks go to Michael Peterson, Penny Graves, Sophy Hernandez, Clara Ramirez, and the Rev. Budu Shannon – they all contributed their kindness and support.

I'm grateful for the support and counsel from Edward Pezzelli and family, Sharon Adler, Diane Metralis, Cheryl Gouveia, Karen Brill, Therese Vezeridis, J. Maggiacomo, Dorothy Gregari, Dr. G. Jackson, Idriss Kay, Rev. N. Friday, Dr. B. Hannah, Dr. Carmen Sanchez, Marino DeLa Cruz, Al Madrid, D. Stewart, W. Sanders, Dr. A Johnson, Dr. D. Disano, Monty and Carol Monteiro, and Jeannine Dugas.

Barbara Morse Silva from NBC Channel 10 became the first to give us media exposure in 2003. That broadcast got Rhode Islanders to discover UDP in a big way. I am grateful to the network and Barbara.

Pat Masters from CBS Channel 12 also helped to get the word on UDP to the New England audience, and I'm deeply grateful.

Deborah Greenspan and the Llumina team were very professional and resourceful.

The entire NESPA team has been invaluable for resources and support.

Thanks, also, for the editorial work of Melissa Chiavaroli from Barnes & Noble.

Finally, the book would not have been completed without the support of family and friends – Carolyn, Chevon, Michael, Genevieve, Rose, Clinton, Sara, Lorina, Hillary,

Bill Johnson

Sylvester, Aman, Evans, Alexie, R. Kekular, T. Beer, O. Barrolle, P. Woodtor, T. Anittye, M. Roberts, M. Tolbert, Dr. R. Sherman, J. Bass, Dr. J. Boyce, Dr. D. Asase, Adelaide, Dr. L. Pham, Ruth Phillips, Dr. K. Allen, Chris Ziplin, Dr. R. Griggs, Dr. D. Mosier, Dr. Rita Luthra, Dr. Kurt Jones, J. Kamara, T. Carter, Clemenceau Urey, Rev. Clinton BobRay and Father Johnson.

Billy C. Johnson, MD, PhD.

# DAN'S ACKNOWLEDGEMENTS

This work has been long in coming and was the brainchild of Dr. Billy Johnson---he deserves my greatest gratitude for this accomplishment. The support and dedication of my wife, Rosa, and our three children was invaluable, especially during the winters of New England. A special note of gratitude for Joseph Benedetto, and to all UDP members past, present, and future--- thank you for the privilege of serving you.

Daniel Chong-Jimenez, B.S

# INTRODUCTION

## Finding a Different Path

In the course of my work as an obstetrician/gynecologist, I had very little interest in nutrition and its impact on health and weight – but that all changed over the years. In the beginning, I began to see many patients who were struggling with weight problems. My interest became more personal and urgent when my older brother, who was diabetic, suddenly died from a heart attack. Shortly afterwards, I learned that I too had diabetes, high cholesterol, and was twenty pounds overweight.

In desperation and fear of sharing my brother's fate, I began to research my condition extensively. To my surprise, neither my PhD. in molecular biology nor my MD. had prepared me to clearly understand how my physical activity and food choices affected my weight, mood, personality, concentration, and overall health.

Over the last five years, I have learned a great deal – and my life has changed quite a bit. My cholesterol is normal without medication and I only occasionally need minimal medication for my blood sugar. My weight and percent body fat are within the normal, healthy range. My energy is great and stress level is low.

I have applied my knowledge and understanding to help my patients lose weight and improve the quality of their lives. Now, I want to share this unique experience with you.

When I started to develop this program five years ago, I wanted something that would be so simple and safe that even a child could understand. This program would be designed to solve the problems of craving, compulsive eating, and, at the same time, guarantee long-term success. First and foremost, the program needed to be centered on improving health as well as effective weight loss that can be maintained for life. And it should not be expensive to maintain either.

The program should focus on proper nutrients and antioxidants instead of just calories. And, most importantly, it should help people tailor food and carbohydrate intake to the individual level of activity.

I wanted a program that addressed the real needs of ordinary people of different ethnic backgrounds so that everyone could still eat foods that taste good without the feeling of being on a diet. To achieve this goal, participants should be encouraged to have direct input in the development of their own individualized program.

I wanted a program that had no rigid guidelines to follow and was simple and flexible enough that the individual felt good and wanted to maintain it for life. I envisioned a program that was not a fad diet or a quick fix or a one-size-fits-all approach. It was to be a program of integrity that taught a proper way of eating that an entire family could benefit from, including the children. It was to be a total lifestyle program that integrated proper nutrition, physical activity, and stress reduction. More importantly, I wanted a program that could help to prevent or halt the medical complications of Syndrome X, diabetes, heart disease, high blood pressure, and other serious chronic degenerative diseases that could affect the quality of life.

I wanted to design a better program that had the best chance of succeeding, allowing even those who had failed other programs to succeed. It had to be flexible, yet well-structured and individualized enough that a person could get the one-on-one attention and support and counseling that so empowers.

I wanted a program in which people could eat and enjoy real grocery foods anywhere they chose: at home, in restaurants, or even in fast food places. The program could not be restrictive and needed to give the individual broader latitude to choose the foods they liked to eat. They should not feel the need to diet to succeed. Above all, the program was to teach people new and better ways to eat (such as how to make a better breakfast and also improve the quality of foods they normally eat).

All of these and more is what the UDP Weight Loss and Wellness program represents.

## Carbohydrates and the Weight Loss Connection

Our brain and muscle cells depend on carbohydrates for fuel. Without adequate amounts of carbohydrates, our muscle tissue is replaced by fat, which slows down our metabolism, spurs inflammation, and weakens the body's immune system. Also, our ability to think and focus is impaired.

Our body converts carbohydrates into blood sugar (glucose), which is used to fuel the body's energy need. Insulin aids the entry of glucose into muscles and body cells, thereby regulating the expenditure and storage of fat. Under normal conditions, there is a healthy balance between fat stored and fat burned. For instance, muscle tissue that is physically active is able to burn calories and carbohydrates more quickly and efficiently, so only a minimal amount of fat is stored. In contrast, physically inactive muscle tissue burns calories and carbohydrates slowly. As a result, large amounts of fat are stored.

Furthermore, the muscles and cells of people who are physically inactive resist insulin's signal to absorb glucose from the blood, causing high and dangerous levels of glucose in the circulatory system – a condition that can encourage the body to store fat. This condition is known as insulin resistance syndrome or Syndrome X. Syndrome X predisposes an individual to the development of diabetes, heart disease, and cancer.

In this book, you will learn that the capacity of your body to use calories and carbohydrates is regulated by your muscles and body cells, which, in turn, depend on your level of physical activity. As you might expect, the more active you are, the more calories and carbohydrates you need and vice versa. A change in your activity level must be followed by appropriate adjustments in your calories and carbohydrate intake on a daily basis. This is the core of the UDP program. It is very easy to do and is fully discussed in Chapter 14.

## Low-Carbohydrate Diets Promote Short-Term Weight Loss

There is no question that low-carbohydrate diets promote short-term weight loss but studies show that most people on low-carbohydrate diets begin to regain the weight they have lost after six months. This may be due to the fact that when they start eating carbohydrates again, they are not tailoring their intake to their level of activity. As a result, carbohydrate is readily converted into fat, which leads to weight gain. Studies comparing the low-carbohydrate diets and the traditional low-fat, low calorie diets also show that in the long run, it is calories that matter. These findings are consistent with the UDP eating plan. But we go even further and promote nutrients and antioxidants first and calories second.

## Too Restrictive

Low-carbohydrate and high-carbohydrate diets are too extreme and are based on the one-size-fits-all approach, which assumes that every individual is the same. They are severely restrictive and limit the amount of carbohydrates you eat regardless of your level of physical activity and special medical conditions. This is the simple reason why most people fail.

Low-carbohydrate diets that are not in line with your level of activity may in fact pose obstacles to high-energy performance and physical activity, both of which have many health benefits, including the development of healthy bones, muscles, and joints. Restricting carbohydrates can cause intense cravings and fatigue as well as emotional and psychological problems. The feeling of deprivation can sabotage your best efforts to reach your goal weight.

## Tailor Carbohydrates to Your Level of Physical Activity

The ultimate solution is to tailor your food, particularly carbohydrate intake, to your level of physical activity – as this will solve the problem most people face on strict low-carbohydrate or high-carbohydrate diets. Throughout this book, I will talk about the connection between physical activity and food, particularly carbohydrates.

It is not required that you eat the same amount of carbohydrates at each meal, but that you adjust your carbohydrate intake on a meal-to-meal basis according to your level of physical activity. Making these appropriate adjustments on a consistent basis will allow you to eat the carbohydrates of your choice (such as bread, pasta, rice, and fruits) and feel satisfied, not deprived. This is what makes the UDP approach superior to the low-carbohydrate or high-carbohydrate diets that encourage you to eat a specific amount of carbohydrates, regardless of your level of physical activity. As a result, most of us either eat too many carbohydrates or too few.

## The Glycemic Index

It is not enough to choose low glycemic carbohydrates. The glycemic index (GI), which measures how quickly carbohydrates turn into blood sugar, can be misleading. It does not differentiate between foods that have nutritional value and those that do not. For example, white bread has a higher glycemic index than sugar, with very little nutritional value. To solve this problem, the glycemic load (GL) was introduced, but it too has a problem. The glycemic load takes into consideration the carbohydrate content in a serving of food, but it cannot accurately separate the good carbohydrates from the bad ones consistently. Neither does it address the amount and quality of fat in foods – all of which can influence the GL. For example, the glycemic load of a baked potato is 26 and that of ice cream is 8. Does this mean that ice cream is better for you than a baked potato? Definitely not!

## More About the UDP Program and Its Individualized Approach

Finding your own level of comfort and the best means to reach and maintain a healthy weight and optimum health takes a personal level of commitment and challenge. The UDP plan meets this challenge by involving you in every aspect of the program (such as participation in creating a shopping list, the development of a meal plan, and the inclusion of your own recipes). In addition, you will receive support that will enable you to individualize the program into a format that is best for you.

## A New Way to Make Grocery Foods Better (Designing a Better Quality of Foods)

The UDP program is designed to help you eat and enjoy food again *(Most people are not born with food issues, they develop them)*. It empowers you so that you can control what you eat, how much you eat, and enables you to choose the foods that you prefer. Most grocery foods, including packaged and canned foods, are not nutritionally complete. If they are complete, they are usually not satisfying. In this book, you will learn how to take your favorite grocery foods and redesign them into foods that are healthier and more satisfying. The process begins with breakfast – you will see how it's done in Chapter 2.

## 30-Day Meal Plan

You will have at your convenience a detailed shopping list of food choices (including ethnic foods) that can be found in your local grocery store. In Chapters 15 and 16, we provide a 30-day meal plan consisting of delicious recipes, some of which were submitted by our patients and local restaurants for makeover. We also include recipes by Chef Dan to make your experience a culinary delight. The meal plans are designed to meet your energy and nutritional needs, to balance macronutrients (carbohydrates, fats, and proteins), to attain a healthy ratio of Omega-6 to Omega-3 fatty acids, and to provide an adequate amount of antioxidants, phytonutrients, vitamins, minerals, and fiber while keeping the levels of saturated fats, trans fats, cholesterol, and sodium low.

**No Deprivation**

The UDP program emphasizes good carbohydrates, good fats, lean proteins, Omega-3 and Omega-6 fatty acids, vegetables, fruits, and legumes. Unlike other programs, we do not eliminate certain types of foods that are considered "bad." You can incorporate them occasionally (or whenever you choose) even at the initial stages of the program. Eating only smaller portions in combination with healthier foods can greatly enhance their nutritional quality. The result is that you maintain the flavor and taste while eating the foods you like.

**No Starvation**

Food is what keeps us alive and functioning. We need to eat more healthy foods that provide nutrients, antioxidants, and fiber. Starvation does not only cause fat storage, but low energy, fatigue, and poor concentration. It also causes muscle loss, which, in turn, depresses body metabolism. For some of you that have been afraid to eat, the UDP program will teach you to begin eating again. Food provides enormous gratification. It does not only satisfy our energy needs, but it also provides for our emotional needs as well. That's why you are encouraged to eat to fullness and not be bogged down with counting calories.

**Vitamins**

Vitamins and minerals are necessary if you are not eating a vast variety of foods, especially vegetables and fruits. The basic ones we recommend are: good multivitamin and mineral supplements, Omega-3 fatty acids (fish oil and flaxseed oil), and a B-complex.

**Success Stories**

In Chapter 18, you will read the stories of people who have lost and gained weight so many times in the past and have finally found the solution to permanent weight loss and optimum health. Some have successfully reduced or completely come off medications with harmful side effects for various medical problems (such as diabetes, high blood pressure, arthritis, high cholesterol, high triglycerides, high inflammatory markers, and high hemocysteine levels). All have found a new and personal way of eating and have a great new look and energy to show for it. Nothing helps results like being able to see them in your mirror.

## Starting the UDP Program

Cravings and emotional eating usually improve within the first few weeks. The UDP program focuses on maximizing fat loss and preservation of muscle mass. As a result, physical appearance as well as energy is greatly improved within a short period of time.

You are now ready to start the UDP program.
Remember, the results will last a lifetime.

Billy C. Johnson, MD, PhD.
March 2006

# Chapter 1

# The Essentials

This chapter deals with the A-B-C's of losing weight and maintaining your weight loss. You will need a basic blueprint in order to develop your personalized plan using the tools you will learn from the UDP program.

This chapter explores the recommendations that I make when patients begin the UDP program. The more closely you stick to these recommendations, the better the results will be. I advise you to read this chapter over and over and to consult other references for in-depth information. After reading this chapter, you should be on your way to controlling your weight and improving your health. Your energy will soar and you will feel good.

The process of losing weight and maintaining the weight loss begins with a desire to make healthy lifestyle changes. This should involve changing bad habits, such as smoking or excessive drinking. The bottom line is that you must make some sacrifices. Anyone who promises weight loss without lifestyle changes is lying to you. Remember, the weight did not creep up on you overnight and it is not going to disappear overnight. There are no quick fixes. If you are not ready and willing to make the lifestyle changes required in order to get the results you desire, you will not succeed. I can promise you, however, that if you follow my recommendations, your weight loss will be impressive.

Let's begin!

## The Basics You Need to Succeed

Normally, you lose weight when you burn more calories and energy than you take in. But, in reality, it is more complex than that. The same formula does not work for everyone. No two people are alike. No two people have the same problems. However, there are some basic things that anyone can do to increase his or her chance of losing weight and keeping it off. These include:

- **Proper Nutrition:** Make proper food choices most of the time – the right food choices can boost metabolism, whereas the wrong food choices can depress it. You also need to eat food, particularly carbohydrates, in line with your level of physical activity. And eat your biggest meals when your metabolism is up (breakfast and lunch) and less when your metabolism is down (dinner).
- **Exercise:** Keep physically active most of the day (exercise or physical activity raises metabolism and prevents fat storage and loss of muscle and bone when tailored to food intake).

- **Relaxation and Meditation:** The stress hormone cortisol is a major factor in fat storage and weight gain. Reduction of cortisol through relaxation and meditation can benefit both the body and mind.

Now, let's explain these recommendations:

## Proper Nutrition

The foundation of healthy weight loss is proper diet. Approximately 80 percent of successful weight loss and maintenance depends upon eating right, which means making the right food choices – foods that satisfy and nourish the body and increase metabolic rate. Most importantly, it is vital that you eat food, particularly carbohydrates (the body's primary energy source), in line with your level of activity on a meal-to-meal basis. Once you get accustomed to making these adjustments, it is then possible to eat the right amount of food that satisfies your physical and emotional needs.

The UDP program is designed to help you develop your own individualized meal plan based on your own weight loss goal and medical conditions. To ensure your success, you are provided with a shopping list that includes a preferred list of foods that are anti-inflammatory and non-fattening. There are also those foods that are cautionary and are potentially inflammatory and fattening.

If you enjoy cooking, you will find delicious recipes packed with flavor and nourishment for making meals that are healthy and delicious while at the same time helping you to lose weight. Planning ahead makes it easier to select foods that are low in calories and unhealthy fats but rich in nutrients and antioxidants.

Eating in restaurants, including fast-food restaurants, requires some thought and knowledge. Chapter 13 will guide you to make better choices when eating out.

Controlling your portion size is vital to weight loss. Too many calories, even from healthy foods, can cause fat storage and weight gain. Likewise, too few calories are not compatible with health. Therefore, it is only by eating the right amount of food that your body needs that can help you lose weight. Various techniques have been employed in this book to help you control your portion sizes so that you get the maximum amount of nutrients that your body needs.

The right vitamins, essential fatty acids (Omega-3 and Omega-6), and mineral supplements can help transform food into energy and repair and revitalize your body. They can help you accomplish your weight goal, burn fat, increase muscle tone, and restore stamina, memory, and libido. Some vitamins, such as E and C, are powerful antioxidants. They can help destroy free radicals that damage cells.

## Exercise

A regular level of physical activity or exercise can help you lose weight, decrease stress, boost the immune system, reduce risk of certain diseases including heart disease, stroke, diabetes, high blood pressure, and certain cancers, such as breast cancer and colon cancer. It also helps to develop healthy bones, muscles, and joints.

Exercise has a positive effect on our brains and virtually every cell and organ in our bodies. Inactivity, on the other hand, is a major cause of fat storage, weight gain, loss of muscle and bone, decreased energy, and poor health. Chapter 14 describes in detail a simple plan for incorporating regular exercise into your life and, most importantly, it outlines how to tailor your caloric and carbohydrate intake to your level of physical activity on a meal-to-meal basis. In this way, even a small amount of regular exercise can produce significant results that encourage you to stay the course.

**Relaxation and Meditation**

Stress is a normal part of life, but it is abnormal to have chronic stress or a feeling of anger, fear, nervousness, or resentment over a prolonged period of time. It can trigger excessive amounts of cortisol, which can cause food craving, insulin resistance, fat storage, weight gain, and inflammation. Cortisol is a powerful stress hormone that can increase appetite and, along with insulin, store fat in the belly area, causing a greater risk of heart disease and diabetes. Prolonged high levels of cortisol can weaken the immune system, which may increase your risk of illness.

Chronic stress raises abnormal levels of cortisol that can affect virtually any part of the body, leading to severe mental and emotional breakdown – headache, dizziness, aches, heart palpitations, fatigue, indigestion, and problems with concentration and sleeping.

*Dorothy, who had type 2 diabetes, soon realized that she was unable to control her blood sugar levels or more or less lose weight the weeks she was under severe stress. She ached all over and had difficulty sleeping. Interestingly, she gained body fat but lost muscle tissue. Cortisol is a well-known hormone that is released in large amounts in the body during severe stress. It can trigger a cascade of chemical reactions throughout the body, causing the release of sugar from muscles and tissues into the blood stream. It can also trigger the appetite and overwork the internal organs, including the brain, liver, and digestive systems. Dorothy understood better when she knew the physical reaction her body was having anytime she was under too much stress. She had much better success when she learned to deal with stress.*

*For instance, any time she felt bad and depressed and didn't let it bother her to the point of negativity, she realized that she could rebound quicker and move on. This, in turn, rewarded her with normal blood sugar readings.*

Researchers also believe chronic stress can lead to poor lifestyle habits, such as smoking, drinking, eating too much, or failing to exercise. All of which can lead to weight gain as a result of emotional eating and the too-busy-to-exercise lifestyle under high levels of stress.

You should recognize what causes your stress and avoid or eliminate these factors completely instead of devoting all of your time and energy to them. Also, learn to cope or reduce the intensity of your emotional reaction to stress – meaning, don't overreact. A practical way to reduce your stress is to learn how to relax in a quiet environment with music. We also promote using meditation tapes. Other methods to resolve stress include deep breathing, exercise, self-hypnosis, or walking away from the situation (just to name a few).

Meditation and simply learning to relax can help you to manage your daily stress more effectively. This will help you to lose weight and keep it off for good. Remember, you may fail to lose weight or to maintain your weight loss if you fail to deal with stress properly. Your health could also be compromised.

## Metabolism

Metabolism is the key. In basic terms, metabolism is the process through which the body converts food and nutrients into energy that is used for various functions, such as bodily repair, walking, talking, etc. Some people are born lucky with a fast metabolism, whereas others are born with a slow metabolism. One thing is certain, the more fat you have in your body, the lower your metabolism. On the contrary, the more muscle tissue you have, the higher your metabolism. Since muscle consumes more energy than fat tissue, people with a lower percent body fat can afford to eat more and not gain weight. On the other hand, it is very easy for an obese person or someone with a higher percent body fat to gain weight if they eat only slightly more than their body requires, especially if they are inactive.

You can assume that your metabolism is slow if you always feel tired, cold, or your skin is dry, pulse is slow, blood pressure is low, and your energy is low most of the time. However, these symptoms could be due to a medical condition that needs attention, rather than a slow metabolism.

The good news is that you can improve your body metabolism by keeping physically active and eating foods that are rich in healthy fats and unprocessed carbohydrates that give a favorable blood sugar and insulin response.

Eating increases metabolism, whereas fasting and extreme dieting decrease it. That is why skipping meals or crash diets often fail to lower body weight permanently. Although you may lose weight initially, this weight loss is due largely to breakdown of muscle tissue rather than fat. As a result, your metabolism drops significantly and a slower metabolism makes it difficult to keep the weight from returning.

Our body metabolism also slows down with age under the influence of cortisol and insulin. Cortisol levels are elevated during chronic stress, starvation, and inactivity, whereas insulin levels are raised by diets high in refined carbohydrates and simple sugars, such as sodas, white bread, white flour pasta, chronic stress, and inactivity.

### Focus on Losing Fat and Not Weight

There are subtle physical signs that would suggest that you are losing muscle instead of body fat: sunken eyes, saggy skin, loss of skin tone and radiance, loss of hair, and brittle nails. And in general, you may look worn out, tired, and not feeling healthy due to lack of energy and sleep. This is the reason why it is important for you to measure your body fat, along with your muscle mass and total weight, weekly to see first-hand the direction in which your body is changing. Remember, your weight consists of both body fat and body mass (muscle, bones, and organs). And losing muscle, instead of excess body fat, is probably the number one reason people regain lost weight so quickly.

You should be concerned if you are losing muscle and gaining fat, as this can depress your metabolism and cause more weight gain. On the other hand, you should not be concerned if your weight changes very little but there is a significant reduction in body fat while muscle mass remains the same or increases (see Tony's testimonial in Chapter 18). This concept is difficult for people who are used to relying on the scale alone to understand and appreciate their progress. One of the best and most accurate ways to measure your body fat is the Bioelectrical Impedance Analysis (BIA), which you can purchase in health stores.

## Other Aspects of a Successful Weight-Loss Formula

### Setting Goals

Setting realistic goals will help you reach your ideal weight and also improve your health. It does not pay to reach your goal weight and compromise your muscles, bones, and other organs in the process. Be sensible about your weight loss. Your health is more important than the number on the scale. Have both short and long-term goals. For example, a short-term goal might be to lose 1 to 2 pounds a week, to flatten your belly, or to fit into a favorite dress. A long-term goal might be to control your blood pressure, reduce your cholesterol, control your blood sugar, reduce elevated inflammatory markers, or get off medications with adverse side effects.

### Positive Attitude

You must maintain a positive attitude, especially when your weight plateaus. You must engage yourself mentally and physically and maintain an environment that will help you make the lifestyle changes that will enable you to lose weight. Doubting your capabilities can only lead to frustration and failure. Initially, you may not see the results that you anticipate on the scale – because of muscle growth (this is a good thing). You may even know someone who has seen more dramatic results. You should not be discouraged. It may take a little longer for you, but you will reach your goal. Research has shown that even those who have tried many other diets can be successful.

## Know Your Reasons

It is very important to know the reason or reasons why you are trying to lose weight and never lose sight of them. This will give you the motivation to make the necessary lifestyle changes. Your reason could be to improve your overall health, decrease your cholesterol level, and control your blood pressure or combat diabetes. You may be doing it to improve your self-esteem or to improve your energy level and concentration. When faced with temptation, remind yourself of why you are doing this and you will be more likely to make better choices, rather than give in to temptation.

## Recognize the Root Cause of Your Weight Gain

Recognizing the reason or reasons why you are overweight will give you insight into what to do to change your situation. For example, genetic factors play a role in the development of obesity in many people. However, the extent to which genetic factors predispose one to obesity depends upon environmental influences. In other words, just because you're genetically predisposed to obesity does not necessarily mean that you are going to be obese.

When we remove the genetic factors, there are three classes of obese people: those who clearly eat too much, those who eat relatively normal diets but who are not active, and those who eat too much and are also inactive. Some people eat more than they think they do and exercise less than they believe. This may not be a deliberate deception. Most often, these individuals believe their resistance to weight loss is genetic and not due to their own behavior. However, if they were to take the time to record their food intake and physical activity, the truth would be revealed. Such knowledge can help one recognize his or her weaknesses and change behavior if he or she truly wants to succeed.

Some people overeat because of emotional and psychological trauma. Dealing with the trauma can help one make the lifestyle changes that can lead to weight loss. Emotional eaters habitually self medicate with food and, as a result, their choice of food is often poor and their caloric intake is more than what their body can tolerate. They also sabotage their own progress and often develop negative thoughts instead of positive, healthy, and empowering thoughts. Moreover, they see themselves as failures.

If you are an emotional eater, find non-food substitutes for celebration or coping, such as relaxation exercises or reading. Identify emotional triggers and develop practical strategies to deal with them, such as eating a healthy breakfast and mid-afternoon snack instead of skipping meals. Low energy and fatigue can trigger emotional eating.

## Develop a Strategy

Have a plan for getting from Point A to Point B. Your plan should be modified as conditions change and should be updated frequently. This will help you to stay on course.

Plan your meals and daily activities in advance and you will find yourself in control and confident about your choices. For example, prepare a large batch of vegetable soup over the weekend and refrigerate it. Take 1-2 servings to work, add multigrain bread, fruit, vegetables, and a lean, low-fat protein source (tuna, chicken, turkey, or meat) – you have a delicious lunch.

There is danger in going to a party or a restaurant without carefully planning what you intend to eat or drink. When you're invited to a party or to a place where you have no control over what you eat, it is wise to eat at home before you leave. All too often, people find themselves in situations where it is too late to make the right choices.

**Accountability**

Successful weight loss requires a system of accountability; otherwise it is easy to get off course. Keep a daily journal. It may seem like a difficult task but it is necessary for you to take the time to record your daily food intake (portions, frequency of meals, etc.), physical activity, energy, and emotional changes, especially during the first four to six weeks of your program. You will become aware of your strengths and weaknesses and, if you are honest with yourself, you will make the necessary adjustments to help you reach your goal. In a nutshell, behavior modification starts with the daily recording of your food intake and physical activity and the elimination of inappropriate triggers and cues that lead to cravings and overeating.

**Support**

You need a positive environment both at home and at work in order to succeed. Trying to lose weight alone without the support of those close to you is extremely difficult and you are more likely to fail. Having support helps behavior modification, builds confidence, and motivates you to work towards your goal. Having someone to talk to – especially a friend or family member – can truly help you. In an office situation, such as the one UDP provides, the weekly one-on-one counseling and support system is highly beneficial. The involvement of family members and friends is also highly beneficial and worthwhile.

**Limit Alcohol Consumption**

Alcohol plays a major role in fat storage and weight gain. Alcohol, including wine and beer, may be good for the heart, but may not be good for weight loss. Several studies have linked alcohol with health benefits, including preventing heart disease. But the benefits are outweighed by the risks, such as liver disease, high blood pressure, stroke, breast cancer, and brain damage.

Alcohol depresses metabolism and can stimulate your appetite. It also causes mood swings and depression. Yet, most people believe alcohol relieves stress and is good for them. Drinking to reduce stress can become habit-forming, creating alcohol dependency and even more stress.

Social drinking or consuming as little as a half bottle of wine each day can cause memory loss, poor balance, impair mental agility, and even reduce intelligence. Studies involving over 200,000 women showed that social drinking two to five drinks a day can increase the risk of breast cancer by over 20 percent compared with non-drinkers. Other studies showed that drinking two or more beers a day increases the risk of developing gout. Gout is a condition that causes inflammation of the joints, often starting in the feet and toes.

Alcohol (beer, wine, etc.) is a highly refined carbohydrate similar to sugars, candies, and white flour that may raise blood sugar and insulin levels, leading to increased inflammation throughout the body. Inflammation increases your risk of major health problems, including obesity. This will be discussed in detail later.

If you must drink, limit the amount to a few drinks and on weekends. Also, eat some food before you drink as this will help to slow down the absorption of the alcohol into your bloodstream.

## Medications

Some common drugs that most of us consider safe are among those with negative side effects that may cause weight gain and fat storage. These include some medications used to treat depression, anxiety, blood pressure, seizures, and diabetes. Others are steroids, such as prednisone and cortisol, birth control pills, injectable progestin only contraceptive (Depo-Provera), excessive food sweeteners (such as fructose and high fructose corn syrup) that are used in many processed foods, such as sodas, juices, and ice cream.

If you can't lose weight despite honest and consistent effort at eating a proper diet and keeping active, you may have a medical condition that needs professional attention. Perhaps adjustments of your current medications or new ones prescribed by your physician can help you get back on the right track towards your goal weight.

For example, if you are on a high dose birth control pill, ask your gynecologist to prescribe one with lower dose of estrogen and progesterone. Anti-depressants like Celexa are known to cause weight gain, where as Wellbutrin does not. In fact, Wellbutrin is known to promote weight loss in some patients who have been treated with the medication for depression. In addition, Wellbutrin does not depress sexual function like some of the other anti-depressants.

## Motivation

You need to be motivated to succeed at losing weight and keeping it off. I always ask all of my patients what motivates them to want to lose weight. Some give me very poor reasons, but most of them have very sound reasons. For example, a patient who is 58 said she wanted to be around to enjoy her children and grandchildren. Another person said he was concerned about heart disease and diabetes, which was common in his family.

You are more likely to succeed if you are motivated for the right reasons – health, energy, and a desire to enjoy a better quality of life. If you are not motivated, you can be by creating some realistic goals for yourself. State your goals clearly and work towards them. Write your goals in your daily journal and state how you will achieve them. For example, it is more realistic to plan to lose thirty pounds in 3-4 months at a rate of 1-2 lbs a week, instead of 1-2 months at a rate of 5 lbs a week. Some people can do it. But are you willing to push yourself that hard? Unrealistic goals bring failure and sabotage motivation.

# Chapter 2

# The UDP Shopping Guide: Food Labels

## Be Well-Informed

My patients are always asking me to tell them what foods are good for them. What they actually want is a list of the foods they should eat. The purpose of this chapter is to give you the background you need in order to make the right food choices for yourself on a meal-to-meal and day-to-day basis. Remember, the food choices you make can directly affect your mood, energy level, sleep, sex drive, memory, and the overall state of your mind and body. Food can make you feel good and happy or it can make you feel depressed and sick. Knowing the foods that provide the macronutrients your body needs can be a potent weapon in the battle against fat accumulation and inflammation. You need to be familiar with what you are putting into your body day after day.

To help you get started, I will focus on the foods that you need to eat in order to lose body fat, increase your metabolism, strengthen your muscles and bones, elevate your energy level and mood, and repair vital organs. But I want you to know that even the best list of foods is partial. Only by investing the time to experiment on your own will you find the foods that will help ensure weight loss and improve health. Your goal is to personalize your meals as well as your grocery list. In later chapters, you will learn how easy it is to do this. But, before you get to the list of foods in Chapter 3, you need some basic guidelines, which are presented in this chapter. A thorough understanding of food labeling is important in making the right food choices.

## Pay Attention to Food Labels

Federal law requires food manufacturers to provide nutritional information on food labels. This helps you to make healthy food selections. Indeed, this can be the road map to steer you toward the goal of healthy and enjoyable eating. People cannot shop intelligently without knowing how to read food labels, just as they cannot drive safely without the ability to read road signs and maps. Reading and understanding labels will help you reduce your shopping time and prepare the meals on your new diet plan.

When you read food labels, pay close attention to the serving size, the total number of servings per container, the calories in a serving size, and the amount of total fat, saturated fat, cholesterol, sodium, fiber, and sugar. Compare the nutritional facts in the products you select with similar items and select the one that has the best qualities – the lowest number of calories, the lowest amount of saturated fat, cholesterol, sodium, and sugar, and the highest amount of fiber. Use figure 2-1, which is a label for a common breakfast cereal, to practice interpreting food labels. You will find it easy to read and understand.

**Serving Size**

Pay close attention to the serving size and to the number of servings per container. You don't necessarily have to eat the amount of food stated. The amount that you eat should be based on your activity level. I will show you how to figure that out later.

**Calories**

Select foods that are low in calories, but dense in nutrients (whole foods and lean proteins have more nutrients and fiber than refined and highly processed foods). In addition, eat calories in line with your activity level. This is the key to losing weight and keeping it off for good, as well as staying healthy.

**Total Fat in Foods**

You should select products containing 5 grams or less of total fat per ounce when shopping for meat and meat products. For example, a 3-ounce portion of white chicken breast contains about 2 grams of fat, where as pork spareribs of equal portion size may contain 26 grams of fat. This is the reason why it is not all right to choose fatty meat, whole fat dairy products, poultry with skin, and high-fat processed products, particularly if you have high cholesterol or a history of breast cancer, diabetes, and heart disease. Leaner and low-fat cuts of meat have less saturated fat (top round steak, eye round, chuck arm, sirloin loin steak, tip round steak, bottom round steak, and tenderloin steak) and are healthier for you.

Fish and seafood, on the other hand, contain fats that are healthy – and it is all right to have fatty fish like salmon, tuna and mackerel. Their health benefits (including how they help us to lose weight) will be discussed later.

However, it is very important to keep the fat portion in your meal within the range that your body can safely handle. Eating an excessive amount of fat can be counterproductive and cause weight gain. You can prevent this by following simple guidelines: For a 1,300-calorie diet, you should aim for no more than 19 grams of fat per meal and for a 1,600 calorie diet, about 23 grams or less per meal. However, this does not mean that you can't have meals that are a few points above your upper limit of fat intake. The key is to eat foods that are high in fat only once in a while. Then to aim for a lower fat intake most of the time without depriving your body of essential fatty acids that are critical for body functions, including weight loss.

Pay close attention to the fat content of foods and food products. Read food labels to see the amount of fat in a given serving size. This will help you to keep your fat intake within a healthy range.

Considering that some of our favorite foods are loaded with fat makes keeping your fat down a real challenge. For example, a bacon, tomato, and cheese sandwich has about 30 grams of fat; 2 slices of pizza has 21 grams; a grilled porterhouse steak has 29 grams; and Buffalo wings (6) have 33 grams.

**Saturated Fat in Foods**

This type of fat raises cholesterol levels and should be limited. The sources of saturated fat are meats, eggs, butter, and other whole dairy products like yogurt, ice cream, and cheese. Other sources include lard, palm kernel oil, and coconut oil.

Saturated fat intake should be no more than 10 % of total caloric intake per day: About 5 grams or less per meal for a 1,300 calorie diet and about 6 grams or less for a 1,600 calorie diet. A very simple practice that will help you to keep your saturated fat down is to select foods with 7 grams or less of total fat per serving. The higher the total fat of a food item, the more likely it is that the saturated fat will be high. This rule may not apply to fish and seafood because their flesh contains healthy fats. A good thing to always keep in mind is the relationship between fat and portion size. For example, a 6-ounce portion of baked chicken thigh with skin contains twice the amount of total fat and saturated fat (26 grams total fat and 8 grams saturated fat) compared to a 3- ounce portion with skin (13 grams total fat and 4 grams saturated fat). Another important consideration is the location of the fat. The skinless chicken breast usually contains less fat (2 grams per 3-ounce serving) than the wings (17 grams per 3-ounce serving). It is easy to lower your cholesterol if you keep your portion size of meat down, particularly beef and chicken with the skin, and also choose sections of meat that are low in fat.

**Trans Fat (Hydrogenated or Partially Hydrogenated Oils)**

Check the fine print for trans fat, which raises cholesterol levels, and decreases HDL (good) cholesterol. It is probably the type of fat that is most harmful to our bodies. Limit foods made with trans fat or partially hydrogenated oils, such as stick or hard margarine, cookies, processed foods, and fast foods.

New government regulations now require companies to list the amount of trans fat present in food beginning this year. But, you can also estimate the amount of trans fat by adding up the saturated fat, monounsaturated fat, and polyunsaturated fat and then subtracting that amount from the total fat.

**Protein**

The leaner the protein source, the greater the health benefits. The best choices are fish and shellfish, chicken, and turkey breast without the skin, wild game, very lean meats and legumes, such as beans, peas, lentils, and soy. Soy protein is low in cholesterol and saturated fat – and you should aim for at least 25 grams (1 scoop or 3 tbsp soy protein powder) per day to help lower cholesterol and burn body fat. There are some controversies about the role of soy protein isoflavones in breast cancer. The overwhelming body of evidence supports a protective role. However, if you have concerns about breast cancer, you should consult with your physician before using soy products.

You need adequate protein intake to ensure satiety, energy, and muscle integrity. Fish and seafood contain a higher quality of protein than chicken and beef for any given weight. In addition, their flesh is the richest source of essential fatty acids.

To give you an idea, for healthy weight loss and wellness, you will require 24-38 grams of lean protein per meal if you are eating a 1,300-calorie diet. This is the equivalent of 3 to 5 ounces of meat (chicken, turkey, eggs, beans, and beef) per meal. For fatty fish like salmon, this translates to about 3 to 4 ounces and, for lean fish like flounder, 3-6 ounces per meal will suffice. Similarly, for a 1,600-calorie diet, you will need around 24-48 grams of lean protein per meal. This is the equivalent of 3 to 6 ounces of meat per meal (chicken, and beef), and about 3 to 8 ounces of fish per meal. Keep in mind that eggs, soy and beans are also lean protein sources that you can include in your meals.

**Carbohydrates**

Select minimally refined or unprocessed carbohydrates over highly refined ones. If you are inactive, you should select items with less than 45 grams (about 3 serving sizes) or less of carbohydrates per serving most of the time. If you cannot find items that meet your needs, have only half of an equivalent serving. For cereals, select unsweetened whole grain, oats, or oat bran cereals with 5 grams or fewer of sugar per serving and higher than 5 grams of total fiber. For example, a breakfast cereal with 25-30 grams of carbohydrate per serving is a better choice for a sedentary person, than one with 40 grams of carbohydrate. Cereals with soluble fiber are better quality than those without. Choose those with 2 or more grams of soluble fiber per serving. If constipation, reflux, or digestive problems are your concern, cereals with a high amount of insoluble fiber would be best for you.

Breads made with 100% rolled oats, oat bran, multigrain, or 100% whole-wheat are better choices than highly refined white flour bread (Italian, French, croissant, wheat, and hamburger buns). When choosing bread, look for those with 3 grams of fiber or more. The higher the fiber, the better the nutrient quality. You will notice that multigrain breads, 100% whole grain and oat bran usually have more fiber than white flour breads. Also, read food labels carefully for deceptive advertising. For instance, check the ingredient list for words like “whole” or “oats”. A whole grain product should read “whole wheat flour” and not “wheat flour.” Other phrases like “stoned wheat,” “cracked wheat” may not contain whole grain as indicated.

Eat carbohydrates according to your activity level. For a sedentary to slightly active individual on a 1,300-calorie diet, keeping carbohydrate intake around 15-35 grams (1-2 servings) per meal will probably prevent significant insulin spikes and excessive fat storage. For a 1,600-calorie diet, 15-45 grams (1-3 servings) per meal will suffice for those with sedentary to slightly active lifestyles. It is imperative to keep your intake of carbohydrate in the lower range whenever your level of activity is low, and metabolism is down (gradually increases when activity is boosted). This is further explained in Chapter 14.

### Sugar

Sugar is definitely problematic, but there is an easy way around it. Select items with 10 grams (2 teaspoons) or less per serving. Diabetics, pre-diabetics, and sugar-intolerant individuals – such as those with Syndrome X or insulin resistance – should select foods with an even smaller amount per serving. Sugar substitutes like Splenda and Stevia are available and safe. But don't abuse!

### Fiber

Fiber holds the key to cravings, feelings of fullness, and more. Eat more foods containing fiber and you will solve your weight loss problem for good. Look for foods that are high in fiber as opposed to foods that are deficient in fiber. You need 20-35 grams of fiber per day not only to lose weight but also to help reduce cholesterol levels and fight cancer and heart disease. Not all fibers are equal, however. The soluble type (found in a variety of foods such as oat bran, broccoli, Brussel sprouts, asparagus, turnip, cabbage, okra, carrots, grapefruit, oranges, pears, kidney beans, navy beans, black beans, pinto beans, and white beans) binds food like a paste and slows down stomach emptying. The net result means keeping your blood sugar and insulin levels even keel, reducing cholesterol, and reducing craving and hunger between meals – and this leads to a faster and more efficient metabolism.

To reap this benefit, you should aim for at least 3-5 grams of soluble fiber per meal. Besides eating foods that contain soluble fiber, you can have 1 tbsp of Benefiber (*Novartis*) or 2 tsp of Clearly Fiber (*DaVinci Laboratories*) with your meals. 1 tbsp of Benefiber dissolved in liquid delivers 3 grams soluble fiber and 2 tsp of Clearly Fiber delivers 5 grams of soluble fiber. Occasionally gas and bloating may be a problem when using fiber supplements for the first time. Starting with smaller doses initially or using products like Beano and Mylanta may prevent this.

Insoluble fiber (or roughage) is also found in a variety of foods (wheat bran, cabbage, green beans, okra, green peas, kale, spinach, turnip, carrots, peaches, raspberries, strawberries, sweet potato, mushrooms, red beans, lentils, pinto beans, and black-eyed peas). This type of fiber creates bulk that keeps us full – a process that distends the stomach and sends a signal to the brain, curbing the sensation of hunger. In addition, foods that are high in insoluble fiber can provide tremendous relief to those suffering from bowel problems, including constipation and irregularity. The active ingredient in Metamucil is insoluble fiber.

In general, you will probably get enough of the different types of fiber if you eat a variety of plant-based foods that are not overly processed – vegetables, fruits, whole grains, legumes, mushrooms, and high-fiber cereals (such as Fiber One, All-Bran with Extra Fiber, and GOLEAN). Meat, poultry, and dairy products contain no fiber.

**Sodium (Salt)**

Sodium is found mostly in processed foods and fast foods. Select items below 500 mg per serving or below 800 mg per meal or reduce the portion of food that is the main source of sodium. You may even have to lower your salt intake if you have high blood pressure, swelling of the extremities, or premenstrual syndrome (500 mg per meal or 1,500 mg per day). For the average person, the recommendation is no more than 2,300 mg of sodium per day or 1 teaspoon of salt.

**Cholesterol**

This is found mostly in meat, poultry with skin, and whole dairy products. The recommendation is no more than 300 mg daily (the equivalent of one medium egg – which derives its cholesterol from the yellow yolk). To meet this goal, you have to pay attention to the sources of cholesterol, particularly if you have high cholesterol or a history of high blood pressure, diabetes, heart disease, or stroke. In addition to watching foods that contain high amounts of cholesterol, be aware of the other significant sources of cholesterol – foods that are high in saturated fats, refined carbohydrates, and simple sugars.

In fact, only about 30% of the cholesterol in our bloodstream comes directly from the foods that are high in cholesterol. It may surprise you to know that about 70% of our body cholesterol is made in our liver using saturated fats and excess blood sugar derived primarily from bad carbohydrates, such as sweets and refined carbohydrates.

Whole eggs are high in cholesterol, but it is generally believed that their contribution to our blood cholesterol is minimal in comparison to eating meat, cheese, ice cream, whole milk, and butter. If you're at risk, eat eggs from free-range chickens, whose Omega-3 fats are much higher than those found in most commercialized facilities. *Eggland's Best* eggs are reported to be high in Omega-3 fats. However, if your cholesterol remains high even while you are on medication, practicing a proper diet, and exercising regularly, you might want to consider limiting eggs in favor of egg substitutes or soy products.

**How to Pick a Cereal That Is Suitable for Your Body Metabolism**

In this section, I will lead you through the process that I use to select some favorite cereals that will be appropriate for various situations (such as someone who is sedentary or suffers from obesity, Syndrome X, diabetes, heart disease, arthritis, or high blood pressure).

To help you understand the importance of choosing the right breakfast cereals, I will give you some simple examples of cereals with low fiber: *Wheaties* and *Kellogg's* Corn Flakes are quite suitable for athletes and active individuals, but may not be for sedentary individuals. In contrast, *Kellogg's* All-Bran with extra fiber and *Kellogg's* Bran Buds are good for you if you are sedentary because they breakdown to sugar slowly. On the other hand, if you are sedentary and choose to eat breakfast cereals that are quickly digested, such as the Corn flakes or *Wheaties*, you may risk converting carbohydrate into fat and raising your blood cholesterol, including cellular inflammation.

Putting high-octane fuel in a car requiring a regular fuel can certainly destroy the engine. It is not any different for our bodies. People who are sedentary or obese should pick cereals that do not turn to energy quickly and flood the body with too much sugar and calories.

My favorite picks for sedentary, obese individuals, or those with high cholesterol are the oat bran and 100% whole grain rolled oats (such as *Old Fashioned Quaker Oats* and *Hodgson Mill* Oat Bran – not the instant). They are low in sugar and high in total fiber – including soluble and insoluble fiber. As a result, they break down to sugar slowly and thereby provide a steady flow of energy. By contrast, the instant oats that are highly refined break down rapidly and do not provide sustained energy.

A serving of ½ cup uncooked Old Fashioned *Quaker Oats* or Old Fashioned Oats cereal contains 27 grams carbohydrates, 7 grams total fiber (of which 2 grams is soluble fiber). Soluble fiber is responsible for the reduction of cholesterol and the maintenance of a stable blood sugar. However, the fat and protein fractions are low (fat is 2.5 grams and protein is 5 grams). As you can see, the carbohydrate portion is several times higher than the fat or protein. In other words, even though the cereal meets healthy standards, it is still not nutritionally balanced. This is not a very serious problem, however, and I will show you simple tricks to improve the quality of some of your own favorite cereals.

*Kellogg's Raisin Bran* and *Post Shredded Wheat* break down very quickly, causing a blood sugar surge even though they have high fiber. This is one of the reasons why you should not pick a cereal solely based on fiber. For instance, it may contain no soluble fiber. Cereals that are lacking soluble fiber may not be suitable for you if you are physically inactive, obese, or at risk of diabetes and heart disease. To add to the confusion, some cereals with soluble fiber may contain other ingredients that may not necessarily be good for your health.

*Kellogg's Smart Healthy Heart Cereal* is made of oat bran and has 5 grams total fiber and 2 grams soluble fiber. But is it really suitable for those who are obese, sedentary and with medical problems? Let's dissect it: A serving size is 1¼ cup with 49 grams carbohydrates, 17 grams sugar, 2 grams fat, and only 6 grams protein. In addition, it has high fructose corn syrup, corn syrup, polydextrose, and partially hydrogenated soybean oil (these ingredients should alert you about possible health risks). While this may be considered an unhealthy cereal, *Kellogg* does have other brands of cereals that are highly recommended (see Chapter 3).

People often make the mistake of choosing a breakfast cereal based on the fact that it may contain an ingredient known to be healthy. A good example is *Nature's Path Organic Optimum Power Cereal* with flaxseeds. A serving of 1 cup contains 40 grams carbohydrate and 16 grams sugar. If your primary interest is flaxseeds, get a better cereal that contains low sugar and carbohydrate and add 1-2 tbsp of ground flaxseeds.

In the shopping list in Chapter 3, you will have a complete list of recommended breakfast cereals. If you like a cereal that I did not include, use the criteria that is listed in this book to assess whether it meets your nutritional need. Most importantly, you can customize and enhance its nutritional quality. Below is a presentation of a breakfast cereal and the exercise should help you learn to read food labels as well as pick higher quality cereals.

## Reading Nutritional Labels

**Nutrition Facts**

Serving Size: 3/4 cup (30 g)
Servings Per Container: about 12

| Amount Per Serving | Cereal | Cereal + 125 ml of fortified skim milk |
|---|---|---|
| **Calories** | 100 | 140 |
| Calories from fat | 15 | 20 |
| | **% Daily Value**** | |
| **Total Fat** 1.5 g* | 2% | 2% |
| Saturated Fat 0 g | 0% | 0% |
| Polyunsaturated Fat 1.1 g | | |
| Monounsaturated Fat 0.5 g | | |
| **Cholesterol** 0 mg | 0% | 0% |
| **Sodium** 190 mg | 8% | 11% |
| **Total Carbohydrate** 22 g | 7% | 9% |
| Dietary Fiber 7 g | 28% | 28% |
| Sugars 6 g | | |
| **Protein** 4 g | | |
| Vitamin A | 0% | 6% |
| Vitamin C | 0% | 0% |
| Calcium | 2% | 16% |
| Iron | 15% | 15% |

* Amount in cereal. One half cup of skim milk contributes an addtional 40 calories, 65 mg sodium, 6 g total carbohydrates (6 g sugars) and 4 g protein.
** Percent Daily Values are based on a 2,000 calorie diet. Your Daily Values may be higher or lower depending on your calorie needs.

| | Calories: | 2,000 | 2,500 |
|---|---|---|---|
| Total Fat | Less Than | 65g | 80g |
| Sat Fat | Less Than | 20g | 25g |
| Cholesterol | Less Than | 300mg | 300mg |
| Sodium | Less Than | 2400mg | 2400mg |
| Total Carbohydrate | | 300g | 375g |
| Dietary Fiber | | 25g | 30g |

Calories per gram:
Fat 9 • Carbohydrate 4 • Protein 4

A basic analysis will simplify the process of selecting a breakfast cereal that is right for you (Figure 2-1).

**Serving Size**

Serving Size = ¾ cup (a unit of measurement and not necessarily the amount you should eat). Depending upon your energy needs, you may need to eat more or less than the serving size. Understanding this concept is important in controlling your calories and weight. There are 12 servings (units) contained in this package.

**Calories:** Total calories = 100 per serving. When ½ cup of skim milk is added the total calories = 140 per serving.

**Total Fat** = 1.5 g

**Saturated Fat** = 0 g

**Cholesterol** = 0 mg

**Sodium** = 190 mg

**Total Carbohydrate** = 22 g

**Dietary Fiber**= 7 g

**Sugar** = 6 g

**Protein** = 4 g

** **Percent Daily Value:** This is a reference value used on labels that shows you how much of the recommended amount the food provides in one serving. For example, if you are eating 2000 calories a day, one serving of this food gives you 7% of your total carbohydrate and 8% of your total sodium recommendations (see inside box).

*This section lists the recommended daily amount for each nutrient for a 2000-calorie diet and for a 2500-calorie diet. For example, if you're eating 2000 calories, your total fat should be less than 65 grams a day.

**Ingredients:** This section should be checked for items, such as partially hydrogenated oils / trans fat, sugars, fructose, or additives. The ingredients that are listed on top of the list are in greater amount than those listed below.

The example given above is *Nature's Path Organic Flax Plus* – a multi-bran cereal that meets the criteria for a very good cereal. It is made of wholegrain, is high in fiber, low in sugar, and has no synthetic additives or preservatives. I would have liked to know how much of the total fiber is soluble fiber. In spite of that, it's one of the best cold breakfast cereals on the market. The good news is that we can make it even better, so that it is balanced in protein, carbohydrates, fats, and even the all-important soluble fiber. You can apply the same ideas to other foods of your choice once you learn the basic principle discussed below (see Chapter 16 for more information).

## How to Make a Balanced and Healthy Breakfast Cereal

In this exercise, I will demonstrate how easy it is to enhance the nutritional quality of some of your favorite cereals – later, you will see more of this within the meal plans in Chapter 16. The first thing that you should know is that even the best breakfast cereal is incomplete in terms of basic nutrients and macronutrients (such as protein, healthy and essential fatty acids, soluble, and insoluble fibers). Therefore, the practice and technique of making your breakfast cereal as balanced and healthy as can be is a very important one – and can be highly beneficial and rewarding.

For instance, you can increase the protein fraction of any breakfast cereal by adding an ounce or slice of low sodium, lean, smoked salmon, turkey, or chicken breast; ½ scoop of soy protein or whey protein; ½ cup low-fat cottage cheese or mozzarella string cheese; whole egg, 2-3 egg whites, or ½ cup egg beaters. The portion of healthy fats (Omega-3 and Omega-6 fatty acids and monounsaturated fats) can be enhanced by adding 1 tbsp of flaxseed oil, 2 tbsp ground flaxseeds, extra virgin olive oil, macadamia oil, cold-pressed canola oil, 1 tbsp of chopped nuts (such as walnuts, almonds, peanuts, and pecans), or peanut butter.

You can increase the fiber portion by adding 1-2 tbsp of oat bran and wheat germ; 1-2 tbsp unprocessed wheat bran, unprocessed bran or 1-2 tbsp ground flaxseed and fruits (such as berries and apple slices). Fiber supplements, such as Benefiber and Clearly Fiber are also helpful for those not getting enough soluble fiber from whole foods.

The portion size of breakfast cereal that you eat must be based on your activity level and not necessarily on the recommended amount listed on the food label. In other words, you could eat less or more depending upon how active you are at that specific time. This strategy will help prevent carbohydrate overload and excessive insulin release. I have already touched on this subject earlier and Chapter 14 will elaborate further.

Use the shopping list in Chapter 3 to choose the best types of cereals – oat bran or whole grains that are high in fiber (especially soluble fiber), low in sugar and that break down slowly. Eating a good quality cereal that is balanced will help you control food craving and mid-morning mood swings. As a result you will lose weight, body fat, lower your cholesterol, control blood sugar, and increase energy.

## Fat-Free or Low-Fat Foods

The words "fat-free" or "reduced-fat" appearing on a label does not mean that the food in question is calorie free. This is an area of confusion that has led many innocent people to indulge in food items that they never would have used had they known better. Most of us tend to eat a larger quantity of fat-free or low-fat foods assuming that they are low in calories. But it might surprise you that the calories are about the same as in the higher fat product – and, in some cases, they are higher in the reduced fat foods.

**Fat-Free vs. Regular Fat Foods**

| Fat-Free or Reduced Fat | Calories | Regular Fat Foods | Calories |
|---|---|---|---|
| Baked Tortilla Chips, 1 ounce | 110 | Regular Tortilla Chips, 1 ounce | 130 |
| Fat-Free Caramel Topping, 2 Tbsp | 130 | Butterscotch Caramel Topping, 2 Tbsp | 130 |
| Fat-Free Fig Cookie | 70 | Fig Cookie | 50 |
| Premium Nonfat Frozen Yogurt, ½ Cup | 190 | Regular Ice Cream, ½ Cup | 180 |
| Reduced-Fat Breakfast Bar, 1 bar | 140 | Breakfast Bar, 1 bar | 130 |
| Reduced-Fat Chocolate Chip Cookie | 128 | Chocolate Chip Cookie | 136 |
| Reduced-Fat Croissant Rolls, 1 roll | 110 | Regular Croissant Roll, 1 roll | 130 |
| Reduced-Fat Granola Cereal, ¼ Cup | 110 | Granola Cereal, ¼ Cup | 130 |
| Reduced-Fat Ice Cream, ½ Cup | 190 | Regular Ice Cream, ½ Cup | 180 |
| Reduced-Fat Peanut Butter, 2 Tbsp | 190 | Peanut Butter, 2 Tbsp | 190 |

Source: Obesity Research, Vol. 6 Supplement 2 – September 1998

Food manufacturers add sugar and other synthetic sweeteners to compensate for the reduction in fat. Otherwise, the food would be bland and unappealing. Some synthetic sweeteners, like fructose, can stimulate the appetite and make you consume more calories. The more calories you consume the more work you have to do to burn off the calories, otherwise you store fat and gain weight.

A very popular trend today is the low carbohydrate foods that have permeated the marketplace. You have to be very careful with these items too – I will say more about them in Chapter 9. For now, it suffices to say that some of these items may not be as good for your health in the long run as the regular foods. They are often high in unhealthy synthetic sweeteners and fats and are low in fiber.

## Added Sugar in Foods

Pay close attention to the amounts of added sugar in foods. A moderate amount of sugar in your diet is nutritionally healthy, but excessive intake of sugar can lead to tooth decay and weight gain, especially for a person with a sedentary lifestyle. Sugar gets into your diet through many sources, most of which you may not even be aware of. Sugar is added in many forms. White sugar, brown sugar, dextrose, corn syrup, high fructose corn syrup, modified cornstarch, and honey are all alternate names for sugar. While these foods supply "pure energy," their nutritional value is low. Unfortunately, these items are used indiscriminately in processed foods. They are usually included in the ingredients list in very fine print.

Sugar is found in a variety of foods that we consider healthy and consume on a regular basis. For example, some concentrated orange juices have 28 grams of sugar per serving.

Grape juice has 40 grams of sugar per 8 fluid ounce serving and apple cider (which is 100% juice) has 30 grams of sugar per 8 fluid ounces. But if you shop around and read nutritional profiles, you would find the same types of items with reduced sugar content – and these items are certainly better. For example, unsweetened pure cranberry juice (*Mountain Sun*), 100% juice has only 8 grams of sugar and no chemical additives. In contrast, light cranberry juice (*Ocean Spray*) has 10 grams of sugar and other chemical additives, such as fructose and acesulfame potassium. The health implications of these additives will be discussed later.

As a rule, use foods containing more than 10 grams of sugar per serving (the equivalent of 2 teaspoons) sparingly, unless of course you are very active and don't run the risk of storing fat. This condition obviously excludes a large segment of our population. A sedentary person whose metabolism is sluggish runs the risk of converting most of what they eat into fat.

Too many refined carbohydrates and simple sugars in your diet can slow down your metabolism and increase your risk of inflammation. Sub-clinical inflammation that lingers on for a prolonged period of time can substantially increase your risk of heart disease, stroke, diabetes, cancer, and even obesity.

It is vitally important that you limit the intake of simple sugars and refined carbohydrates, as well as fats and calories. Simple sugar and refined carbohydrates have minimal to no enzymes, vitamins, or minerals to aid in their metabolism and digestion. As a result, they take nutrients away from other parts of the body. An excessive amount of these foods can raise blood glucose and insulin levels. In fact, the blood insulin levels rise higher than even the glucose levels. This has the effect of lowering your metabolism and makes it difficult to lose weight, especially fat, even if you are exercising.

Now, you are ready to become familiar with the shopping list, so that you can learn more about the foods that offer the best chance of raising body metabolism and burning fat.

# Chapter 3

# UDP Food List

**Low Calorie and Low-fat Shopping List**

Your shopping list should include foods that are low in calories but dense in nutrients (antioxidants, phytonutrients, vitamins, minerals, and fiber). It is vital to make a list and to eat before you do your grocery shopping. Otherwise, items that you did not intend to buy, and that do not meet healthy standards, might end up in your shopping cart.

The foods we eat contain macronutrients, such as carbohydrates, proteins, fats, and micronutrients, such as antioxidants, phytonutrients, vitamins, and minerals. They also contain essential elements, such as water and fiber. Sources of the macronutrients – carbohydrates, fats, and proteins – are listed below:

**Sources of Carbohydrates**

Grains (rice, cereals, barley)
Breads
Pasta
Sugar, Syrup and Honey
Dairy Foods (milk, yogurt, milk products)
Fruits
Starchy Vegetables (potatoes, corn, cassava, yams, plantains)
Juices
Alcoholic Beverages
Soda
Bakery Products
Legumes (beans, peas, lentils, soy)

**Sources of Fats**

Butter and Margarine
Vegetable Oils
Olive and Canola Oils
Palm Oil
Coconut Oil
Flax Oil
Flaxseeds
Meats
Whole Milk and Whole Milk Products
Nuts and Seeds
Fish (the richest source of healthy Omega-3 fats)
Whole Eggs (yolk)
Avocado

**Sources of Protein**
Meat
Fish
Poultry
Egg Whites
Egg Substitute
Milk and Milk Products (cheese, yogurt)
Legumes (beans, peas, lentils, soy)
Whole Grains
Nuts

## Carbohydrates: Our Primary Energy Source

Carbohydrates, starches, and sugars are the basic sources of our energy but not necessarily of the nutrients that our bodies need. The distinction between energy (calories) and nutrients needs to be clear. Calories make you fat and sluggish if you eat more than your body can burn. This happens when you are physically inactive. On the other hand, nutrients can help you to lose weight, increase your stamina and strength, and improve your concentration and overall health and well being. Carbohydrates are found in a large number of foods (see shopping list below). This makes it easy to overload on poor quality refined carbohydrate foods even when you are being careful.

All carbohydrates and starches are metabolized into blood sugar (glucose) and used as the primary energy source for the body. When the muscles do not immediately use glucose, it is converted by the liver and stored as fat.

Scientists have found a semi-reliable way to predict the behavior of carbohydrates in our bodies. The low-glycemic carbohydrates (unrefined flour and products made with it, such as brown rice and multigrain whole bread, oats, beans, peas, lentils, spinach, broccoli, apples, grapefruits) are broken down slowly and do not cause a rapid rise in blood sugar and insulin levels. As a result, they are likely to be non-fattening and anti-inflammatory. In contrast, the high-glycemic carbohydrates (highly refined foods, such as sugar, pastries, white flour, white rice and white flour pasta, potatoes, and corn) are broken down rapidly and produce a spike in blood sugar and insulin levels. These are more likely to be fattening and inflammatory, particularly when used by people who are physically inactive.

**Breads (High Fiber and Multigrain)**
**(Non-Fattening and Anti-Inflammatory)**

Choose unrefined whole grain or oat bran bread containing 3 or more grams of fiber per slice, such as 100% whole-wheat bread, oat bran, multigrain bread (7 or more grains), pumpernickel bread, sourdough bread, oat bran/whole-wheat flour tortillas *(Joseph's)*, oat bran/whole-wheat flour pita bread (*Joseph's*), multigrain or whole-wheat crackers (*Carr's*), The low carb breads are fine if they have enough fiber and are made of 100% whole-wheat, 100% multigrain, or oat bran. Some examples are given below:

- *Stop & Shop* Natural Commit multigrain ( 1 slice: 100 cal, 21g carb, 6g fiber)
- *Pepperidge Farm* Natural whole grain bread (1 slice: 110 cal, 20g carb, 3g fiber)
- *Joseph's* Oat bran/whole wheat tortilla (1: 70 cal, 11g carb, 6g fiber)
- *Joseph's* Oat bran/whole wheat pita (1: 60 cal, 10g carb, 5g fiber)
- *Arnold* whole grain 12 grain bread (1 slice: 110 cal, 19g carb, 2g fiber)
- *Thomas' Hearty Grains 100% whole wheat (*1: 120 cal, 23g carb, 3g fiber*)*
- *Thomas' Bagels 100% whole wheat (*1: 140 cal, 23g carb, 7g fiber*)*
- *Brownberry Natural Oatnut bread (*1 slice: 90 cal, 3g fiber)

Note that some bread labels make you think the bread is high fiber, when in reality it is not (such as the *Arnold* whole grain 12 grain bread).

**Cereals**

Avoid cereals that are made with highly refined flour, sweetened with sugar, or made with puffed rice, puffed wheat, caramel, honey, raisins, rice flakes, or corn flakes –these will probably raise your blood sugar and insulin quickly and cause fat storage and inflammation. Look for unhealthy ingredients, such as high fructose corn syrup and partially hydrogenated oils or trans fat. Some good choices are (reasonable carbohydrate load, high fiber, low sugar and 100% whole wheat or multigrain or oats):

**High Fiber, Whole Grain Breakfast Cereals**
**(Non-Fattening and Anti-Inflammatory)**

- *Kellogg's All-Bran with Extra Fiber* (½ cup, 22g carbs, 13g fiber, 50 cal)
- *General Mills Fiber One* (½ cup, 24g carbs, 13g fiber, 60 cal)
- *Kellogg's Bran Buds with Psyllium* (1/3 cup, 24g carb, 13g fiber, 80 cal)
- *Kellogg's Original All Bran* (½ cup, 23g carbs, 10g fiber, 80 cal)
- *Post 100% Bran* (1/3 cup, 23g carbs, 8g fiber, 80 cal)
- *Kashi Seven Whole Grains and Sesame* (3/4 cup, 8g fiber, 90 cal)
- *Barbara's Organic Soy Essence* (3/4 cup, 25g carb, 5g fiber, 100 cal)
- *Rice Bran (*1/2 cup dry, 131 cal, 21g carb, 9g fiber)
- *Kellogg's Special K (1 cup, 110 cal, 23g carb, 1g fiber)*
- *Quaker Oats*, 100% whole grain/rolled oats cereal (½ cup, 27g carbs, 4g fiber, 150 cal)
- Oatmeal, old fashioned, cooked (avoid instant oatmeal: will spike your blood sugar and cause fat storage and inflammation)

- *Quaker* Oat Bran Hot Cereal (½ cup, 25g carb, 6g fiber, 3g soluble fiber, 150 cal)*
- *Quaker* Instant Oatmeal Weight Control Hot Cereal (1 packet, 29g carb, 6g fiber, 4g soluble fiber, 160 cal)*
- *Muesli* (low-fat and low carb varieties, check label)
- *Kashi Good Friends, Original* (3/4 cup, 24g carbs, 8g fiber, 90 cal)
- *Kashi Good Friend, Granola (*2/3 cup, 43g carb, 12g fiber, 170 cal)
- *Kashi Good Friends, Cinna-Raisin Crunch (*1 cup, 39g carb, 10g fiber, 150 cal) – Compare the three *Kashi Good Friends cereals* with brand names that are very similar and can be confusing. The *Original* brand is a better choice for people with obesity, sedentary lifestyles, diabetes and heart disease.
- *Nature's Path Organic Flax Plus Multibran* Cereal (3/4 cup, 22g carbs, 7g fiber, 100 cal)
- *Nature's Path Organic Optimum Slim* Cereal *(*1 cup, 38g carb, 11g fiber, 180 cal) – contains soy isoflavones
- *Kashi GOLEAN* (1 cup, 30g carbs, 10g fiber, 140 cal). Note: ¾ cup may be appropriate for most sedentary individuals eating a 1,300- calorie diet.
- *Uncle Sam Cereal (*low glycemic and contains flaxseeds. 1 cup, 38g carb, 10g fiber, 190 cal). Sedentary individuals may require less, such as ½ - ¾ cup.
- *Hodgson Mill All Natural Bulgur Wheat With Soy Hot Cereal (*¼ cup dry, 22g carb, 3g fiber, 115 cal)
- *Hodgson Mill All Natural Oat Bran All Natural Hot Cereal (*¼ cup, 23g carb, 6g fiber, 3g soluble fiber, 120 cal)*
- *Mother's* 100% Natural Oat Bran Creamy Hot Cereal (1/2 cup, 25g carb, 6g fiber, 3g soluble fiber, 150 cal)*

**Cereals with 2 grams or more of soluble fiber*

**Pasta**
**(Non-Fattening and Anti-Inflammatory)**

- Whole-Wheat Pasta (Bionaturae: tender fettuccine and spaghetti, Organic fusilli; DeCecco: linguine)
- Multigrain pasta (Barilla Plus)
- Spaghetti, whole grain
- Protein-Enriched Pasta (make sure the protein is high)
- Vermicelli pasta noodles
- Fettucini
- Tortellini
- Macaroni (whole-wheat)
- Capellini

The landscape of pasta is changing fast. The unappealing whole-wheat pasta is a thing of the past. In recent years, pasta is made with whole-wheat flour that is not only nutritionally superior to conventional white flour pasta, but comes in different shapes and sizes and with texture that is (for all purposes) identical to white flour pasta, as well. In addition to whole-wheat flour, you can find pastas made with brown rice, buckwheat, spelt, farro, kamut, and quinoa.

The key to handling pasta safely is to keep your portion small and pair with abundant non-starchy vegetables and low-fat sauce. Limit the amount of cheese you use (low-fat varieties of cheese are better choices). The approach of mixing some whole-wheat pasta with regular white flour pasta is also a great idea. Whole-wheat pasta is one way to increase fiber intake and provide a healthier substitute for many of the regular pastas. It is also high in protein. Barilla Plus is a well-liked enriched multigrain pasta that is made from a blend of grain and legume flour to provide high fiber without an overly strong flavor and tough texture. Look for these in your local grocery or health food store.

**Grains**
**(Non-Fattening and Anti-Inflammatory)**

- Bulgur
- Brown Rice
- Basmati Rice
- Wild Rice
- Rice Bran
- Pearled Barley
- Buckwheat Groats
- *Uncle Ben's Converted Rice* (original). Avoid or limit short grain white rice, especially the instant varieties (they release their sugar rapidly).
- White rice, long grain (again, avoid the short grain)
- Parboiled rice that is not instant (long grain)

**Dairy**
**(Non-Fattening and Anti-Inflammatory)**

*This is a major source of saturated fat and extra calories in the American diet. Check the label to make sure it is low in fats, trans fats, sodium, and sugar.*

- Low-fat (1%) or Fat Free (skim) Milk with 10g or less sugar per serving
- *Soymilk Original* (fewer than 10g of sugar per serving)
- Low-fat or Reduced Fat Cottage Cheese
- Low-fat Cheeses (such as mozzarella sting cheese)
- Reduced Sugar, Low-fat Yogurt (examples: *Dannon Light 'n Fit*, *Yoplait Ultra* or *Hood Carb Countdown*) – all excellent sources of calcium

- Light or Diet Margarine (tub, squeeze or spray)
- Margarine made with Canola or Olive Oil (tub preferred to stick)
- *Smart Balance Omega Plus* (lowers cholesterol)
- *Smart Balance Omega Natural* Peanut Butter (2 tbsp, 190 cal, 16g fat, 2.5g saturated fat, 0 trans fat, 6g carb, 1g sugar, 7g protein, 2g fiber)
- Reduced Fat or Fat Free Sour Cream
- Fat Free Cream Cheese
- Egg White/Eggbeaters
- Soy Butter (2 tbsp, 1.5g saturated fat, total fat 11g, 170 cal)
- *Eggland's Best Grade A Eggs* (or eggs from free range chickens)
- *Benecol* (lowers cholesterol)
- *Take Control* (lowers cholesterol)

**Low-Starchy Vegetables**
**(Non-Fattening and Anti-inflammatory)**

You should eat abundant low-starch vegetables that contain 10 grams or fewer carbohydrates per serving. They are low-glycemic, nutrient-dense, and low in calories. Develop your food template with dark green leafy vegetables in combination with other colored vegetables. The more colorful your plate, the more phytonutrients and antioxidants you are eating and the greater the health benefits will be. You should have a serving or more of these before each major meal. Remember, your goal is to provide your body with enough nutrients, antioxidants, and phytonutrients to protect you from free radical attacks and to help repair damaged tissue and organs. Free radicals are compounds that are made in our body and some come from the food we eat and can cause oxidative stress. They can damage DNA and other vital compounds and increase inflammation (see Chapter 5). The simplest way to understand oxidative damage to our bodies is to recognize that a similar process takes place when iron is exposed to the air or oxygen – the iron rusts and loses its function. Our bodies undergo a similar process in which highly charged oxygen molecules can cause oxidative damage to vital organs and molecules. Antioxidants found in foods (vegetables and fruits) help to prevent the oxidation of vital compounds in our bodies and thereby maintain their integrity. You will learn more about this life-saving process in Chapter 7.

The suggested serving size is ½-1 cup of cooked leafy vegetables or 1-3 cups of raw leafy vegetables eaten before each meal or at least twice daily. You can "turn your vegetables into soup" or eat your vegetables raw, steamed, grilled, baked, or stir-fried in a small amount of olive oil or canola oil. Good choices of vegetables are asparagus, artichokes, lettuces (romaine, red leaf lettuce, butterhead, and arugula); broccoli, Brussel sprouts, cabbage, cauliflower, chard, Bok choy, spinach, watercress, Eggplant, Chinese cabbage, cassava leaf, cauliflower, celery, collard greens, eggplant, endive, escarole, kale, mustard greens, potato greens, spinach, turnips, and other non-starchy ethnic greens (see shopping list). Iceberg lettuce has very little nutritional quality and should be substituted in your salads with romaine or arugula.

Other low-starch vegetables can be treated as complementary vegetables and added to your food template in order to enhance nutrient density and variety. They also add flavor and color. You can also use some of these as part of your basic food template, if you so desire. They include, cucumbers, garlic, ginger, horseradish, mushrooms, okra, onions, peppers, beets, carrots, kohlrabi, seaweeds (arame, dulse, shushi nori, wakame), bean sprouts, tomatoes, yellow squash, zucchini, green beans, green snap, yellow snap, and Chinese green peas.

**Starchy Vegetables**
**(Fattening and Pro-Inflammatory)**

Unlike low-starch vegetables, vegetables high in starch will cause a rapid rise in blood sugar levels and an intense insulin response that will cause fat storage. This can lead to weight gain, even if your caloric intake is not excessive. These vegetables are more likely to be pro-inflammatory and should be treated as pure starch instead of vegetables. Even those considered low-glycemic are no exception. It is not necessary that you omit them from your diet because some of them are a valuable source of vitamins, minerals, and fiber. The important thing is to eat them in small amounts and in combination with other foods that will help prevent a rapid sugar release.

Vegetables that are high in starches include cassava, broad beans, corn, eddoes (root yam found in Hawaii or the west coast of Africa), farina, legumes, green peas, parsnips, plantains, white potatoes, sweet potatoes, pumpkin, rutabaga, yam, and squash (winter: acorn, butternut, hubbard). Sweet potatoes, yams, beans, soybeans, and green peas are relatively high in starch, but should be part of a healthy meal without fear because their sugar is released slowly. The key is to watch your portion size and eat according to activity level on a meal-to-meal basis.

Carrots, beets, and squash (summer) are high glycemic, but their starch content is low. You can eat them in moderation. Better yet, have them in combination with other foods that have a low glycemic index in order to decrease the overall glycemic load. It is often believed that cooking carrots causes the sugar to be released quickly, a fact that may also be true for ripe plantains as well. Therefore, eat carrots raw and plantains green (boiled or baked). However, you can still eat cooked carrots as long as you keep the portion size small (about ½ cup).

Legumes, such as beans, lentils, soybeans, and soy products, are low in fat and a good source of protein. Most people exclude this group from their meal plan because of their high starch content. But this should not discourage you from incorporating one of the readily available nutrient sources in your meal plan. They are high in fiber, including soluble fiber, which is partly responsible for releasing their blood sugar slowly.

Beans and lentils are rich sources of folic acid, potassium, iron, magnesium, and phytonutrients that help fight heart disease, stroke, diabetes, and cancer. They are anti-inflammatory and are a good substitute for processed and highly refined carbohydrates that are pro-inflammatory. Except for broad beans, baked beans, and Fava beans, most beans and lentils can help to boost metabolism. Eating beans, lentils, or soy can actually help you lose weight as well as reduce cholesterol levels. For example, chana dal, a lentil that is very popular in India, has very low glycemic index (GI 8). About ½ cup of this delicious lentil can be added to salads, soups or side dishes to help lower blood sugar and cholesterol levels. You can buy chana dal in Middle Eastern stores or Indian stores.

In spite of the health benefits, you should still eat beans in moderation (½ cup cooked 3-5 times per week.). Navy beans, split peas, canned chickpeas/garbanzo beans, cowpeas, black-eyed peas, lima beans, Cannellini beans, black beans, Great northern beans, red kidney beans, mung beans, and soybeans are all relatively high in starch, but you only stand a greater risk of carbohydrate overload if you eat too much at once. This is also the case when there is another carbohydrate source. In this instance, reducing the serving of your other favorite carbohydrate source will help to give a better metabolic profile. You should try to include (as a side dish) beans that are known to be high in soluble fiber, such as Navy beans, kidney beans, and lima beans.

Add beans and lentils to vegetables or side dishes. Both canned and dried beans are recommended. Use low-salt or salt-free canned legumes if you have high blood pressure, swelling of the extremities, or fluid retention. Wash the beans several times even if no salt is added in order to remove chemical additives.

Soybeans are unique among plants in containing all of the essential amino acids, just like meat. In addition, they also contain isoflavones (genistein and daidzein) that help fight osteoporosis, muscle loss, and cancers (breast, ovary, uterus, and prostate). The isoflavones in soybeans can actually counteract cancer-promoting estrogen by binding to estrogen receptor sites in the breast in much the same way as the drug tamoxifen. Soybeans and soy products also help to alleviate symptoms of menopause (hot flashes, mood swings). About one cup of cooked soybeans or edamame a day, or three tablespoons of soy protein isolate powder, is sufficient to provide most of these health benefits.

Beans, lentils, and soy are delicious, yet most of us are missing out on these nutrient-rich foods because we are either not familiar with them or we simply don't know how to incorporate them into our meal plan. Here are a few suggestions to help you incorporate them into your meal plan:

- Soak and rinse legumes carefully before cooking.
- Soak dried legumes overnight before cooking or boil them in water for about 5 minutes and then soak for about an hour before cooking (split peas and lentils do not require soaking).
- Wash canned beans thoroughly before cooking.
- Add beans to soups, stews, casseroles, or salads (see recipes).
- Substitute beans, such as tofu, for meat.
- Use pureed beans, such as hummus, for dips, sauces, and spreads (see recipe).
- Substitute tofu for eggs in omelets (see recipe).
- Substitute soy flour for white flour.
- Make delicious soy smoothies for breakfast or a snack (see recipe).

**Fruits**

Like starchy vegetables, fruits are a major source of starch and sugar in our diet; and this should be taken into consideration when planning your meals. This means that their overall contribution to the carbohydrate load at each meal (and the entire day) should be accounted for. Such practices will help you to stay within the range of carbohydrates that can be safely handled by your body.

Fruits are also an important source of fiber, vitamins, minerals, antioxidants, and phytonutrients. Some fruits like olives and avocado are high in monounsaturated fat (the same healthy fat found in olive oil) whereas coconut and palm kernel are rich in saturated fats that raise cholesterol levels.

When you eat fruits, especially as a snack, balance it with proteins or healthy fats to keep blood sugar from surging, even if the fruit is high in fiber or low-glycemic. Eat fruits with the outer skin. The skin or outer coat contains most of the nutrients and fiber. Generally, choose fresh fruits instead of dried ones, which are a concentrated source of sugar and fructose. Avoid fruits canned in sugary syrup. Those canned in water or light syrup are better choices if the sodium content is low.

Juices are high in sugar and contain virtually no fiber. Their consumption should be limited, except for freshly squeezed juices. Occasional use in moderation should not be a problem, particularly if you balance them with proteins or fats. Aim for at least two fruits a day, preferably as snacks and generally not with your meals as this can easily create a carbohydrate overload that could cause a strong sugar response. However, there is no reason why you can't have fruit with your meal if your total carbohydrate intake is within the range that does not overburden your body.

You should opt for those fruits that are not only low in sugar, but also release their sugar slowly: apples, apricots, avocados, blackberries, blueberries, cherries, cranberries, grapefruit, grapes, kiwi, lemon, lime, oranges, peaches, pears, plums, strawberries, raspberries, tangerines, and tomatoes. Avoid frozen strawberries and frozen raspberries that are sweetened. Fresh fruits have only a modest amount of sugar and fructose.

Sweet tasting tropical fruits like overripe banana, mango, papaya, oranges, nectarine, and dried dates are a real challenge to someone with a sweet tooth. These are typically high in sugar and could pose a hindrance to weight loss. However, the rise in blood sugar level and its effect on you is weak if you eat only a small amount in combination with proteins, fats, or other low glycemic foods, such as lemons or vinegar. Avoid eating overripe bananas – they are mostly sugar and could stimulate your appetite. One way to enjoy these fruits is to incorporate them into a fruit smoothie with soy protein powder or a fruit cocktail (see recipes).

Other fruits like raisins, watermelon, cantaloupe, and pineapple have low to average sugar content, but they release their sugar very quickly. However, it is believed that these fruits only cause a weak blood sugar and insulin response, with the exception being raisins. Be aware that raisins are widely used to sweeten a host of food products, including some popular brands of cold cereals. Again, if you have cantaloupe, watermelon or any of the other fruits in small portions and in combination with other foods that will help balance and stabilize the carbohydrate content, you should have no feelings of guilt or worry about their effect on you. There is nothing worse than being deprived of foods you enjoy and cherish. Cantaloupe, for instance, is rich in potassium, a mineral that helps to lower blood pressure.

## Proteins: The Builder

### Common Protein Sources

Proteins are the backbone of every organism. They provide the basic building blocks of our cells and are involved in building and repairing our entire bodies, including muscle, bone, and organs (liver, heart, kidney, skin, hair, and nails). They are used to build enzymes and antibodies that help us fight disease. The stuff of life, DNA, contains protein and without it the replication and transcription of DNA would be impossible.

All of the proteins we need are made from 22 amino acids, of which 9 are essential for life and must be provided through the diet. If any of the essential amino acids are missing, the protein that is made will be nonfunctional or defective. This can lead to diseases, such as sickle-cell anemia.

**Common Protein Sources**

| |
|---|
| Animal: Fish, Shellfish, Meat, Poultry, Eggs, Cheese, Dairy |
| Plant: Legumes (soy, beans, peas, lentils) |
| Nuts (almonds, walnuts, peanuts, pistachios) |
| Whole Grains |

Protein foods that provide all or enough of the essential amino acids are meat and other animal products and are said to be complete proteins. These include fish, shellfish, beef, turkey, chicken, pork, lamb, egg whites, milk, and milk products. Some protein foods do not supply all of the essential amino acids and are said to be incomplete proteins. They include grains, fruits, vegetables, and legumes (except soy). Vegetarians can combine foods to include all of the essential amino acids and get complete proteins.

Most of us get our proteins from sources that are high in unhealthy fats, such as meat, poultry with skin and whole fat dairy foods. For example, a slice of American cheese, provolone cheese and Swiss cheese contain 8-9 grams of total fat and 5 grams of saturated fat. Cheeses are the hidden sources of fat that pose health risk and weight gain. They are widely used for snacks and sandwiches. Eating meals laden with saturated fats will not only lead to high cholesterol, fat storage, and weight gain, but will also cause inflammation. To prevent this from happening to you, use protein sources that are low in unhealthy fats.

Without an adequate supply of good quality protein, the body breaks down muscle and tissue, including the heart, which can lead to serious health problems as well as a sluggish metabolism. Exercising or losing weight improperly without adequate protein intake can also lead to muscle breakdown. An inadequate protein intake may cause you to age faster, lose your hair and nails, and, most importantly, store fat.

Proteins are very important and I will elaborate further later. They help to control cravings, make you feel fuller so that you eat less, increase your body's metabolism, and burn more calories. Sometimes, we use this knowledge wrongly and go to extremes to get our protein. I do not advise that you follow unhealthy practices, all of which would only hurt you in the long haul.

In my practice, I have often seen patients who eat high-protein supplement bars to help them lose weight. This is unfortunate because these protein meal replacements are often very high in simple sugars, fat and proteins and are lacking in antioxidants and other vital nutrients found in vegetables, fruits, and other whole foods. Furthermore, these high calorie protein bars are not appropriate for average people living a sedentary lifestyle. They may be suitable for body builders and athletes who can quickly burn up the calories because they are active. Think about these things before you indulge in another protein bar. Instead of helping you, they may in fact work against you.

**Your Choice of Protein is Key**

The best choices of protein are fish, egg whites, skinless chicken and turkey breast, lean meat, wild game, and legumes. These are better choices of protein because they are low in saturated fats and other unhealthy fats. You should have a serving or two at every meal (for example, 3-6 oz lean fish or 3-4 oz fatty fish, 3-5 oz chicken breast, 3-4 oz lean meat, 25 mg soy protein, or ½ cup cooked beans or lentils).

If you are not accustomed to eating fish, when you start eating fatty fish you will notice a sensation of hunger, usually very early in the morning. It is a different type of hunger and is an indication that your metabolism is operating in high gear. Your body is burning fat, instead of storing it.

Our bodies do not store protein well, so it must be replaced at each meal. When you do not have adequate protein in your diet, your body will pull it from muscle. When weight loss plateaus or you feel hungry a few hours after a meal, it may be due to inadequate protein intake. Another serious mistake people often make is eating an inadequate amount of carbohydrates, while at the same time dramatically increasing protein sources that are high in fat. Unfortunately, most are not aware that they are inadvertently increasing fat as well as calories – far beyond what they had intended.

To help you get started on your fish, seafood, meat, and poultry list, here are a few suggestions:

**Anti-Inflammatory Protein Sources**

- Fish and seafood are a rich source of B-vitamins and trace minerals (calcium, magnesium, potassium, zinc, iodine, sulfur, phosphorus, selenium, copper, and fluorine). Fish is high in protein but low in saturated fat and cholesterol. By comparison, even high-fat fish typically contains less fat than red meat, including beef, veal, lamb, and pork. Fatty fish, such as salmon, tuna, or mackerel, are high in Omega-3 fatty acids – a type of fat that has potent anti-inflammatory activity and may help to lower your risk of heart disease and stroke. Shellfish, such as shrimp, have moderate amounts of cholesterol, but it is less harmful than the cholesterol from meat. Shellfish are also lower in saturated fat than poultry or meat.

- Eat 3-4 oz of fish at least four times a week and eat different types of fish, including those that are not fatty, so that you are not bored. All fish are good. Avoid frying fish. Bake, steam, grill, or sauté fish in a small amount of olive, canola oil, or cooking spray.

**Fatty Fish (Excellent Source of Protein)**
**(More than 1 g of Omega-3 Per 3 oz serving or ½ Cup)**

| | | |
|---|---|---|
| Albacore Tuna | Sablefish | Blue Fin Tuna |
| Bluefish | Chinook(King)Salmon | Atlantic Halibut |
| Atlantic Salmon | Yellow Fin Tuna | Pacific Herring |
| Lake Whitefish | Lake Trout | Mullet |
| Mackerel | Swordfish | Dogfish |
| Shad | Caviar* | Sardine |

* 1 tbsp serving size

Note: *3 oz skinless cooked portion (Atlantic/Coho Salmon) contains 7g fat, 1g saturated fat, 22g protein and 50 mg cholesterol. Eat healthy and keep portion size of fatty fish in line with level of activity to prevent storing excessive fat. For example, a 9 oz portion of Atlantic salmon will contain 21g fat and 150 mg cholesterol. A 3-4 oz serving of fish or seafood from this group will meet your daily requirement of Omega-3 fatty acids.*

**Lean Fish (Excellent Source of Protein)**
**(Less than 0.5g of Omega-3 per 3 oz Serving or ½ Cup)**

| | |
|---|---|
| Low-fat Tuna Fish | Haddock |
| Fresh Water Bass | Pacific Halibut |
| Lingcod | Cod |
| Flounder | Grouper |
| Croaker | Whiting |
| Shark | Snapper |
| Sole | Pollock |
| Shrimp | Catfish |
| Crab | Other Seafood |
| Clams | Lobster |
| Frog Legs | Pike |
| Oysters | Scallops |
| Snails | Squid |

Note: *3 oz skinless cooked portion (Flounder/Sole) contains 1.5g fat, 0.5g* saturated fat, 21g protein and 60mg cholesterol. To get the daily-required amount of Omega-3, you will need to eat about 5- 6 oz portions.

**Alternate Fish and Other Lean Protein Foods**

Very lean meats and meat substitutes that are low in saturated fat, cholesterol, and calories are also good sources of protein. These include chicken or turkey (breast or white meat, no skin) and the rest are listed below.

**Very Lean Meats and Meat Substitutes**
**(Good Source of Protein)**
**(Low in Saturated Fats, Cholesterol, and Calories: 0-1g Fat and 35 Calories per Ounce)**

- Poultry: Chicken or turkey (breast or white meat, no skin), Cornish hen (no skin)
- Game: Duck or pheasant (no skin), Venison, Buffalo, Ostrich
- Cheese with 1 gram or less fat per ounce: Nonfat or low-fat cottage cheese, fat free cheese
- Processed Sandwich Meats with 1g or less fat per ounce (such as deli thin shaved meats, chipped beef, turkey ham) – choose those low in sodium
- Egg Whites
- Egg Substitutes (plain)
- Hot Dog with 1g or less of fat per ounce
- Sausage with 1g or less of fat per ounce
- Beans, Green Peas, Lentils, Soy, and Soy Products

Note: *3 oz skinless cooked portion (chicken breast) contains 2g fat, 0.5g saturated fat, 24g protein, and 70mg cholesterol.*

Poultry is a healthier choice than beef for the simple reason that it has less saturated fat and, therefore, leaner protein per ounce of meat. The leanest poultry is white meat from the breasts of either chicken or turkey with the skin removed. Other lean choices include ground breast meat or low-fat ground chicken or turkey. Eat 3-4 oz of white meat four or more times a week (roughly ¼ chicken breast is 4 oz). Cut off the skin and visible fat before cooking poultry. If you are roasting a whole chicken or turkey, remove the skin after cooking but before you carve the meat. Most of the fat is in the skin. To avoid salmonella poisoning, wash your hands thoroughly. Be careful not to contaminate other foods or cutting boards and cook meat until it is well done.

Eat eggs without the yolk frequently. Egg whites are rich in proteins and they are very inexpensive. They are good in omelets with vegetables, such as spinach, green peppers, and tomatoes. It is best you limit whole eggs to a few times (less than three) per week if you have high cholesterol, diabetes, heart disease, or high blood pressure. However, eggs from chickens domesticated on vegetables and algae or free ranging have a healthier profile of fats (more Omega-3) and you can have them more often.

Legumes (beans, peas, lentils, soybeans, and products), as you already know, are good sources of low-fat protein that can either replace meat protein or add variety. Eat about ¼ -½ cup cooked with either your lunch or dinner. Choose low-salt varieties or dried beans.

Processed sandwich meats and hot dogs could have high sodium content of over 800 mg. So, eat these less frequently if you have high blood pressure or water retention. Also, read the labels carefully when buying processed foods. Especially look for unhealthy fats in the ingredient list – and keep portion sizes small. Unprocessed or whole foods are by far preferred to highly refined ones. However, you may find certain processed foods handy and convenient. It is all right to have them as long as you keep portion size small and eat them infrequently. Then, you won't have to worry about your health.

## Fatty Meat: Source of Inflammation: Eat Less of It

Meat is a very good source of the vitamin B12 and iron, which are necessary for energy and vitality. However, meat and meat products are a major source of saturated fat, which raises cholesterol levels. They are also a source of arachidonic acid (AA), a compound, which is converted into very powerful inflammatory compounds in our body. Obviously, the cuts of meat with more fat pose more health risk. That's why you should choose the leanest cuts of meat available. For beef, this means round tip, top round, eye of round, chuck arm, sirloin, tenderloin, or top loin, including extra-lean ground beef. For pork, the leanest cuts are tenderloin, center loin chops, top loin roast or top loin chops. In general, choose the USDA Choice or USDA Select grades of beef, which have less fat content than the USDA Prime. Choose ground meat with the lowest percentage of fat by weight, (15% fat or lower) and avoid meat that is heavily marbled, which means it is high in fat. Also avoid chicken or turkey skin and beef fat, including cooking with palm kernel oil and coconut oil.

Always thaw meat completely and cook immediately after defrosting. For healthy, low-fat cooking, bake, roast, grill, stir-fry, or broil meat after trimming away all visible fat. Keep portion sizes about 3-4 oz and eat beef no more than three times a week. In order to prevent E. coli contamination, cook meat to 160-180°F. The list below will guide you to select healthier choices of meat and meat products:

**Lean Meats and Meat Substitutes**
**(Average Source of Protein)**
**(Contains About 3g of Fat and 55 Calories per Ounce)**

- Poultry: Chicken, Turkey (dark meat, such as leg and thigh, no skin), Chicken (white meat or breast, with skin), Domestic Duck, or Goose (drained of fat and no skin)
- Game: Goose (no skin), Rabbit
- Veal: Lean Chop, Roast
- Lamb: Roast, Chop, Leg
- Pork: Lean Pork, Fresh Ham, Canned, Cured, or Boiled Ham, Canadian Bacon, Tenderloin, Center Loin Chop

- Beef: USDA Select or Choice grades of Lean Beef trimmed of fat [Round, Sirloin, and Flank Steak, Tenderloin, Roast (Rib, Chuck, Rump), Steak (T-Bone, Porterhouse, Cubed), Ground Round (extra lean ground meat)
- Cheese: 2 % fat Cottage Cheese, Grated Parmesan, Cheeses with 3g or less fat per ounce
- Hot Dogs with 3 grams or less fat per ounce (Chicken, Turkey)
- Processed Sandwich Meats with 3 grams or less fat per ounce (Turkey, Pastrami, or Kielbasa)

Note: *3 oz cooked portion (chicken thigh, no skin) contains 7g fat, 2g saturated fat 25g protein, 80 mg cholesterol. Loin Tenderloin Steak (3 oz portion, trimmed of visible fat) has 9g fat, 3g saturated fat, 24g protein, and 70mg cholesterol.*

**Moderately Fattening and Pro-Inflammatory Meats**
**(Average Source of Protein)**
**(Contains 5g of Fat and 75 Calories per Ounce)**

- Poultry: Chicken (dark meat or leg and thigh, with skin), Ground Turkey or Ground Chicken, Fried Chicken (with skin)
- Veal: Cutlet (ground or cubed, not breaded)
- Lamb: Rib Roast, Ground
- Pork: Top Loin, Chop, Boston Butt, Cutlet
- Beef: Most beef products fall into this category (Ground Beef, Meatloaf, Corned Beef, Short Ribs, prime grades of meat trimmed of fat, such as Prime Rib)
- Cheese: with 5 grams of fat per ounce (Feta, Mozzarella, Ricotta, Goat Cheese)
- Whole Eggs (high in cholesterol, limit to 1-3 per week except *Eggland's Best* and eggs from free range chickens)
- Sausage with 5 grams or less fat per ounce

Note: *3 oz cooked portion (Top Loin Steak, 1/8" fat trim) contains 15g fat, 6g saturated fat, 22g protein and 65 mg cholesterol. When trimmed of visible fat the steak now contains 8g fat and 3g saturated fat. Ground Beef with 27% fat (3 oz portion) has 17g fat, 6g saturated fat, and 85mg cholesterol, whereas Ground Beef with 10 % fat has only 11g fat, 4 g saturated fat.*

**Highly Fattening and Pro-inflammatory Meats/Products**
**(Poor Source of Protein; High in Saturated Fat, Cholesterol, and Calories)**
**(8g of Fat and 100 Calories per Ounce)**

- Pork: Spareribs, Pork Sausage, Ground Pork
- Cheese: All common domestic full fat cheeses (American, Monterey Jack, Cheddar, Swiss)
- Peanut butter (1 tbsp smooth contains 8g fat and 2g saturated fat)
- Processed Sandwich Meat with 8 grams or less fat per ounce (Bologna, Pimento Loaf, Salami)

- Sausages (Bratwurst, Italian, Knockwurst, Polish, or Smoked)
- Hot Dog with full fat (Beef, Pork, Turkey, or Chicken)
- Bacon

Note: *3 oz cooked portion (Rib Roast, Large End, 1/8" fat trim) contains 24g fat, 10g saturated fat, 20g protein, and 70 mg cholesterol. Also note that 3 oz Pork Spareribs contains 340 calories, 26g fat, 9g saturated fat, 25g protein, and 105mg Cholesterol.*

When you make a conscious effort to eat healthy, it's all right to occasionally indulge in some of your favorite foods that may be considered bad. This approach would help to reduce anxiety that is often associated with deprivation. You should always have the freedom to have some "bad" or "forbidden" foods, but it must be on your own terms – make sure that you know what you are getting into, you have a plan, and had thought about other important things, such as the portion, other foods that may help to neutralize their harmful effects on your body, the best time to have them, and so forth. Of course, you are well aware that the less frequently you eat bad foods the better your health. As a rule, you should increase the portions of healthy foods (Omega-3 fatty acids, non-starchy dark green leafy vegetables, or legumes) whenever you have bad foods.

You can cause serious damage to your body if you ignore healthy practices and constantly make bad choices, especially having large portions. It's even worse if you omit healthier choices of food that could help to protect your body. Again, it's not practical and really necessary to completely eliminate bad foods from your meal planning. Sometimes, they can help to satisfy your emotional needs that could sabotage your best efforts if they are not taken care off. On the other hand, if you are a very disciplined person and have no real concern about completely eliminating some bad food choices, that's fine too – as long as it is your decision.

## Fats: They're Not All Bad

Over the years, we have learned that not all fats are bad. Our problem has been that we eat too many unhealthy fats and too little of the healthy ones, particularly the Omega-3 fats from fish, flaxseed oil, and leafy green vegetables. The simple reason for this disparity is that most of our fats are from animal sources, such as meat, butter, milk, cheeses and other whole dairy products, and processed foods. The types of fats we eat can have either a positive or negative effect on our health and weight:

- Saturated fats (very bad)
- Trans fats (Partially Hydrogenated Oils) (very bad)
- Triglycerides (good and bad)
- Cholesterol (good and bad)
- Monounsaturated fats (good) – olive and canola oils, nuts, and avocado
- Polyunsaturated fatty acids (good) – fats from fish, flaxseed oil (Omega-3), and vegetable oils (Omega-6)

Get into the habit of checking food labels and choose products with a fat content of less than 5 grams per ounce, except for fish and shellfish. Saturated fat content should be less than 10% of the total calories you consume per day. For example, in a 1,300 and 1,600 caloric diets, saturated fat intake should be no more than 14 grams and 18 grams per day, respectively. Limit consumption of products with hydrogenated fats, such as hard or stick margarine and other processed foods. Fat intake should be limited to about 20-35% of calories consumed.

I do not recommend low-fat diets (10% of calories) because they are not healthy and can be harmful to the body. When your intake of fat is too low, your liver just makes more bad fats – saturated fat and cholesterol. Your liver is a fat-making machine that is able to make more than twice the normal cholesterol per day, especially when the diet is deficient in fats. That is one good reason you need to eat adequate amounts of healthy fats.

Low-fat diets are also likely to be deficient in essential fatty acids. This can have several health repercussions involving skin, hair, nails, memory, mood, depression, and the ability to mount an adequate defense against infection and disease. Vitamins that are fat-soluble, such as A, D, E, and K, are not absorbed easily and this can lead to serious health problems. A low-fat diet can also lead to unexpected weight gain. This happens when the fat is replaced by excess sugar and sugar substitutes.

**The Very Bad Fats (Downright Ugly): Saturated Fats and Trans Fats**

Saturated fats, trans fats, and cholesterol raise blood cholesterol levels and increase the risk of heart disease and inflammation. Other health problems associated with the consumption of saturated fat are diabetes, breast cancer, colon cancer, immune disorders, and obesity.

Most people interested in lowering their cholesterol pay close attention to their cholesterol intake and literally forget about saturated fat and trans fat. The irony is that the latter two are the main sources of cholesterol in the body and not cholesterol per se. Therefore, if you really want to lower your body cholesterol, pay attention to the sources of saturated fats and trans fat in your diet as well as sources of cholesterol. Also, cut back on carbohydrates that are quickly digested (refined grains, white flour pasta, and potatoes), since they are easily converted into fat.

Trans fats, or partially hydrogenated oils, also pose a more serious health risk than even saturated fats. These fats not only raise blood cholesterol but also lower the level of HDL (good) cholesterol, thereby increasing the risk of heart attack and stroke. Trans fats are found in foods that you may not even suspect, such as baked goods, snack foods, and mixes. Check food labels and the fine print for hydrogenated or partially hydrogenated oils.

You can cut down on the amount of saturated fat and trans fats in your diet by eating smaller portions of meat (3-4 oz per meal) and limiting your intake of butter, salad dressings, hard margarine, cheese and whole dairy products, commercially fried foods, and most processed foods. Cutting down on palm kernel oil, coconut, coconut oils, and cocoa butter will also help to reduce the saturated fat content in your diet.

As a rule, eat all fats in moderation. Eating a large amount of any fat adds calories. Fat contains 9 calories per gram, compared to 4 calories per gram for carbohydrates and proteins.

### Triglycerides

The fat in the foods we eat is broken down into triglycerides and used for energy or stored. In fact, body fat is stored as triglycerides. The body also makes triglycerides from other sources, such as highly refined carbohydrates. Your triglyceride level rises steadily after a fatty meal only if muscle and other organs do not use up the fats immediately. A high triglyceride level means an increased risk of heart attack and stroke, even though your total cholesterol level may be normal. High levels of triglycerides can also lead to an inflammation of the pancreas. If unchecked, this condition can cause pancreatitis, an enlarged liver, spleen, and fatty deposits in the skin called xanthomas.

### Cholesterol

Most people are familiar with the word "cholesterol" and assume that it's bad for their health. But that is far from the truth. In fact, the body uses cholesterol as a backbone for making many important compounds and molecules, such as estrogen, progesterone and testosterone. Cholesterol comes from food, but it is also formed in the body. In fact, the body makes most of the cholesterol that it needs. For example, the liver can manufactures about 800-1,500 mg of cholesterol per day, which contributes much more to the total cholesterol than the dietary source. The liver can also make cholesterol from carbohydrates (particularly refined grains), fat or protein. Cholesterol is found only in animal foods, such as meat, cheese and milk.

The problem is when cholesterol builds up in the blood vessels it can increase risk of oxidation causing the buildup of plaques on the walls of arteries (a condition called atherosclerosis)---thereby triggering inflammation and damage to the artery carrying blood to the heart and other organs. When a plaque forms in coronary arteries, blood flow to the heart is slowed or completely blocked--- leading to a heart attack. It may surprise you that the damage may start as earlier as in your teens and manifests itself in your adult life. The good news is that you can prevent this by keeping daily cholesterol intake to not more than 300 mg/dl, the amount in a medium egg.

Reading food labels will help to identify foods that are high in cholesterol (such as meat, eggs, poultry, shrimp, squid and organ meat). It's the combination of these foods and the large portions often consumed that is responsible for the build up of dietary cholesterol. Reducing foods high in saturated fats and trans fat will help keep blood cholesterol down, but most importantly, will help burn body fat. Refined carbohydrates (white flour pasta, white flour bread and sugary deserts and cookies) are all converted to saturated fats and eventually to cholesterol by the liver.

### Monounsaturated Fatty Acids (MUFAs)

These are healthy fats. They are found in olive oil, olives, canola oil, avocados, most nuts, and peanut butter. MUFAs help the body get rid of newly formed cholesterol as well as reduce cholesterol deposits in the walls of arteries. They also reduce blood cholesterol (provided the overall dietary consumption of saturated fat is low).

The well-studied Mediterranean diet is rich in monounsaturated fats from olives, olive oil, and canola oil. This is one of the main reasons for the lower risk of heart disease, breast cancer, and colon cancer in this population, but only when their diet is the typically original Crete diet (high in antioxidants, leafy dark vegetables, whole grains and fish). Monounsaturated fatty acids make up about 80 percent of the daily fat intake recommended in the UDP program.

**Polyunsaturated Fatty Acids (PUFAs)**

These are made up of two families – Omega-6 and Omega-3 fatty acids. Both are essential fatty acids that the body cannot make and must be obtained from food. Omega-6 fatty acids are found in vegetable oils, such as corn oil, peanut oil, sunflower seed oil, and safflower oil. Omega-3 fatty acids are found in plants and fish. In plants, it is found as alpha-linolenic acid in dark green vegetables, flaxseeds, flaxseed oil, and walnuts. The best source of Omega-3 is fish (salmon, mackerel, and tuna), which has the basic building compounds called eicosapentaenoic acid (EPA) and docosahexaenoic acid (DHA).

Our bodies need an adequate supply of both Omega-6 and Omega-3 fatty acids in their proper ratio of 2:1 or 1:1. From these two essential fatty acids, the longer chain fatty acids, and their derivatives can be made using one set of enzymes that is shared by both. Therefore, when an excess of one family of essential fatty acids is present in the diet, the transformation of the other may be blocked, causing an imbalance in the production of hormone-like compounds called prostaglandin, leukotrienes, and thromboxanes. The family of compounds produced from Omega-3 fatty acids reduces inflammation and causes blood to thin, whereas the Omega-6 family of compounds causes inflammation and blood clotting. These two competing processes are vital to life and getting the right balance of Omega-6 to Omega-3 in your diet is key. Most of us eat a diet that is grossly imbalanced.

Typically, the intake of Omega-3 fats (EPA and DHA) in the American diet is quite low, about 0.15 gram per day, whereas that of Omega-6 is quite high. A deficiency of Omega-3 fatty acids has been implicated in cravings and feelings of hunger that lead to overeating and weight gain.

**Suggested intake of Omega-3 fats**
**(EPA + DHA): 500-1000 mg/d**

A 3 to 4 ounce serving of salmon provides about 1000 mg of EPA and DHA. If you do not eat fish, you can take fish oil capsules (1000 mg) three times daily to give approximately 500-1,000 mg of EPA/DHA combined. Obviously, you may need more if you have heart disease, high blood pressure, or arthritis. This is covered in detail in Chapter 12. Fish oils (such as cod liver oil) are very cheap and provide high amounts of EPA and DHA. However, new and potent Omega-3 delivery medium have been recently developed, such as the Neptune Krill Oil. The Omega-3 in Neptune Krill Oil is in the form of phospholipids that are highly bioavailable and absorbable. In fact, the Krill Oil Omega-3 has more potent antioxidant activity than fish oil Omega-3. For example, the ORAC value for Krill Oil is 378 and that for fish oil is 8. The ORAC is the antioxidant content of foods. Flaxseed oil is also a good source of Omega-3 (1-2 tbsp daily). The following are other ways in which you can close the gap:

- Select foods rich in EPA and DHA, such as fatty fish (salmon, tuna, mackerel).
- Eat more fish and poultry (white meat) and less red meat.
- Eat fatty fish, such as salmon and tuna, at least 3-4 times a week (a 3-4 oz portion per meal gives the right amount of EPA and DHA suggested).
- Take 1-2 tbsp of flaxseed oil daily or a flaxseed capsule (1000 mg) 3 times a day.
- Add ground flaxseeds to cereal, yogurt, cottage cheese, and vegetable salads (1-3 tbsp daily).
- Limit your intake of Omega-6 sources, such as vegetable oils (for your daily requirement of Omega-6 fats, take about 300-500 mg in supplement form or 1-3 tsp vegetable oil, such as safflower oil).
- As you increase your intake of Omega-3 fats in your diet, replace vegetable oils with monounsaturated fats (olive and canola oils) for cooking and salads. This will also help to raise your HDL (good) cholesterol. If your HDL is low (below 40), you could still be at increased risk of heart attack even with normal cholesterol. A high HDL (60 or more) is protective and decreases risk.
- Limit your consumption of high fat meat, whole dairy, processed foods, sweets, and refined carbohydrates.
- As you increase your intake of essential fatty acids, your requirement for vitamin E also increases (take 400 – 800 IU vitamin E supplement if your multivitamin does not have the right amount).
- Non-hydrogenated Omega-3 oils are now incorporated into many foods, such as margarine and low-fat spread, yogurt, milk, and bread.

Because fish and seafood are considerably lower in total fat and saturated fat than meat, substituting fish for meat can help to reduce your cholesterol level and fight heart disease, depression, and arthritis. Eating fish high in fat also helps to improve concentration, focus, and learning ability. In fact, the fats in fish oil and vitamin E, a fat-soluble antioxidant, may help to fight Alzheimer's disease.

In conclusion, when you make your shopping list, remember to include non-fattening and anti-inflammatory food sources, such as leafy green vegetables, whole grains, mushrooms, seaweed, soy, beans, lentils, avocados, canola oil, extra virgin olive oil, red palm oil, fish, fish oils, flaxseeds, flaxseed oil, soft or tub margarine, olives, *Smart Balance Omega Plus*, *Benecol*, *Take Control,* and very lean meats.

Finally, limit the use of fattening and pro-inflammatory food sources, such as simple sugars (table sugar, regular sodas, fatty desserts, and fruit juices), refined carbohydrates, bacon grease, butter, coconuts, coconut oil, egg yolks, lard, stick or hard margarine, regular mayonnaise, meat fats, whole milk, regular cheeses and yogurt, palm kernel oil, coconut oil, regular salad dressings, shortening, and vegetable oils.

## FIBER

Fiber is found in the skin and pulp of vegetables, fruits, seeds, whole grains, legumes, seaweed, and nuts. Soluble fiber is found in foods that contain gums and pectin whereas insoluble fiber is in foods high in cellulose and hemicellulose. Fibers like pectin and guar (from oat bran, oats, beans, carrots and apples) forms gels in water (increase bulk) and prolong the time of transit of food through the intestine. Whereas, insoluble fiber, such as cellulose found in whole grains and wheat bran tend to reduce the time.

For a healthy diet, you need about 20-35 grams of fiber per day. Yet, most of us get an average of 9-13 grams a day due to our poor food choices. Fiber has specific functions and health benefits. They are summarized below:

- Decreases fat digestion and reduces the amount of fat (including cholesterol and saturated fat) that is absorbed into the bloodstream. The reduction of cholesterol levels helps to decrease the risk of heart disease (oat bran and pectin from apples).
- Binds and eliminates bile acids (made from cholesterol in the liver) in the digestive track. As a result, the body uses some of its cholesterol to make new bile acids, thereby lowering cholesterol levels (oat bran and pectin from apples).
- Helps to lower blood sugar, decrease insulin resistance, and boosts metabolism (oat bran and pectin from apples).
- Helps you to lose and maintain weight loss.
- Promotes regular bowel movements (wheat bran, whole grains).
- Decrease the risk for some types of cancers (such as colon)

### Sources of Fiber

| **Non-Starchy Vegetables** | **Amount Fiber (g)** |
|---|---|
| Asparagus, ½ cup | 2.0 |
| Broccoli, ½ cup cooked | 2.0 |
| Cauliflower, ½ cup cooked | 2.0 |
| Iceberg lettuce, 1 cup | 0.5 |
| Kale, chopped, frozen, ½ cup | 3.0 |
| Mixed vegetables frozen, ½ cup | 4.0 |
| Okra, frozen, cooked, ½ cup | 4.0 |
| Spinach, ½ cup cooked | 2.0 |

| **Starchy Vegetables** | **Amount Fiber (g)** |
|---|---|
| Acorn squash, baked, ½ cup | 5.0 |
| Carrots, ½ cup | 3.0 |
| Corn, ½ cup | 2.0 |
| Green beans, canned, ½ cup | 2.0 |
| Green peas, ½ cup | 3.0 |
| Potato, baked w/skin, 1 medium | 5.0 |

| **Fruits** | **Amount Fiber (g)** |
|---|---|
| Apple w/skin, 1 medium | 5.0 |
| Banana, 1 medium | 3.0 |
| Blueberries/Raspberries, ½ cup | 4.0 |
| Grapefruit, ½ large | 2.0 |
| Orange, 1 medium | 3.0 |
| Pear, canned, ½ cup | 4.0 |
| Prunes, dried, 3 med | 2.0 |
| Strawberries, ½ cup | 2.0 |

| **Legumes** | **Amount Fiber (g)** |
|---|---|
| Black beans, ½ cup cooked | 8.0 |
| Chickpeas, ½ cup cooked | 4.0 |
| Kidney beans, ½ cup cooked | 7.0 |
| Lentils, ½ cup cooked | 8.0 |
| Lima beans, ½ cup cooked | 4.0 |
| Navy beans, ½ cup cooked | 7.0 |

| **Grains, Cereals, Breads** | **AmountFiber (g)** |
|---|---|
| All bran cereal ½ cup | 13.0 |
| Bagel 100% whole wheat 1 | 7.0 |
| Bagel plain ½ (3 ½") | 1.0 |
| Barley ½ cup cooked | 3.0 |
| Brown rice ½ cup cooked | 2.0 |
| Bulgur ½ cup cooked | 4.0 |
| Egg noodles ½ cup cooked | 0.9 |
| Multigrain bread 1 slice | 3.0 |
| Oat bran/whole wheat tortilla 1 | 7.0 |
| White flour pasta ½ cup cooked | 0.8 |
| White rice long grain ½ cup cooked | 2.0 |
| White rice short grain ½ cup cooked | 1.0 |
| Whole-wheat pasta ½ cup cooked | 2.0 |
| Whole-wheat pita ½ (6½") | 3.0 |

**Are You Getting Enough Fiber?**

Most Americans are not getting enough fiber and are not coming close to the recommended 20-35 grams of fiber each day. The following tips will help you get the daily fiber requirement:

- Choose breakfast cereals that are high in fiber (5grams or more per serving), such as bran or oats.
- Add 1-2 tbsp of wheat bran, oat bran and bran cereal, wheat germ, or ground flaxseeds to your cereal, vegetables, yogurt, or cottage cheese.
- Increase fiber intake by mixing your favorite cereal with one with high fiber (such as *General Mills* Fiber One, *Kellogg's* All Bran with extra fiber or *Kellogg's* Bran Bud)
- Substitute white bread or refined wheat bread (such as Italian or French breads) with multigrain bread or 100% whole grain bread with high fiber.
- Eat whole grains, such as brown rice or barley, instead of refined white rice.
- Substitute whole-wheat pasta for refined white flour pasta.
- Substitute refined white flour in baking with whole grain flour (wheat germ or whole-wheat flour)
- Add beans, peas, lentils, and soybeans to your meals, including vegetables and salads.
- Make smoothies using soy or whey protein powder, low-fat yogurt, or 1% milk with fruits (see recipes in Chapter 17).
- Eat whole fruits with the skin and choose whole fruits over juices.
- Have fruit as a snack, but don't forget to add protein or fat to balance the sugar.
- To avoid bloating and heartburn, add fiber gradually, and drink enough water each day to prevent constipation or impaction.
- Aim for 7-10 grams of fiber per meal.
- Get about 3-5 grams or more of soluble fiber per meal – fiber supplements like *Benefiber* and *Clearly Fiber* are very helpful if you are not getting enough soluble fiber from dietary sources.

Again, the role of fiber in optimizing health, weight loss, and energy cannot be stated strongly enough. The best way to get your fiber is to eat a variety of foods and not just limit your choices to green vegetables and fruits. The highest concentrations of fiber, especially soluble fiber, are found in beans, lentils, oat bran, oats, carrots, apples, okra, and cactus. Soluble fiber dissolves in water and helps to lower blood cholesterol and sugar levels. The insoluble fiber is the type that does not dissolve in water and is found in oats, wheat bran, whole grains, fruits, and vegetables. It promotes a smooth and regular bowel movement. You need to get an adequate amount of both in the diet and the best way to achieve this is to include foods that are high in fiber. Omitting the high fiber foods in favor of those with low fiber in your meals may cause you to not reach the daily fiber requirement – even though you might have increased your intake of vegetables and fruits. Take a look again at the chart above and it will become clear to you why that is so. With this new knowledge, make sure you have plenty of fiber-rich foods with each meal. It's best that you increase fiber slowly in order to prevent experiencing gas and bloating. Drinking enough water may prevent the stool from being very hard and difficult to eliminate (about eight glasses of water or other uncaffeinated beverages daily).

## Other Things to Remember

### Antioxidant-Rich Foods

Foods rich in antioxidants help to neutralize oxygen-free radicals that are produced when food is metabolized causing oxidative stress. These free radicals can damage DNA, RNA, proteins, carbohydrates, enzymes, and lipids – particularly those that form the cell membrane. Free radicals are a major cause of inflammation that can prime the body for chronic diseases, such as obesity, heart disease, diabetes, immune disorders, and cancer. In order to counteract free radicals, you should eat an abundant supply of foods that are rich in antioxidants with each meal. These include blueberries and other berries, dark leafy green vegetables (spinach, broccoli, kale), lemon, salmon, tomatoes, bell peppers, cantaloupe, avocado, yellow-colored squash, wheat germ, beer yeast, and green tea as well as numerous other foods. Red palm oil is also rich in super-antioxidants.

### Baking

Highly refined sugar, white flour and products made with them are fattening and pro-inflammatory and should be used infrequently, if at all. In cooking or baking, substitute wheat germ, rice bran, oat bran, or rolled oats for white flour. Substitute splenda, stevia, unsweetened apple juice, applesauce, dried fruits, sugar free marmalade, or preserves for sugar. Other common house products include unsweetened cocoa powder or dark chocolate, non-fat dry milk, and unflavored gelatin.

### Condiments, Sauces, and Seasonings

It is important to use these items properly to add flavor, taste, and palatability to foods, which helps to decrease boredom. Experiment with different condiments, sauces and seasonings to find out what you like. Some brands may be loaded with undesirable chemical additives and even trans fat, so be sure to check the labels.

### Beverages

There is no substitute for clean, good, natural water and you should have about six to eight glasses a day in order to be well hydrated and healthy. Water keeps your metabolism up, helping to burn fat and removing toxins from your body. Water is good for your skin, hair, muscles, and digestive system. Tissue and cells depend on water for their survival. Water can also help you control cravings and feelings of hunger. As you increase your intake of vegetables and fruits, you need to drink more liquid to prevent constipation. Inadequate intake of water by itself can cause constipation, impaction, bloating, and abdominal distention.

Green or black tea contains antioxidants and catechins polyphenols (a compound called egigallocatechin-3-gallate or EGCG) that boost metabolism, help burn fat, and neutralize harmful free radicals. Green tea blocks the absorption of saturated fat, which will help lower your cholesterol levels. It can also elevate mood as a result of an amino acid called theonine. There are both caffeinated and decaffeinated teas.

In contrast, drinking coffee (as little as two cups) increases cortisol levels. You will recall in Chapter 2 that cortisol is a powerful stress hormone that adversely affects brain cells, the immune system, and causes fat storage in the belly. Drinking green tea helps with weight loss – and this is not due to the effect of caffeine.

Substitute green or black tea for coffee or reduce your intake to one cup a day. Diet sodas are laden with chemicals and you should use them infrequently. These chemicals can increase the free radicals in your body.

## TIPS ON FOOD PREPARATION

Preparing dishes that are high in nutrients and low in calories is easy and does not require a great deal of time. It is important to learn how some basic ingredients can add calories and fat to your meals. The following are some food preparation tips:

### Cooking Methods

- Avoid or limit the use of high-glycemic carbohydrates, such as breadcrumbs, refined white or wheat flour, most potatoes, white rice, and sweets.
- Use low-glycemic carbohydrates, such as whole grains, legumes, skim milk, non-starchy green vegetables, soy flour, oat bran, or wheat germ.
- Broil, bake, steam, or microwave.
- Avoid frying or breading meats.
- Roast vegetables or poultry (without the skin).
- Grill seafood, chicken, or vegetables.
- Lightly stir-fry or sauté in measured amounts of olive oil, canola oil, low sodium broth, or cooking spray.
- Avoid cooking at very high temperatures.

### Ingredients

- Avoid or limit the use of butter, vegetable oils, palm oil, coconut oil, lard, hard or stick margarine, and Crisco. Soft or tub margarine is preferred to hard or stick margarine.

- Use low sodium lite mayonnaise in place of regular mayonnaise.
- Cook with extra virgin olive oil, canola oil, or a mixture of olive and canola oil (1 to 1).
- For ethnic cooking with red palm oil or coconut oil, dilute with olive or canola oil (1 to 2).
- When using vegetable oil to cook, dilute with olive or canola oil (1 to 2).
- Don't reuse cooking oil (cooking destroys the nutrients and creates free radicals).
- Keep your cooking oil protected from sunlight and heat.
- Add ground flaxseeds to cereal or vegetables.
- Salad Dressings: Avoid regular salad dressings. They are loaded with fat and sodium. Some reduced fat dressings are often high in sodium. For example, *Kraft's Fat Free Oil Free Italian Dressing* has only 5 calories, but has 450 mg sodium in a 2 tbsp serving. Among the better picks in commercial salad dressings are *Diet Italian Salad Dressing (*2 tbsp contains 30 calories, 2 grams carb, 3 grams fat, 9 mg sodium); and *Good Seasons Italian Fat Free Dressing,* dry mix (2 tbsp contains 10 calories, 3 grams carb, 0 gram fat, 290 mg sodium). Some of the best natural dressings that you can prepare on your own are: Lemon juice with your favorite herbs and pepper; Red wine vinegar; Balsamic vinegar, Apple cider vinegar; Sherry vinegar, and vinaigrette (modified to reduce fat: 1-2 tsp extra virgin olive oil + 2 tbsp Balsamic vinegar or Red wine vinegar or Apple cider vinegar with herbs and black ground pepper to taste).

**Flavorings**

- Use a vegetable source to add flavor (salsa).
- Use herbs (basil, oregano, cilantro, sage, rosemary, thyme, parsley).
- Use spices (nutmeg, black ground pepper, paprika, cinnamon, Mrs. Dash).
- Use lemon or lime juice.
- Use red wine vinegar or apple cider vinegar.
- Use fresh or powdered ginger.
- Use horseradish.
- Use low sodium seasoning (soy sauce, *Goya* vegetable seasoning, *Maggi* cubes, chicken broth, vegetable broth)
- Use *Worcestershire* sauce or *Kikkoman* sauce/lite soy sauce (low sodium).
- Sprinkle on a butter flavoring (not real butter).
- Sprinkle with Parmesan cheese.
- Use sodium-free salt substitutes.
- Use mustard.

## Chapter 4

# Making the Right Food Choices - Choose Good Quality Food

Like most of us, perhaps you have wondered why you gain weight or why you lose weight only to regain it despite dieting and exercising vigorously. Perhaps you have even wondered why you feel anxious, tired, or depressed, suffer from frequent headaches, and feel hungry a few hours after eating.

You may be surprised to learn that the answers to all of these questions lie in the food choices we make day after day. We are literally at war with food. Some of the foods we eat today are not only deficient in nutrients and antioxidants, but they are also high in pesticides and other harmful toxins, some of which may be carcinogenic. In order to protect our body, we must make better choices and change the way we think about food and physical activity.

We need to eat more foods that provide adequate antioxidants and phytonutrients. As discussed in Chapter 3, making the food choices that are suitable for our bodies and activity level can boost a sluggish metabolism, neutralize free radicals, and decrease cellular inflammation and catabolic hormones, such as insulin and cortisol. The proper foods can also increase concentration, decrease fatigue, elevate mood, keep skin, muscle and bones toned, decrease body fat, and promote weight loss. This seems like a pretty good incentive if you need a motivation to eat better or exercise.

## The Consequences of Poor Food Choices

Food choices can make all the difference between losing weight and gaining weight and feeling good about yourself or feeling lousy. Once you begin to make the right food choices for your body, you will immediately begin to feel better and see results. Let's take a look at four of my patients who ultimately realized this food and wellness connection.

### Susanna Learned That Food Affected Her Mood and Personality

Susanna, a 50-year-old menopausal homemaker, recently came to me for help with weight problems. She had many other health issues including fatigue, anxiety, depression, and frequent headaches. She also had high blood pressure, high cholesterol, and thyroid disease. She was taking several medications, some of which made her feel worse than the problems she was taking them for. While her case may have been a tough one, her pleasant personality made it easy to work with her.

The first thing that I noticed was that she was eating foods, such as potatoes, pizza, pasta, hamburgers, and sweets quite often. She had no idea that the type of foods she was eating was in many ways responsible for her emotional distress, high cholesterol, and weight.

Susanna was surprised to learn that her medical condition and weight could improve if she made simple changes in her food choices and lifestyle. After the initial evaluation, she began an anti-inflammatory diet consisting of adequate non-starchy leafy vegetables, low-glycemic fruits and carbohydrates, lean proteins (including soy), and healthy fats. She learned to eat these foods according to her activity level. As a result, instead of storing fat, her body burned calories. Within a few weeks, her energy level increased dramatically and she became more physically active. She felt better than she had in years.

In a mere eight weeks, Susanna dropped 15 pounds, of which 13 pounds were body fat. With the weight loss came a change in mood and personality. This all happened as a result of her making the right food choices (anti-inflammatory diet) and maintaining a moderate level of physical activity that is in line with her food consumption. She achieved so much without making drastic and unrealistic alterations to her lifestyle.

*"It's like running your car," she said, "When you put gas into your car, you want to put in the best grade. If you put a low-grade gas into your car, it will run but not as smoothly. I want to make the best choice. If I do it for my car, why not for my body?"*

This reminded me of a patient in my gynecology practice who had hysterectomy for a large fibroid and persistent heavy bleeding that did not respond to conservative management over a long period. After a short, uneventful post-operative period, suddenly, I realized that she was more concerned about her weight than the reasons that I had done a major surgery on her. She had severe depression and lacked self-esteem to the point where she didn't think life was worth living. She had tried to take her own life on multiple occasions, and was on several anti-depressants and potent psychotropic drugs. It wasn't immediately obvious to her doctors that the root cause of her problems was her weight and all the things that were associated with it.

Adding to all the internal pressures and stress, her husband from childhood had abandoned her for a close friend. She turned forty-five few weeks after her hysterectomy—alone she made up her mind to seek help, fearing the inevitable. She reached the decision to get her life back together after a long spiritual counseling with the priest who had convinced her that suicide was against God's will. Losing weight becomes an obsession, suddenly, but in spite of her eagerness, she could not really commit herself to the sacrifice and discipline that was required for a long term weight loss program. As a result, her progress was up and down and going nowhere – until a conversation regarding her dog came up one day. I wanted to know if her dog was in good health. She responded with a nod.

"Is he overweight? I asked.

"No," she replied, beginning, rather painfully, to explain, "I feed him better than I feed myself. I won't give him any junk food, but I can't understand why I give it to myself."

Most of us have pondered issues like this and have come to the realization that we often spend energy and effort taking care of others but pay very little attention to our own needs. I often ask my patients, "Who is taking care of you?" And the answer is always the same – an embarrassing "nobody". It took time and conviction to get Susanna to accept the idea of paying attention to the most important person in her life. That prompted her to take action – making healthier food choices a way of life and maintaining a level of physical activity (breaking sweat five to seven days a week).

Recognizing the negative effect of some foods is a critical step that all of us need to know in order to make the right food choices. The wrong choices can drain our energy, slow our body's metabolism and cause weight gain, while the right foods can increase energy, speed up our metabolism, and help us lose weight. The UDP shopping list and meal plan are high in foods that boost energy and can help to transform a slow metabolism into an efficient fat-burning one.

**Jonathan Experienced Frequent Headaches and Fatigue**

Jonathan is a 42-year-old businessman with a demanding lifestyle. He was frequently tired and suffered from depression. He had classic symptoms of hypoglycemia: headaches, lethargy, hunger pangs, and cravings just a few hours after he had eaten. His cholesterol was high despite the fact that he was on medication. He joined a gym on the advice of his personal physician. When nothing changed in five months, he decided to see me.

Jonathan's day was typical and most of us could relate to it. It started with a stop at the convenience store where he would grab one or two bags of mini muffins (8 per bag), a bottle of water and a diet coke for breakfast. Lunch was a stop at *McDonald's*. His usual meal was a Quarter Pounder with cheese, large fries, and a diet coke. His dinner consisted of a whole plate of pasta with lots of cheese, Italian bread, and sweetened iced tea.

Looking at his diet, it was easy to see why his cholesterol was high and he had so many health problems. First, his diet was high in fat and calories and deficient in nutrients and antioxidants. It lacked adequate fiber – particularly soluble fiber. Remember, soluble fiber slows the absorption of calories and carbohydrates (reducing blood-sugar spikes after meals) and enhances weight loss. His carbohydrate consumption was far more than he needed for his level of physical activity. Instead of burning calories, his body was storing fat. In spite of his best efforts, he was gaining weight.

Jonathan was frustrated and on the verge of giving up when he came to see me. He was very insightful and appeared motivated and willing to do whatever it took to improve his life. His problem was that he was not aware of the extent to which his poor food choices affected his progress and his entire life.

Making the wrong food choices hurts you in more than one way. First, it promotes fat storage. Second, it cancels out any gains resulting from physical activity. Jonathan was not unusual in this respect. Most of us start our day making the wrong food choices and are not truly aware of the consequences. This causes an energy drainage that can lead to cravings and compulsive eating. On the other hand, eating the right balance of carbohydrates that do not convert to blood sugar rapidly can boost energy and help to lower blood cholesterol levels. Like Susanna, Jonathan learned that his food choices had everything to do with the way he was feeling – the cravings, the headaches, the depression, the high cholesterol levels, and the simple fact that he could not lose weight even with vigorous exercise.

**Salvatore Found That Exercise Alone Was Not Enough**

Salvatore was 53 years old and had high blood pressure when he first came to see me. He worked out regularly in order to lose weight and control his blood pressure. He was 35 pounds overweight and had a body fat level of 36 percent (normal: 11-22%). Besides his medical condition, Salvatore was unhappy about his appearance – particularly the fat around his belly. It made him look much older than his age and he was willing to do anything to get rid of it.

Salvatore was also well aware that the risk for heart attack and stroke is higher when fat is stored mainly around the belly area, close to major internal organs. He was very worried because other members of his family had died of heart disease.

Surprisingly, Salvatore was not a big eater and had been on a high protein diet for some time. He had joined a gym and was exercising fanatically. Despite his best efforts, he did not lose weight or lower his blood pressure. His problem seemed to be that he was eating the wrong types of carbohydrates (those that rapidly raise blood sugar levels) and fats that were high in saturated fatty acids.

His typical meal included baked potatoes, hamburgers, high-fat salad dressings, and some low-quality vegetable choices. He thought he was cutting down on calories by skipping breakfast and that was a terrible mistake. Unbeknownst to him, skipping breakfast made him vulnerable to stress and the urge to overeat. By dinnertime, he was out of control and would eat everything in sight. It was no surprise then that he was usually very tired and lethargic after dinner.

Working with Salvatore was not as difficult as working with most people in a similar situation. He was motivated, disciplined, and eager to lose weight and improve his health. He was on three medications for his blood pressure and was hoping to come off of at least one of them. Although he exercised regularly, he had no idea that the high-protein and high-sugar meal replacement bars that he was using frequently were sabotaging his progress. Most people who are exercising make this mistake, assuming that it is going to be beneficial for them. I strongly believe that these high-protein meal replacement bars are only beneficial to serious body builders and athletes – not the average person trying to lose weight.

By changing his diet and making better choices (eating an anti-inflammatory diet), Salvatore was able to decrease his body fat from 36 percent to 26 percent in less than 10 weeks. In total, he lowered his body fat to 16 percent, lost 41 pounds of fat, and gained 27 pounds of muscle. His biggest reward has been a better blood pressure reading and fewer medications. In addition, the belly fat is gone.

Salvatore is very happy with his healthy and toned physique. "I did not realize that making the wrong food choices was my major problem. Now I see how food can affect me," he says. "I plan to do this for the rest of my life." Maintaining his weight and keeping healthy is easier now than it has ever been. Salvatore has maintained his weight loss for over three years. His food choices and tailoring his intake to physical activity have made all the difference (see testimonial in Chapter 18 for complete story).

**Beatrice Used Foods to Self- Medicate**

Beatrice, 36, has Type II diabetes, high blood pressure, and high cholesterol. At 256 pounds and 5'4" tall, she was over 100 pounds overweight. She was feeling quite bad about herself when she first came to see me. She had tried many weight-loss programs and had lost weight just to gain it all back.

Her main issues were controlling her impulses to eat and snacking even when she was not hungry. She had a voracious appetite that nothing could satisfy. "I eat mostly when I'm bored. I use foods to self medicate," she confessed. She was eating more than 3,000 calories a day (50% fat, 33% carbohydrates, and 12% protein).

Her main motivations for trying to lose the weight were her dissatisfaction with the way she looked and her lack of energy. She also wanted to come off the medications she was taking. Even though she wanted help, she wasn't convinced that changing the way she ate was going to work. Her doubt was understandable because she had been through many diet programs.

Even after all her disappointments, Beatrice was willing to give the UDP program a chance. The first thing that she noticed was that she had no desire to eat the way she used to. "I feel more satisfied even though I'm eating fewer calories than I ever did before and that's amazing!" she said. Beatrice lost an impressive 70 pounds in about eight months.

She felt better about herself, which reduced her need to eat when she was under stress.

She also had other things to be thankful for. She was taken off her blood pressure medication and no longer needed medication to control her blood sugar. "The most important thing that I learned is how to plan ahead, how to make the right food choices, and how much to eat when I'm exercising or not exercising." she said. "I also learned how to feed my body what it really needs and not necessarily what I like to eat, which are the kinds of foods that made me eat more and become out of control in the first place."

**What They All Have in Common**

They all made improper food choices on a consistent basis and, most importantly, eating disproportionately to their level of physical activity. But this is not unique to these four individuals. The obesity epidemic seen in this country within the last 20 years is definitely a result of our poor food choices and other bad choices we make day after day – such as a sedentary lifestyle and the pursuit of self-gratification (which could raise our level of stress).

We cannot simply blame our genes, which have remained unchanged over the last ten thousand years. Yet, the level of obesity that we know today was absent in the last two to three generations. By now, you must know that the foods we eat provide not only calories but also essential nutrients and antioxidants that are vital to our mental and physical well-being. It is imperative that we make the right food choices and also eat portion sizes that are in line with our level of physical activity. This is the only way to reduce the chance of converting calories into fat instead of energy. The food choices that you make form the foundation for your health and happiness.

## The Rewards of Good Choices

### Ellen Defeated Her Stress and Anxiety

Ellen, 65, had worried about being heavy and sluggish. Over the years, she had lost and regained weight and was tired of that routine. "Stress and anxiety usually make me lose control," she painfully admitted.

She had good reasons to be concerned. She had been very thirsty and urinating frequently in the past months. All of this came at the time when her weight soared. She had gained 30 pounds within the past few years. Since diabetes runs in her family, she was afraid that she could also develop the disease.

Before her retirement, Ellen was an active person. More recently, she had begun leading a sedentary lifestyle. Worse yet, she ate a diet high in fat and highly refined carbohydrates. The good news was that she was willing and eager to change her lifestyle and to eat a proper diet. Her transformation really centered on making the right food choices and keeping physically active in line with her food intake.

Ellen's new anti-inflammatory diet was low in calories and unhealthy fats and high in soluble fiber. The fiber made her feel full and also helped to reduce the number of calories she absorbed. But making the proper food choices was only part of the answer. She incorporated exercise into her lifestyle, getting about 30 minutes of aerobic and strength training about five days a week. Sometimes she walked. When she was not physically active, she decreased the amount of calories she ate. Her efforts paid off and, to her surprise, she lost 21 pounds in two months with a reduction in body fat from 44 percent to a healthy 35 percent.

"I never thought I could lose weight at my age. I've been trying for so long," she said with a big smile. Since she was lighter, she found her exercise routine easier to do. "I feel very good and energetic," she said, "But the most important thing that I'm proud of is the fact that I am eating a proper meal and I don't miss the bad foods that I used to like."

Ellen not only shed pounds, but she also probably halted the progression of insulin resistance syndrome (Syndrome X) into full-blown diabetes. Early in the UDP program, her blood profile showed her sugar levels in the range considered to be pre-diabetic. I will explain this later.

One summer, Ellen learned another important lesson that I always stress to my patients. Like many grandparents, she found herself busy trying to organize the family reunion and was not able to maintain her exercise routine. Imagine that you are Ellen and caught in this situation.

What would you have done – eat more calories, eat the same amount of calories, eat fewer calories, or eat smaller portions? The correct thing to do is to eat fewer calories and to choose your carbohydrates carefully in order to prevent elevated levels of blood sugar and insulin. This was what Ellen did and the reward was that she lost body fat and gained lean muscle mass in circumstances where most people would have gained weight (see Ellen's testimonial in Chapter 18).

We are all bombarded with foods that are low in nutrients but high in calories. We have been sold the idea that we have to eat a specified amount of calories to lose weight, regardless of our activity level. This is a serious mistake. The key to weight loss is to get the nutrients and antioxidants that are critical for our bodies to function properly and our brains to perform at maximum capacity. Above all, the greatest benefit is abundant energy and optimal health. We can easily achieve this goal if we tailor our food intake to our activity level on a regular basis.

The wrong food choices, such as the typical American diet that includes large amounts of calories and unhealthy fats and starches, not only causes weight gain but also promotes cellular inflammation and damage to skin, muscles, bones,, and arteries. It also promotes emotional problems and continual cravings that sabotage our best efforts to lose weight and improve our health.

## Are You Making Bad Choices?

By now, it shouldn't surprise you that a study done at the Harvard School of Public Health showed that more than 70 percent of the top 20 carbohydrate foods Americans eat today consist of the types of carbohydrates that are rapidly converted into blood sugar and body fat. I have listed some examples of such high-glycemic foods below. The low-glycemic foods listed on the left hand side are preferred options to the high-glycemic foods, which are ones we should limit.

| Low GI foods | High GI foods |
|---|---|
| Apples | Baked potatoes |
| Jam (no sugar added) | Bananas |
| Oranges | Candy |
| Skim Milk | Coca-Cola |
| Whole-wheat Pasta | Cranberry Juice (sweetened) |
| | French Fries |
| | Fruit Punch (most have sugar added) |
| | Mashed potatoes |
| | Most cold breakfast cereals |
| | Muffins |
| | Pancakes |
| | Pizza |
| | Refined Pasta |
| | Table Sugar |
| | White Bread |
| | White Rice (refined) |

Source: Dr. Simin Liu, Harvard University School of Public Health. ''Top 20 sources of carbohydrate in the American diet". Quoted in Brand-Miller, Jennie et al. The Glucose Revolution: The Authoritative Guide to the Glycemic Index. New York: Marlowe & Co., 1999.

In my opinion, carbohydrates are not bad foods. Problems arise when people whose bodies are unable to convert the calories into energy efficiently consume excessive amounts of carbohydrates, especially the refined types. As a result, instead of being burned, they are converted into fat, which leads to weight gain and health risk.

Sedentary people eating an excess of high-glycemic carbohydrate foods (carbohydrates that are digested quickly) are guaranteed to gain weight and to compromise their health. In contrast, people are more likely to lose weight and decrease cholesterol and blood sugar levels if their diets consists of low-glycemic carbohydrates (carbohydrates that are digested slowly) and are not rapidly converted into sugar. Low-glycemic carbohydrates in the right amounts are probably more suitable for the metabolic profile of sedentary individuals, whereas high-glycemic carbohydrates appear to be more appropriate for physically active individuals.

The Harvard Nurse's Health Study also found that most Americans do not eat adequate amounts of leafy green vegetables, beans, and whole fruits. These are foods that can balance our intake of nutrients and ensure an overall favorable low-glycemic load. In this respect, the typical American diet is a recipe for disaster.

Eating the wrong foods cause our muscles and body cells to work below capacity. Instead of burning calories, the body stores fat. We feel hungry in spite of the extra calories we consume and the huge stock of fuel we have stored in fat cells. Our bodies appear to be confused and in an assumed state of starvation and famine.

Our bodies hold on to fat instead of burning it for energy. Our appetites are stimulated and we eat more. Our muscles are forced to give up some energy by breaking down vital muscle tissue to provide proteins, which are converted into amino acids and then to more blood sugar for energy.

This happens because our brain and body cells solely depend on certain critical nutrients and their deficiencies could pose serious health risks and intense craving. In most cases, the symptoms and signs we later experience are indications that the brain and body cells are trying to communicate to us. Perhaps, trying to alert us that the environment is hostile and help is urgently needed: more nutrients and antioxidants and less carbohydrates, fats, and calories.

Muscles tissues and proteins are broken down at a faster rate than we can replace them and all of these are communicated through the only language that we understand – fatigue, low libido, and aches and pain. The question is, are we really listening?

The more our body fat increases, the slower our ability to burn calories and body fat and, above all this, we tend to eat more because we feel hungrier. As the body fat increases, so do the levels of insulin, cortisol, blood sugar, cholesterol, triglycerides, and inflammatory compounds that can virtually destroy every organ and tissue in our bodies – including the brain and heart.

The good news is that we can truly halt the progression of these bad things that drain our energy and make us vulnerable to disease – and I will show you how to do it. But, first of all, a brief review of some of the medical consequences of our poor food choices and lifestyle will help us to grasp the concept more affirmatively (see Chapter 5).

# Chapter 5

# The Medical Consequences Are Real

## Diabetes: The Silent Killer

### How Gloria and Dorothy Learned to Take Control

Gloria is living with type 1 diabetes that she developed when she was 18. She was tired, had an unquenchable thirst, and urinated frequently. She spent three weeks in the hospital before her blood-sugar level stabilized. She was told that she would have to take insulin injections for the rest of her life.

That was 30 years ago. Even though treatment has improved considerably, there is still one major aspect of the treatment plan that she still has to master: eating right and keeping physically active in order to help the muscle and body cells clear the sugar from the blood. Unfortunately, like most diabetics, Gloria depends solely on the insulin to clear her blood-sugar levels. This common mistake will be explained in detail later.

Dorothy is learning to live with type 2 diabetes. Dorothy, 69, is a retired teacher who has settled down to a life of inactivity. She gets fatigued after walking just a block. She has difficulty sleeping and suffers from anxiety. She struggles with her condition and, even with medication, her blood sugar and hemoglobin AIC are high. Hemoglobin AIC tells how well a diabetic is doing in keeping glucose and insulin under control over the previous three months. A high number like Dorothy's predicts a greater chance of future problems.

Dorothy also suffered from high blood pressure and high cholesterol, which were both elevated even though she was on several medications. Heart disease and stroke run in her family and she was well aware that diabetics with high blood pressure and high cholesterol are more susceptible to a heart attack (see her testimonial in Chapter 18).

### A Fast Growing Disease

It is estimated that worldwide about 150 million people have diabetes and the number is expected to double by the year 2025, according to the World Health Organization. This disease is one of the most challenging health problems of our time. In America, an estimated 15 million people have the disease and over 500,000 new cases are diagnosed each year and, worst of all, millions have the disease but don't even realize they have it. About ten percent of the adult population in Canada has diabetes. And up to four percent of the Swede population has the disease.

Diabetes is rapidly growing in developing countries that have adopted westernized diet and lifestyles (such as India, Indonesia and various African countries).

## What Causes Diabetes?

Diabetes is a chronic disorder in which there is too much sugar in the blood. Type 1, or insulin dependent diabetes, is the form that occurs most commonly in children and young adults. It is also the form that Gloria lives with. It accounts for about 5 percent of all diabetes cases. The major difficulty in this form of diabetes is that the pancreas produces little or no insulin.

Type 2 diabetes affects nearly 90 percent of people with diabetes and typically occurs in adults like Dorothy who are over 40. Now, let's try to answer the question of what causes this form of diabetes.

In the case of someone like Gloria, who has type 1 diabetes, it is often an unfortunate circumstance in which a person's immune system attacks the insulin producing beta cells in the pancreas. Viruses, poisonous chemicals, and certain drugs could trigger the attack. The cause of Gloria's diabetes was never established, except for the fact that her grandmother on her father's side had died from complications related to the disease.

Type 2 diabetes, like Dorothy has, is at an epidemic level worldwide and is often associated with weight gain, a sedentary lifestyle and a diet laden with large amounts of fat and refined carbohydrates. Unlike type 1, this disease is preventable. At the very least, its onset can be delayed – and I will show you how shortly.

When Dorothy retired and all her children grew up and left home, she found herself eating high-calorie foods and getting little or no exercise. She also had close family members with diabetes, placing her at a higher risk but not necessarily making her destined to develop the disease. While genes are important, our lifestyles and food choices are perhaps far more important in the development of diabetes.

There are now several studies that confirm this. For example, recent studies at Harvard University's School of Public Health involving 70,000 women and 50,000 men revealed that diets with low fiber and high-glycemic carbohydrates increased the risk of developing diabetes by as much as two-to-three times. Several other studies are supporting the usefulness and value of exercise. Both walking and vigorous activity have been found to substantially reduce the risk of type 2 diabetes in women.

## Children With an Adult Disease

About three years ago, my computer specialist asked me to help his daughter, Natasha, who was 8 and weighed a whopping 133 pounds. She was shy, introverted, and doing poorly in school. Classmates teased her and she had no friends, she said.

Her father's main concern was that his daughter might develop type 2 diabetes. The disease ran in his family and he had it too. Natasha fit the profile perfectly. She had abdominal obesity with 45 percent body fat, she was sedentary and she loved fast food, sodas, and sweets. Later, you can learn more about her story in Chapter 18.

Twenty years ago, type 2 diabetes was primarily an adult disease, but that is changing. Doctors are now seeing the disease in children. Close to half a million children in the United States alone are now diagnosed with the disease. Why the increase? Though genetic predisposition is partly responsible, the real culprits are weight (belly fat) and sedentary lifestyle. About 80 percent of young people with type 2 diabetes are overweight. The number of obese children has doubled in the past 20 years to roughly one-third of the children in this country. Being overweight or obese in the womb and childhood increases the likelihood of being overweight in adulthood (see Chapter 6). If this trend continues, it could compromise the health and productivity of future generations.

**What Accounts for This?**

Being born to a mother who had gestational diabetes or a woman who gained too much extra weight during pregnancy increases a child's chance of developing diabetes (see Chapter 6). Also, eating habits and activity patterns have changed over the past 20 years. More and more people are relying on soft drinks and fast foods that are high in fats, highly refined carbohydrates, and simple sugars as staples in their diets. This is all happening at a time when there has been a marked reduction in physical activity in schools and homes. Educating children, especially those who are at risk, to stay away from junk food and to get involved in recreational activities, such as sports, will help to slow the number of cases of type 2 diabetes diagnosed each year.

**Are You At Risk?**

You are at risk if one or more of the following is true:

- You are overweight with belly fat.
- You gained 11-18 pounds in a short time (this can double your risk).
- You are over 40.
- You have a family history of diabetes.
- You are living a sedentary lifestyle.
- You are eating a poor diet containing large amounts of fat and refined carbohydrates (fast food and take-out).
- You have high blood pressure.
- You have diabetes during pregnancy (gestational diabetes).

Fortunately, you can reduce your risk by eating a healthy diet, increasing physical activity and keeping your weight down, particularly body fat. Even a modest weight loss of 10-20 percent has been shown to have significant health benefits.

## How Can I Tell If I Have Diabetes?

There are warning signs, even though they are not specific to diabetes, which may help to keep us alert and force us to seek medical help. The symptoms most people report to their doctors are excessive thirst, frequent urination, fatigue, mood swings, and, in women, chronic vaginal yeast infection.

The definitive diagnosis can be made in a simple procedure that involves fasting overnight and having the blood sugar level checked before breakfast the following day. Blood sugar under 110mg/dl is normal; between 110 and 125 is pre-diabetic or insulin resistant; and 126 is considered full-blown diabetes. A fair number of the people with weight issues whom I see in my clinic fall into the pre-diabetic state or Syndrome X (insulin resistance syndrome). Syndrome X predisposes one to diabetes – but with proper diet, nutritional support, and regular exercise, it is possible to control or halt the progression of the disease.

## What Is Syndrome X (Metabolic Syndrome)?

In order to fully understand diabetes, heart disease and many other chronic health problems, you need to know a little bit about Syndrome X, also known as metabolic syndrome or insulin resistance syndrome. It is estimated that about 30 percent of the adult population in the United States suffers from Syndrome X. It is a precursor to diabetes and heart disease that can predate the onset of these diseases by a decade or more.

Syndrome X is actually a cluster of conditions that include high blood-sugar levels, high cholesterol and triglyceride levels, high blood pressure, increased blood clotting, abdominal obesity, and insulin resistance. If left unchecked, Syndrome X frequently progresses to type 2 diabetes and also increases the risk of heart disease.

Syndrome X occurs when one consumes too many carbohydrates, especially the refined types, forcing the body to produce more insulin to move the blood sugar into the muscles and cells. But, without exercise or a significant level of physical activity, the muscles are unable to absorb and burn off the excess blood sugar.

The body tries to deal with the problem and clears out the excess sugar by converting it to fat. The more fat the body stores, the more the muscle and cells become resistant to insulin. As a result, the blood sugar and insulin levels can be raised to dangerously high levels. This, in turn, can lead to the formation of destructive free radicals that can trigger inflammation. You will learn more about inflammation later. The high blood sugar and insulin can also cause your body to make more cholesterol and triglycerides, increasing your risk of stroke, heart attack, or sudden death.

To deal with the high level of blood sugar, the pancreas may react by producing more insulin. As the years pass by, however, the pancreas becomes incapable of keeping up the demand and exhausts itself. It is at this point that full-blown diabetes develops. As noted previously, some people don't even realize they have the disease until after a severe health crisis.

## The Dangers of High Insulin

Our trillion body cells and muscles need insulin for glucose to enter the cells and be used as fuel. This is a good thing. Without this hormone, dangerous levels of sugar would build up in the blood and our cells and muscles would literally starve. This is one reason why diabetics frequently suffer from low energy and fatigue.

A healthy pancreas keeps blood sugar levels stable by releasing just the right amount of insulin as glucose levels rise after a meal and fall between meals. The liver also helps to keep the blood sugar level stable by storing excess glucose in a form called glycogen. It then releases the glycogen back into the bloodstream when the levels of glucose fall critically low between meals or in a state of starvation.

Both the pancreas and the liver ensure that blood-sugar levels and insulin levels are kept stable throughout the day. Because when sugar and insulin levels build up in the blood, inflammation increases and it is a health hazard that could lead to Syndrome X, diabetes, heart disease, and many other chronic health problems.

An obese person with Syndrome X or early stages of Type II diabetes can produce significantly higher amounts of insulin than a healthy person as a result of excessive blood sugar. A high level of blood insulin causes fat storage in the belly area and makes it difficult to lose weight. So, as long as Gloria was injecting a high dose of insulin, the weight loss was slow and so was the reduction in body fat. Increasing foods high in nutrients, antioxidants, and soluble fiber and boosting metabolic rate through exercise solved the problem. High levels of insulin not only raise inflammation levels, but may cause the liver to produce more cholesterol, as well. High levels of oxidized LDL (bad cholesterol) can stick to the walls of arteries, causing the build-up of plaques. The plaques can attract inflammatory cells that are trying to ward off the attack.

With time, the plaques grow larger as excess blood sugar and inflammatory cells attach to them, clogging and damaging arteries, vessels, and nerves. This increases the chance of heart attack, stroke, dementia, and damage to the eyes (the primary cause of blindness in America). High insulin and sugar levels can also affect the kidneys and cause fluid retention that may lead to high blood pressure.

If the trend is left unchallenged, the end result can be catastrophic. It explains why two-thirds of diabetics die of complications related to cardiovascular disease (heart attack, stroke, and kidney failure). It also explains why the mortality rate is two to four times that of the normal population. The irony is that diabetes is a severe disease, though the early symptoms are relatively mild and the disease may go unrecognized for years until the damage is already done. Hence the name: the silent killer!

## Diabetes Is Manageable

In spite of this grim reality, there is good news. It is within your power to control or halt Syndrome X, as well as diabetes, by making better food choices and healthy lifestyle changes including decreasing excess abdominal fat. Remember, the onset of diabetes actually occurs

10 years or more after Syndrome X, which can be reversed by eating low-glycemic index foods and high-fiber foods that are low in saturated fats, trans fats, and Omega-6 fats, as was the case with Evelyn.

Gloria and Dorothy, who already had diabetes, were better able to control their blood sugar, cholesterol, and blood pressure by eating appropriate portions of foods high in fiber and low in saturated fats. In addition, they both became active and engaged in regular exercises at least five days a week.

Gloria lost nearly 50 pounds and was able to decrease her insulin dosage from around 90 units to about 40 units daily. Dorothy lost 35 pounds and reduced her fat percentage from 45 percent to a healthy 34 percent. Her blood sugar stabilized and she was able to use a low-dose oral medication with minimal side effects. Both women have more energy and a very positive attitude towards life. They are well aware that diabetes cannot be reversed; therefore, it is wise to follow a simple common sense approach of exercise and a good diet, including proper stress management.

Later, you will meet other ordinary people who have gained some considerable degree of knowledge about the illness that is bothering them, and are better able to care for themselves as well as relatives. It should be stressed that even as you gain the knowledge to improve your own health, you should always consult and work with your physician. Most physicians would be very appreciative caring for a patient that is anxious to learn and know more about their diseases. In fact, this might open a window of opportunity to develop a stronger relationship and trust with your physician.

**Treating Diabetes**

Drug companies are constantly working to find new and more effective medications to regulate blood sugar and enhance the body's use of insulin. However, these drugs are not without side effects. For example, Rezulin was recently withdrawn from the market because of liver toxicity. Perhaps drugs are not a panacea or the ultimate solution. "Prevention is better than a cure" is a cliché that still holds true.

In my view, insulin should never be the first line of defense because of its side effects. High levels of insulin can affect every organ system in our bodies, particularly the muscles. The heart is made of muscle and it too is vulnerable. Paired with cortisol, insulin can break down muscle tissue and promote the storage of belly fat. It's very difficult to lose weight or burn body fat when one is injecting into their body high amounts of insulin and, in most cases, people end up gaining weight and storing belly fat.

*Insulin is an appetite stimulator that causes cravings and overeating. The bad news for those trying to lose weight is that when the levels of insulin are high, the body is instructed to hold onto its fat reserve. As a result, the body burns muscle tissue instead. This could be one reason why the majority of people who are diabetic and are on high doses of insulin find it hard to lose weight or body fat.*

*The irony is that these people need to lose weight, particularly body fat, in order to decrease insulin resistance and subsequently use less insulin. Ideally, a smaller dose of insulin is far better than a higher dose.*

*Therefore, the goal for better diabetic control should be to aim to decrease insulin dosage while at the same time maintaining fairly normal levels of fasting and postprandial blood sugar readings. The bottom line is that insulin should not be taken lightly. What then, should you do?*

## Educate Yourself

When considering treatment or weight loss, you must take full responsibility for your own care and learn all you can about the disease and treatment. Even though you may be under the care of medical professionals, you are still in charge – and no other person knows your body better than you. Regardless of how good a treatment is, it's bound to fail without your total involvement and commitment. Therefore, try to know everything possible about the disease, including the foods that will help you to control your blood sugar better. The more you learn about the disease, the better you will be equipped to manage your health and increase the prospect of living a longer and healthier life. Most of the useful information that you need to help you manage diabetes or lose weight won't be found in pamphlets and books. It will come from your own personal experiences in due time. You benefit and gain competence by paying attention and being observant. This calls for patience and curiosity. Below are some basic recommendations:

## Limit Simple Sugars, Refined Carbohydrates, and Animal Fats

Limiting sugars, refined carbohydrates, high-glycemic starches, and animal fats is crucial in the management of Syndrome X, diabetes, and obesity. They increase the need for insulin – which, as we have already seen, is a powerful appetite stimulator and fat storage hormone. High blood-insulin levels frequently lead to low blood-sugar levels (hypoglycemia) that can cause headaches, anxiety, low energy, sweating, confusion, loss of consciousness, and even death. Very often, dealing with low blood sugar requires taking foods that will cause your blood sugar to overshoot. And then you're back to square one, which forces you to take extra insulin or oral medication in order to stabilize the blood-sugar levels. The vicious cycles of high and low blood-sugar levels are not healthy.

Both Gloria and Dorothy are familiar with these experiences, which are sometimes very frightening and distressing. For Dorothy, the main cause of hypoglycemia was eating bagels with cream cheese and orange juice for breakfast. One morning, a few hours after eating one of these carbohydrate loaded meals, she had a bad reaction that left her shaking, sweating, and feeling like she was going to pass out. She thought she was having a heart attack, while in reality her body was in shocked due to the sudden and rapid drop in blood sugar (hypoglycemia). You will learn more about this phenomenom in other chapters.

You too can prevent the frightening experience Dorothy went through by simply avoiding the consumption of refined or high-glycemic carbohydrates. Elevated sugar in the blood stream, as you already know, can stress the body by raising free radicals that can be harmful to many organs. People with diabetes are particularly prone to cataracts, blindness, and problems with blood circulation that often lead to leg amputation. You should also minimize the consumption of alcohol, including beer, which can cause a sudden drop in blood sugar.

Limit foods high in animal fat, especially full fat cheeses and fast foods that are dense in calories and fat. The higher the body fat, the more inflammation is triggered unnecessarily, increasing the risk of heart disease, cancer, and so many other diseases. Also, the more body fat you have, the more your muscles and body cells become resistant to insulin. This means you have to take higher insulin doses to keep your blood-sugar level in a healthy range. Unfortunately, high insulin levels promote more fat storage as well as stimulate the appetite.

## Can You Eat Too Many Carbohydrates?

You certainly can – particularly if your main staples are refined and high glycemic carbohydrates. The tendency is for your body to release blood sugar faster than it can use it. This is what happens when you eat a diet that is high in saturated fats and refined carbohydrates, such as regular pasta, sweetened breakfast cereal, or white rice.

The current recommendation for low-fat and high-carbohydrate diets (50-65 percent of total calories) is definitely not suitable for many diabetics or even people who lead sedentary lifestyles. Several studies have touched on this subject, including those by Dr. Ann Coulston and her colleagues at Stanford University. Their research shows that eating a low-fat and high-carbohydrate diet might hurt, instead of help, diabetics.

The high-carbohydrate diet was found to increase blood levels of sugar and triglycerides while lowering HDL (good) cholesterol. You can easily see how such a diet may increase the risk of heart attack instead of preventing it. But this may not be the case if you choose the whole grain carbohydrates and in addition eat them according to your level of physical activity.

When this rule is applied to all carbohydrates, including whole grains, it's possible to have a better control of your blood sugar levels. Most often, we fall into the trap of eating more food, including whole grains, simply because they are considered healthy and safer. But that is far from the truth since too much of even good quality foods can cause weight gain or destabilize your blood sugar.

## Snacking Stabilizes Blood Sugar

Gloria's habit of checking her blood-sugar level before snacking almost cost her her life. One afternoon, she was driving home after checking her blood sugar. She did not have a snack because she believed her blood sugar was normal and didn't need one. About 20 minutes later, as she was in a heavy traffic, her blood sugar suddenly dropped so low that it seemed her brain was not getting enough glucose. Unable to figure out what was happening to her, somehow, she managed to get out of traffic and safely park on the side of the road, where she was later found semi-conscious and disoriented.

Serious incidents like this can be prevented by snacking between meals, instead of depending on blood-sugar checks, which are not always reliable. Gloria learned a hard lesson and she now snacks regularly between meals. Snacking helps to stabilize blood-sugar levels and also promotes healthy weight loss by helping to reduce the amount of food you eat during meals, especially dinner.

**Exercise Stabilizes Blood Sugar**

Over and over in this book, you will see the UDP mantra: maintain a regular level of physical activity throughout the day. Every little bit of activity matters. For instance, you will burn more calories if you take the stairs than if you use the elevator or walk short distances instead of driving. At the end of the day, if you have accumulated a minimum of 60 minutes of physical activity, you are on track as long as you don't sabotage your effort by eating extra calories.

Gloria and Dorothy realized that it was easier for them to control their blood-sugar levels with less medication if they exercised regularly. Gloria went to the gym with her son about three times a week – in addition to exercising on the treadmill in the morning. Dorothy liked brisk walking and went bowling three times a week. Regular physical activity, besides helping these women control their blood sugar and decrease insulin resistance, also helped them cope with stress in addition to losing weight and body fat.

**Foods to Include in the Diet**

Ideally, you should have fish (particularly fatty fish like salmon and mackerel) 3-5 times a week, chicken and turkey breast, lean meat, egg whites, egg beaters, and soybeans or other legumes. Soy is a high quality, low-fat protein source that increases insulin sensitivity and may even help to reduce the amount of insulin you are taking.

Soy also protects against kidney damage and increases metabolism. Both soy proteins and high-fiber carbohydrate foods are not easily converted to fat. Eat low-glycemic carbohydrates and whole grains (such as multigrain bread, brown rice, sweet potatoes, whole-wheat pasta, barley, and oats). Include low-glycemic fruits (such as apples, peaches, plums, and grapefruits), lots of dark, leafy, green, non-starchy vegetables (such as collards, spinach, and kale), cruciferous vegetables (such as broccoli, Brussel sprouts, and cabbage), colorful vegetables (such as raw carrots, turnips, tomatoes, red and green peppers, cactus, and okra), onions, garlic, kelp, mushrooms, berries (blackberries, blueberries, and strawberries), flaxseeds, flaxseed oil, and extra virgin olive oil, and drink plenty of water and green tea regularly.

In my own experience, you will find it very easy to control your blood sugar by doing simple things like: adding ½ cup of lightly steamed broccoli florets, chana dal lentil, cactus, or okra along with other vegetables during lunch and dinner. You can also have these vegetables separately at breakfast. These can be added as side dishes, vegetables dishes, or delicious vegetable soups. Other fiber sources that you can add to enhance fiber density include 1-2 tbsp of oat bran, ground flaxseeds, Benefiber, or Clearly Fiber.

**Supplements That Help**

In addition to eating a diet rich in non-starchy vegetables, fruits, soy, fish, lean meat, and whole grains, I recommend using supplements. Supplementing your diet with the right nutrients can substantially improve your chance of not developing diabetes or better controlling the disease if you have already been diagnosed with it. Supplements can help stimulate immune functions and protect healthy body cells against the damaging effects of elevated blood and insulin levels. Those to include on a daily basis for Syndrome X or diabetes are as follows:

- Broad-spectrum multivitamin/mineral.
- Vitamin E 400-800 IU (antioxidant) daily (d-alpha-tocopherol together with other tocopherols). The delta-tocotrienol vitamin E derivative found abundantly in red palm oil has more potent super-antioxidant activity than the standard vitamin E tocopherol.
- CoQ10 (antioxidant) 60-120 mg daily (improves metabolism, stabilizes blood-sugar levels, protects against cardiovascular disease and increases energy).
- Omega-3 or fish oil capsules, especially DHA, and fortified eggs (1000 mg 3 times a day). About 2 grams DHA per day has been shown to help reduce the risk of type 2 diabetes in people with Syndrome X.
- 1 tsp of ground cinnamon daily (sprinkle over cereals, sweet potatoes, vegetables, salads, or hot drinks) lowers blood sugar, triglycerides, and cholesterol.
- Soy protein powder (1 scoop has 25 grams protein and about 85 mg isoflavones). Add to foods, cereal, or mix with any fluid. Studies have shown that it helps people with diabetes control their blood sugar as well as some prescription drugs. Also drink soymilk with low sugar.

**Monitoring Your Blood Sugar**

Carefully monitoring your blood sugar and seeing how it changes with food, physical activity, and stress is very important. This sort of thing can be learned only over time through trial and error. So, never overlook the monitoring of your (fasting) blood sugar before breakfast and two hours after each meal. You are doing well if your fasting blood sugar is below 110 and the level two hours after a meal is below 150. Maintaining a normal blood sugar most of the time can help to prevent the harmful effects of high blood sugar.

For example, Gloria found out by careful monitoring that a certain variety of apple raised her blood sugar and Dorothy learned that stress caused her blood sugar to shoot up.

"One thing I learned that makes a big difference in controlling my blood sugar is how to listen to my body," Dorothy said.

Before coming to me, both Gloria and Dorothy had high blood-sugar levels. This was not because they were not getting enough insulin or medication but because they were not eating a proper diet (anti-inflammatory diet) or tailoring their food consumption to their physical activity level, and were definitely not managing stress properly. They were also accustomed to check their blood sugar before meals in order to gauge the dosage of insulin to administer. This method of monitoring did not offer them the benefit of knowing how various foods affect their blood sugar. It posed some serious drawbacks because it was difficult to accurately determine the dose of insulin appropriate for a given amount of food. Monitoring blood sugar this way can be effective in the initial stage of controlling brittle diabetes, but it's not the best choice in the long run.

*A much more reliable approach would be to check the blood sugar increase between fasting and two hours after a meal. This simple approach will enable you in a very short time to actually know the foods that increase your blood sugar versus those that don't. After a couple of trials, you will have a library of foods that in your own experience can affect your blood sugar either positively or negatively.*

*You can see how this can be empowering. In other words, you can control your blood sugar more accurately and hopefully cut down your dependence on insulin significantly. The added bonus is that you will be spending less on medications and, if you are employed, your employer will be cutting medical cost to boost the bottom line.*

*For example, Rosalyn was on the program for less than four weeks when she had to reduce her dosage of insulin from 130 units daily to about 43 units. Not surprising, her blood sugars were reading within the normal range – whereas, before, they were in the 300mg/dl range (see her full testimonial in Chapter 18).*

Both Gloria and Dorothy have become role models for relatives and friends and that is a very good thing. Gloria's teenage son and her husband followed suit and began eating healthy and exercising. Dorothy's daughter (who is a nurse in a prestigious hospital in Boston) was so impressed with the transformation of her mother that she was motivated to try to improve her own life. Dorothy also had the opportunity to care for her older brother, who had had multiple heart attacks. He was also diabetic. She took care of him during the most critical period and nursed him back to health when he was discharged home.

Without the experience with UDP, Dorothy knew she couldn't have been so resourceful, helpful, and confidant doing it at that rate. Not only was she helping her brother monitor his blood sugar and medications, she was also teaching him a better way of eating without deprivation. Sharing her knowledge and experience has even brought them closer together in a way she couldn't have imagined.

Teaching the average person the basic knowledge and skill to take care of some of the medical responsibilities that are received from a trained medical professional has great benefits that could help insurance companies cut cost and deliver efficient health care. It's possible to better manage medical cost in a partnership between the ensurer and ensuree. Dorothy demonstrated that such a program has a place in modern medical care.

## The Syndrome X -- Heart Disease Connection

In the previous sections, we saw how a good number of obese people have a pre-diabetic disease (Syndrome X) for many years before they actually develop diabetes. And, if they lose body fat and not necessarily weight, eat properly, and adopt a healthier lifestyle, they have a good chance of preventing Syndrome X from developing into diabetes. In this section, I will touch briefly on the connection between Syndrome X and heart disease. But first, let's look at the grim statistic:

**Heart disease is America's # 1 killer**
500,000 men and women die each year, but most heart disease can be prevented or reversed with proper diet, exercise and a change in lifestyle.

### What Is Heart Disease?

In brief, most heart disease is caused by hardening of the arteries called atherosclerosis, probably as a result of free radicals, inflammation, and plaque deposits. In most cases, the condition develops gradually and could start from childhood (as observed from autopsies of young people who died in accidents). If it develops slowly, you may even have the disease during your adult life without experiencing any major symptoms. But, in people with high risks (such as smoking, drinking, and sedentary), the condition may develop earlier and cause major symptoms.

Atherosclerosis causes a reduction in the blood flow through the arteries that are affected. When the arteries of the heart (the coronary arteries) are involved, the muscles are deprived of oxygen and nutrients and, as a result, the heart is unable to pump blood effectively. Consequently, the heart works twice as hard to try to maintain normal blood circulation. The increase in workload can cause enlargement of the heart and aorta. If the trend persists, the heart eventually cannot keep up and begins to fail. It is at this point that most people will begin to experience chest pains, shortness of breath (especially during exercise like snow shoveling), and even swelling of the ankles.

In some unfortunate instances, a blood clot or plaque inside an artery can completely block blood flow, causing a heart attack. In the brain, atherosclerosis can cause stroke. A significant reduction in blood flow in elderly people or those with diabetes as a result of hardening of the arteries in the legs can result in poor wound healing, gangrene and leg amputation. In brief, this is the end result of two competing processes that are vital to life –

one that causes blood to clot and another that prevents blood from clotting. Diets high in fatty fish and rich in Omega-3 fatty acids prevent blood from clotting, whereas diets high in vegetable oils and meat that are rich in Omega-6 fatty and arachidonic acid cause blood to clot. I have touched on this subject in Chapter 3 and will go into further details in Chapter 11.

If you're an athlete, you may have experienced muscle cramps or spasm, especially during exercise. This is most likely due to accumulation of lactic acid in a young, active person and probably not related to blood clots as discussed above.

### The Syndrome X – Heart Disease Connection

In the previous sections, I explained that Syndrome X is a condition in which the body becomes insensitive to insulin. As a result, dangerously high levels of insulin are needed to achieve the same effect as in healthy people. We have seen previously that a high level of insulin causes inflammation – a key process in the destruction of arteries and heart muscle. Interestingly, a high number of patients with heart disease have Syndrome X, just like people who are diabetic.

The most obvious connection is that in most cases these people have blood-sugar levels and insulin levels that are higher than those found in the average person. In addition, they may have varying degrees of other problems that are linked to insulin – such as high cholesterol, high triglycerides, high blood pressure, increased clotting, and abdominal obesity (this is the cluster that is classically described as Syndrome X or more recently metabolic syndrome).

### Inflammation Sets the Stage for a Heart Attack

It's only appropriate that I say a bit more in this paragraph about inflammation without going into too much detail. Inflammation has long been considered a normal process – a natural response that protects us. It is nothing more than the body's immune response to injury, cancer, foreign body, virus, or infection. However, more recently it is believed to do more than protect us. There is accumulating evidence that it is the underlying cause of most chronic diseases including heart disease, diabetes, cancer, and even obesity.

The immune system forms an intricate web of defense that protects us at all levels – so that anytime we are injured or attacked by bacteria or foreign chemicals (such as pesticides and other food poison), our body fights back by releasing a host of potent chemical compounds. Activated white cells or macrophages are stimulated to produce a variety of compounds that promote inflammation – such as C-reactive protein (CRP), interleukin-6 (IL-6), tumor necrosis factor-alpha, and prostaglandins. In most of the cases, the invader is engulfed, subdued, and destroyed promptly and the inflammatory response returns to normal without any incidence.

However, in some cases, the inflammatory response lingers on as a low-grade inflammation that silently and quietly destroys the very tissues and organs it is supposed to be protecting. Unfortunately, this destructive process could go on for months or years. It is this painless, chronic low-grade inflammation that is now widely believed to cause heart disease, stroke, diabetes, premature aging, arthritis, Alzheimer's, cancer, obesity, and other chronic diseases.

The challenge now is to detect chronic inflammation early before serious damage is done and, to that end, researchers have developed blood tests that can be cheaply and easily measured like any other lab test. One area in which there has been tremendous progress is the early detection of heart disease. As you know, heart disease kills more people yearly than any other disease in this country.

## Tests to Detect Low-Grade Systemic Inflammation

Since chronic low-grade inflammation silently attacks and destroys the walls of arteries, causing fatty plaques to rupture and trigger heart attacks, a marker that shows an elevated level of inflammation before heart attack strikes would undoubtedly save lives. There is such a marker today and it is called C-reactive protein (CRP) – a blood protein that is not only elevated with inflammation, but also promotes inflammation.

One drawback is that it is not as specific as some physicians would like. Nevertheless, most practioners are already using it routinely to measure inflammation levels in the body. The CRP test is a better predictor of heart disease than traditional tests, such as total cholesterol, LDL (bad) cholesterol, or homocysteine levels. It has the ability to predict heart disease long before any of the older tests. When used in analysis with other risk factors, such as high cholesterol, smoking, diabetes, and high blood pressure, there is no doubt that it is a powerful predictor of heart attack.

Dr. Paul Ridker of the Harvard Medical School found that people with elevated CRP levels were at a greater risk of a heart attack by four and a half times. The second best test was the ratio of total cholesterol to HDL cholesterol – which is the standard test most people are familiar with.

Sharply elevated inflammatory markers (such as C-reactive protein and IL-6) strongly indicate the presence of an underlying inflammatory disease (heart disease, diabetes, arthritis, and other degenerative diseases). Elevated levels of inflammatory markers are also strongly predictive of people who will suffer a heart attack in the near future. Since elevated C-reactive protein and IL-6 predict way ahead of time those people who are at high risk for mortality, it is a good idea to ask your physician to include these inflammatory markers in your routine blood work.

These tests can even predict the risk of stroke, heart attack, sudden death, and vascular disease among those individuals that do not display the classic symptoms or those with no history of cardiovascular disease. Inflammatory markers do not only help to identify impending disease, but they can also be helpful in following the course of disease and treatment.

## Anti-Inflammatory Foods

The good news is that elevated and life-threatening levels of inflammation in the body can be reduced with diets that are high in antioxidants, such as fatty cold-water fish (mackerel, salmon, and herring), extra virgin oil, cold-pressed canola oil, macadamia oil, flaxseed oil, and non-starchy dark leafy green vegetables (kale, broccoli, green beans, cauliflower and spinach). Fruits with anti-inflammatory nutrients are also beneficial (such as prunes, blueberries, blackberries, strawberries, and citrus fruits). You can find a detailed list in Chapter 3.

### Nutritional Supplements With Antioxidant Properties

Another important line of defense includes nutritional supplements that have antioxidant properties, such as vitamin E 400-800 IU daily (as mixed tocopherols and natural form), vitamin C 500-1,000 mg daily, mixed carotenoids 15,00-20,00 mg, coenzyme Q10 60-120 mg, selenium 200 mcg, GLA 1, 000 mg daily (GLA supplements are found in borage oil, evening primrose oil, and black currant oil), 3-6 grams of fish oil daily or flaxseed oil capsules, and 1-2 tbsp wheat germ daily.

### Foods That Promote Inflammation

Cutting back on foods that promote inflammation – such as refined carbohydrates and grains (pasta, white bread, white rice, and high glycemic breakfast cereals) and starchy vegetables (potatoes and corn) – is a necessary step. These foods raise insulin levels, which may, in turn, trigger inflammation and CRP levels.

More directly, diets high in refined carbohydrates and foods that rapidly raise blood sugar and insulin levels can trigger intense cellular inflammation, leading to an increased risk of heart disease and other degenerative diseases. The evidence has come largely from studies reported by Dr. Simin Liu of Harvard Medical School. Middle-aged women whose diet consisted of highly refined breakfast cereals, white bread, muffins, potatoes, and white rice had elevated levels of CRP in their bloodstream – suggesting an increased risk of heart attack. Interestingly, the women who were overweight and were at increased risk of insulin resistance showed the highest inflammation levels.

In Chapter 3, I talked briefly about Omega-6 and Omega-3 fatty acids. Omega-6 fatty acids and its family of compounds are largely pro-inflammatory and are found in vegetable oils, such as corn, peanut, safflower, sunflower, and soybean. They are also found in meats and processed foods made with hydrogenated or partially hydrogenated oils (some margarines are high in Omega-6 fatty acids and trans fats). In contrast, the anti-inflammatory Omega-3 fatty acids and family of compounds are found largely in cold-water fish (salmon), flaxseeds, and flaxseed oil. The secondary sources are seeds, walnuts, butternuts, chestnuts, and leafy dark green vegetables. Olive oil, a monounsaturated fatty acid, also has anti-inflammatory properties.

### Are You At Risk of Chronic Inflammation and Heart Disease?

Obviously, you are at risk if you eat too much refined grains, vegetable oils, animal fats, and processed foods. You are even at a greater risk if your diet is grossly deficient in foods that are rich in anti-oxidants and anti-inflammatory nutrients (fatty fish, flaxseeds, nuts, dark leafy green vegetables, and fruits) that wage battle with free radicals.

Heart disease is a direct consequence of chronic sub-clinical systemic inflammation that can be reduced and thereby improve the outcome greatly. Indeed, it is good news to know that there are simple things that anyone can do to help change or reverse the course of inflammatory diseases that could eventually develop into chronic illness. There is even hope for those who have already developed chronic disease to enjoy a better quality of life and energy.

By now, you know that you will increase your risk of inflammation and heart disease if you have high cholesterol, high triglycerides, high LDL (bad) cholesterol, low HDL (good) cholesterol, and high hemocysteine levels. All of these are late players that are no match for the real inflammatory markers (C-reactive protein and IL-6), which are the root cause of disease.

Other modifying factors that could increase your risk are smoking, high blood pressure, diabetes, abdominal obesity and a sedentary lifestyle. Genetic predisposition also raises your risk, but it probably does so only when one interacts negatively with the environment.

There is undoubtedly a strong link between bad diets (a diet high in animal fats, refined carbohydrates, and high-glycemic foods) and the development of sub-clinical inflammation that triggers heart attack. Therefore, making better food choices, eating an anti-inflammatory diet that is tailored to physical activity, and better stress management should be part of your strategy to beat heart disease and other degenerative disorders that are brought about by chronic low-grade systemic inflammation.

## What You Can Do to Reduce Chronic Sub-Clinical Inflammation

You can reduce systemic low-grade inflammation by doing simple things like eating more fish (salmon, mackerel, herring, sardines, and tuna), cooking with healthier oils (such as olive oil, cold-pressed canola oil, red palm oil and macadamia oil), and cutting back on vegetable oils and processed foods made with them (hard margarine and fast foods). Also eat abundant non-starchy vegetables (such as spinach, kale, broccoli, romaine lettuce, and cauliflower), and other dark leafy green vegetables. They are rich in antioxidants that can neutralize the free radicals that trigger inflammation,

You should cut back on simple sugars, refined carbohydrates (pasta, white bread, sodas, and sweets), and starchy vegetables like potatoes, corn, and plantains. These foods raise blood sugar and insulin levels, which promote inflammation. At the very least, replace the high-energy carbohydrates with whole grains and non-refined carbohydrates (low-glycemic carbohydrates). First, they are high in fiber, which will help to fill you up so that you eat fewer calories. Second, the low glycemic carbohydrates help to reduce the body's resistance to insulin, so that less insulin is needed to achieve the body's normal function. Recent studies have shown that the low-glycemic foods made the tissues of insulin insensitive patients more sensitive after just a few weeks. This can reduce the body's ability to produce inflammation.

**What Else Can You Do?**

If you are a smoker, quitting will decrease your risk. Lowering your blood cholesterol by eating a diet high in fiber (low-starch vegetables, fruits, soy, legumes, and whole grains) but low in saturated fat and getting regular exercise can decrease your risk as well. Again, eating low-glycemic carbohydrates has been shown to reduce the risk of heart disease by helping to improve blood sugar and insulin levels. In the Harvard Nurses' Study, it was shown that those who ate a low-glycemic diet (whole grains) had half the risk of having a heart attack than those who ate a high-glycemic diet (potatoes, white bread, white rice, and pasta). The low-glycemic diets also help to reduce the total blood cholesterol and LDL (bad) cholesterol. Also, people who ate a low-glycemic diet had high levels of HDL (good) cholesterol, which is protective against heart attack and stroke.

Losing weight, especially the extra body fat around the belly area, also improves your chance of beating heart disease and other degenerative diseases (stroke, diabetes, and cancers of the breast and colon). As you already know, being significantly overweight (30 or more pounds above your ideal weight) increases your risk substantially and is associated with diabetes and high blood pressure, both of which increase the risk of heart disease and stroke. So, simply losing weight and body fat can help control blood sugar, blood pressure, and insulin resistance – all of which can decrease your chance of having heart disease or a heart attack. Exercise and stress reduction are fundamentally beneficial and can help to decrease the risk of heart attack and other chronic diseases.

Here is a quick summary of the things you can do to improve your chance of reducing chronic intense systemic inflammation and beating heart disease and other chronic degenerative diseases:

- Lose belly fat and keep a healthy body fat percentage.
- Eat more vegetables, especially non-starchy dark leafy green vegetables (e.g. spinach, broccoli, cauliflower, romaine lettuce, arugula, kale, collard greens, mushrooms, etc.). These contain several anti-inflammatory nutrients and antioxidants that help to neutralize free radicals that trigger inflammation.
- Eat more low-glycemic load fruits with the skin, such as prunes, apples, plums, peaches, berries, and grapefruits.
- Eat more fish. Cold-water fish (salmon, mackerel and herring) are rich in EPA and DHA, which are anti-inflammatory. Fish oil reduces blood pressure, lowers triglyceride levels, prevents abnormal blood clotting and helps to prevent heart attack. Eat fatty fish 3-5 times a week – but if you don't like fish or don't eat enough fatty fish, try fish oil capsules (1000 mg 3 or more times a day or 6-8 grams daily), or Cod liver oil 1 tbsp daily or flaxseed oil (1-2 tbsp daily).
- Cook with healthier oils. Olive oil, walnut oil, macadamia nut oil, and cold-pressed canola oil are rich in monounsaturated fatty acids that help to lower LDL (bad) cholesterol while keeping HDL (good) cholesterol stable. Olive oil also

contains an anti-inflammatory substance called squalene, which is as effective as aspirin, but without the bleeding and stomach ulcers. Red palm oil is rich in potent super-antioxidants that lower cholesterol. Limit vegetable cooking oils and stick or hard margarine, which can be high in Omega-6 fatty acids and trans fatty acids, which are inflammatory. For salad dressings, use those made with olive oil, vinegar or lemon.

- Limit refined and high glycemic carbohydrates: Simple sugars, refined carbohydrates (such as, sodas, white bread, and white pasta), and starchy vegetables (such as potatoes, corn, and plantains) raise insulin levels and increase inflammation. Some of these foods are also low in nutrients and may crowd out good quality foods as well as contribute to excess weight and fat storage in the belly area.
- Supplements: Vitamin E 800-1,200 IU daily; CoQ10 60 -120 mg daily; vitamin B-complex 75-100 mcg daily; vitamin C 1000 mg daily; Folic acid 400 mcg daily; broad-spectrum multivitamin and mineral delivering 1000 mg of calcium and 500 mg of magnesium.
- Increase your consumption of foods rich in soluble fiber, such as oats, oat bran, broccoli, asparagus, beans, carrots, cactus, turnip, apples, and okra. Soluble fiber is effective in lowering cholesterol, blood sugar, and insulin levels.
- Cranberry juice (rich in phenol antioxidants; increases HDL and lowers LDL). Drink 2-3 glasses daily. Choose an unsweetened brand, 100% juice (*Mountain Sun* brand) and not from concentrate.
- Aspirin (81mg or baby aspirin; anti-inflammatory. Thins blood and reduces clots). Take one a day. Consult with your own physician especially if you are taking other blood thinners.
- Green tea (rich in antioxidant and compounds that help burn fat). Drink several cups of green tea regularly.
- Wheat germ. 1-3 tablespoons daily (source of natural Folic acid and vitamin E). Add to cereal or vegetables. 1-3 tsp in low-fat yogurt or low-fat cottage cheese.
- Ground cinnamon. 1-2 tsp is effective in controlling blood sugar (add to cereals, vegetables, teas, smoothies, etc.)
- Eat soy food and other legumes regularly. Experiment with soy protein powder (25-30 grams /day), soymilk, edamame or other soy-based foods (tofu, soy burger, soy nuts, smoothies, etc.).
- Nuts. Eat half-ounce almonds or walnuts a few times per week. Make sure your fat intake from other sources does not exceed your daily requirement, otherwise reduce portion size to 1 tbsp chopped (note that 1 oz serving of walnuts contains 185 calories and 18 grams fat and 1 oz of almonds contains 170 calories and 14 grams fat and it is easy to put on weight if your total fat and calorie intake is excessive).
- Exercise regularly or keep physically active most of the time
- Practice effective stress management (meditation, relaxation, self hypnosis, etc.).

- Cholestsure (*DaVinci Labs*): Dietary supplement to support cardiovascular function and normal cholesterol levels (contains Red Yeast Rice, Beta-sitosterol and Chromium Polynicotinate).

In addition, you need to change negative lifestyle choices, such as smoking and heavy alcohol intake, get adequate sleep, and lower levels of stress (this is only possible if you learn to deal with stress effectively). Following these recommendations, along with those of your personal physician, will help improve your health greatly.

I will end this chapter with a powerful message, " You should educate yourself about the dangers of bad foods". I hope this chapter has helped you to think more about the power of food and the consequences of consistently making bad food choices. Bad food choices (those that provide many calories and very few nutrients and antioxidants) cause fat storage and drainage of energy and vital nutrients. They make you feel anxious, tired, depressed, and constantly hungry. Worst of all, they increase your blood sugar, insulin, and cholesterol levels and make you vulnerable to Syndrome X, diabetes, heart disease, cancer, and even obesity.

On the other hand, you will lose weight and enjoy better health and energy if you make the right food choices most of the time. Foods that provide powerful nutrients and antioxidants – and not just calories – can help your body burn fat and turn calories into energy instead of fat. They can increase your mental concentration, elevate mood and boost energy levels. They can also help to reduce free radicals and inflammation, which in turn help to reduce risk of Syndrome X, diabetes, heart disease, and other chronic diseases (including depression and obesity).

# Chapter 6

# Pregnancy: A Double-Edged Sword

## Pregnancy Holds the Key

In the previous chapter, we saw how the wrong food choices can increase inflammation and the risk of developing diabetes, heart disease, and obesity. In this chapter, I will go even further and explore the possibility that obesity and a sedentary lifestyle could begin in the womb where the developing fetus can be influenced by the eating habits and lifestyle of a woman during her pregnancy. This chapter is also important because most women begin their struggle with weight and chronic health problems during and after pregnancy. For this reason, I am writing specifically for them.

Pregnancy is a double-edged sword. On one hand, it has a beautiful outcome. On the other hand, it may pose a serious threat to you and your new loved one. During my time practicing as an obstetrician, I was concerned with the reasons why women were gaining so much weight during pregnancy, as if the outcome of a healthy pregnancy depended on it. Contrary to popular belief, the more weight you gain, the higher the health risk to both you and your child.

Every pregnant woman can tell you that putting on unnecessary extra pounds made pregnancy miserable: lots of back pain, difficulty sleeping, shortness of breath, ankle swelling, and even pain while walking. However, those women who had managed to keep their weight down will tell you how wonderful their pregnancy was. They didn't experience any of the aforementioned adverse symptoms. This is the kind of prenatal advice and care every woman should yearn for (and should demand) from their obstetrician.

With today's technology and medical advances it seems unthinkable that babies are born that are exceedingly overweight from birth. This trend is likely to continue from childhood into adulthood. In fact, the average size of babies born today is greater than those born twenty years ago. The medical implication is enormous.

## Eating Habits During Pregnancy Have Long-Term Effects

High blood-sugar levels are harmful to you and your unborn child. The extra pounds you gained during pregnancy may increase your risk of diabetes, high blood pressure, preeclampsia (toxemia), and other chronic health problems. Some may appear sooner and others long after the pregnancy. Your growing unborn child may also suffer from low blood sugar, jaundice, or grow too large.

Recent studies with rats suggest that the predisposition to obesity, inactivity, and poor eating habits are linked and may be influenced by the mother's pregnancy. The researchers suggest that the observed association between obesity, metabolic syndrome (Syndrome X), and sedentary behavior and overeating might be due to a common biological cause. Their findings have enormous implications for public health policies in western societies and in developing countries where Western diets and lifestyle are adopted.

My guess is that the common association linking these conditions is insulin and sub-clinical inflammation in the prenatal environment as a result of poor quality foods and maternal inactivity. The inflammation precedes the disease. But, as inflammation leads to disease, a vicious circle of inflammation and disease develops and is fueled by dietary habits, inactivity, and other negative lifestyle activities (such as smoking, anger, stress and alcohol). It is this subject matter that this chapter is going to address. It is my hope that taking preventive measures before, during and after pregnancy will help to change the trend of childhood and adult obesity and its associated medical problems. Now, it is more likely people will wait until serious medical problems develop before intervening.

Let's take a closer look at some of the complications that can be avoided during pregnancy and at some of the best practices for a healthy and happy pregnancy.

**What Is Gestational Diabetes?**

As we saw in the last chapter, diabetes (high blood sugar) is a disease in which the blood sugar can be excessively high as a result of insufficient insulin or defective insulin receptors on muscles and body cells to which insulin binds (insulin resistance).

Just like in the non-pregnant state, high levels of sugar and insulin raise inflammation levels, which can damage the heart or brain cells. It is the fetus, whose cells, tissues and organs are rapidly dividing, that is the most susceptible to the adverse effects of gestational diabetes or a high sugar environment. We can assume that any sub-clinical inflammation acquired by the fetus during pregnancy may persist for a long time, even after birth. It is also possible that it could set the stage for chronic inflammation affecting organs and tissues – including blood vessels and brain cells and probably increasing the risk of diabetes, heart disease, obesity and behavioral problems (such as attention deficit disorder and learning disorders). This could be brought about early in childhood as we see today when the environmental conditions are poor (such as poor eating habits and sedentary lifestyles) or later in adulthood.

The prevalence of this disease makes it worthy of serious attention. It is estimated that 1 in 100 women of childbearing age has high blood sugar before getting pregnant (preexisting diabetes). Another 2 to 5 percent of pregnant women develop high blood sugar during pregnancy (gestational diabetes) yearly, making it one of the most common health problems in obstetrics. In both preexisting and gestational diabetes, it is crucial to control blood-sugar levels in order to reduce the risk both mother and fetus face.

After pregnancy, about 5 to 10 percent of women with gestational diabetes are found to have type 2 diabetes. Also women who have had gestational diabetes have a 20 to 50 percent increased risk of developing type 2 diabetes within the next 5 to 10 years.

## Who Gets Gestational Diabetes?

A number of cases of gestational diabetes occur in women without known risk factors. But the women most at risk include:

- Those who are obese.
- Those who have a family history of diabetes (such as a mother or sister).
- Women over the age of 30.
- Women who previously gave birth to a very large baby (over nine pounds).
- Women whose own weight at birth was greater than nine pounds.
- Women who had a previous pregnancy with high sugar.
- Women who had a significant weight gain in early childhood and during pregnancy.
- Women who had multiple stillbirths.
- Native Americans, African-Americans, and Hispanic women (women of these descents face a greater risk than women of other ethnic groups).
- Women who are pregnant with twins.
- Women who suffer from high blood pressure.
- Women who smoke.

Gestational diabetes also occurs in women who have Polycystic Ovarian Syndrome (PCOS). About 40 percent of women with PCOS get gestational diabetes according to some studies.

PCOS affects 5 million or more American women of reproductive age. It is associated with elevated blood sugar, high levels of insulin, and male hormones. PCOS is not widely understood and frequently goes undiagnosed. The majorities of women with PCOS have infertility problems and should see a reproductive endocrinologist.

The underlying culprit is believed to be insulin, which may cause the ovaries to produce high levels of male hormones that disrupt the menstruation and reproductive cycles. Most women with PCOS develop the condition early in childhood, forcing them to battle weight problems for most of their lives. Often, their weight will continue to soar despite diet after diet, even if they are doing all the right things. PCOS is associated with insulin resistance or Syndrome X, which is familiar to you by now.

## Testing for Gestational Diabetes

Most women with gestational diabetes have no symptoms – although some may experience extreme thirst, constant hunger, low energy, and fatigue. These symptoms are by no means specific to gestational diabetes, but they could raise suspicion.

To make the diagnosis, most pregnant women are screened for blood sugar between the sixth and seventh months of pregnancy. However, if you have risk factors you may be screened earlier. In fact, it is important to have your blood sugar tested before you try to get pregnant. If it is high, you must bring it under control before you try to conceive.

High blood sugar at conception and in the early weeks of pregnancy is strongly associated with serious birth defects, miscarriages and stillbirths. In 1991, John L. Kitzmiller, M.D. and others at the University of California, San Francisco, showed that controlling blood sugar before pregnancy in women with previously high blood sugar significantly reduced the risk of birth defects.

There are a number of tests for gestational diabetes. The most common include the fasting blood-sugar test and the blood-sugar test two hours after a meal (postprandial blood-sugar test). There is also the glucose tolerance test. This test involves taking a sample of your blood after an overnight fast and one hour after consuming a drink of 50 grams of glucose. HBA1C is also useful and maybe predictive even when other tests are unproductive.

When gestational diabetes is diagnosed during pregnancy, most women will control their blood sugar with diet and sometimes with insulin injections. Blood sugar usually returns to normal after delivery and, in most cases, no further action is taken. This is a mistake, since these women have an increased risk of diabetes and other serious health problems, as well as an increased risk of becoming overweight.

Evaluating women with gestational diabetes and their infants (during the prenatal, gestation, and post delivery periods) can provide useful scientific information (such as monitoring hemoglobin A1C, fasting blood sugar, and insulin, inflammatory markers like C-reactive protein, interleukin-6, body mass index or BMI, and body fat percentage). It will also be useful to measure these markers in pregnancy and during childhood and adolescence to try and understand how the maternal environment could have short and long term medical consequences on a woman and her child. For example, Metzer and Freintel in their research used the amniotic fluid insulin to determine fetal obesity.

Investigative tools like Doppler, sonogram, amniotic fluid, and simple non-invasive tests like fetal movements can produce useful information. The amniotic fluid during pregnancy can tell us quite a bit about the fetal environment and only a small amount of fluid is needed for analysis. This procedure is routinely done today under sonographic guidance and it is safe. Evaluations of fetal cord, placenta, amniotic fluid, and fetal cord blood can also help to shed light on this subject.

## Why All This Concern About Gestational Diabetes?

A persistent high level of sugar in the bloodstream is potentially harmful to many organs, as well as the baby. In spite of this, most babies born to women with gestational diabetes seem relatively healthy. But is that really true? We don't really have all of the answers at this point. What is known is that when blood sugar is poorly controlled during pregnancy, especially in those who already have diabetes, there is an increased risk of miscarriage, high blood pressure, preeclampsia (toxemia), excessive amniotic fluid (polyhydramnios), pre-term labor, pre-term delivery, and even death of the fetus (stillbirth).

And it doesn't stop there. Painless, silent and unsuspecting low-grade inflammation may linger in both mother and baby for years. It may eventually destroy brain cells; damage the heart, the pancreas, and cause insulin resistance syndrome.

Women with high blood sugar during pregnancy are also more likely to need a Cesarean delivery. This can mean more pain, infection, and a longer hospital stay. Even though Cesarean sections are routinely performed today, they still carry a 10 percent higher mortality rate than vaginal deliveries, especially in multiple repeat C-sections. Also, women with high blood sugar during pregnancy are likely to gain extra weight and become diabetic later in life. None of this is good news.

## Fetal Complications

Fetal complications are serious and include birth defects, such as heart defects or defects of the brain or spinal cord (neural tube defect), miscarriage, and stillbirth. High blood sugar triggers excessive growth and fat accumulation in the baby. It is not unusual today *(this is a new trend)* to see babies who weigh 10 pounds or more. The medical term for this phenomenon is macrosomia (meaning large babies).

These babies grow extremely large because of the excessive amount of sugar in the mother's blood that crosses the placenta and goes directly to the fetus. The fetus's pancreas responds by producing extra insulin, which helps to convert the sugar into fat. The extra fat usually accumulates around the shoulders and trunk, making it harder to deliver these babies vaginally. Labor and birth are often long and difficult and may put the baby at risk for injuries.

In addition, babies born to women with high blood sugar face a greater risk of breathing difficulties (respiratory distress syndrome), low blood sugar, jaundice, and low calcium. They have an increased risk of being obese later in life, which can lead to other serious health problems. They are also more likely to get insulin resistance syndrome (Syndrome X), high blood sugar, or diabetes.

## Why Are Pregnant Women Gaining so Much Weight?

### Eating for Two

Most pregnant women are asked to eat an extra 300 calories each day. This daily intake could amount to 2,200-2,500 calories or more a day. Combined with an inactive lifestyle, this could increase your chances of adding extra pounds and developing abnormally high blood-sugar levels.

Encouraging you to eat more, regardless of your activity level, is wrong and has no scientific basis. This recommendation is based on the idea that during pregnancy you should gain between 25 and 35 pounds in order to support a healthy pregnancy. It does not take into account your pre-pregnancy weight, which actually should be the determinant factor. If you are overweight or obese at the onset of pregnancy, you should gain less weight or not gain any weight at all. Following the 1990 Institute of Medicine recommendation concerning maternal weight gain will help women to avoid the problems associated with excess weight gain during pregnancy.

The Institute of Medicine committee based maternal weight gain on a woman's BMI (body mass index) at the time of entry into prenatal care. For example, for a woman whose BMI is greater than 29, the total weight gain should be less than 13 pounds. For a BMI between 26-29, the suggested weight gain is 15-25 pounds and for women of normal weight, a BMI between 19.8-26, it is 25-35 pounds. The big question is: how many women have healthy weight at the time of entry into prenatal care? Probably one in three is a good guess considering the fact that over 30% of the adult population is overweight or obese. It is my opinion that even these recommendations do not go far enough. A more reliable approach would be to have a healthy range of body fat before and during pregnancy, since this is more predictive of health than the BMI.

You should always pay close attention to your level of physical activity. If your food and caloric intake are based on your level of physical activity, you will not have to worry about maternal weight and retention gain ever again.

Ideally, you should not gain more than 20 pounds. The fetus, uterus, blood volume, breast tissue, amniotic fluid, and placenta account for about 13 to 17 pounds of the normal weight gain in pregnancy. Any weight beyond this is mostly undesirable maternal fat. The only exception to this is if you are considered underweight before getting pregnant or having twins. A BMI less than 19.8 is underweight and gaining 28-40 pounds is quite reasonable under this circumstance. If you have gained excessive weight in a previous pregnancy, it is very likely because your activity level was far below your needs for your caloric intake. The following section will help you to plan ahead for a much more enjoyable pregnancy with your next child.

**Plan Ahead Before You Get Pregnant**

To prevent excessive weight gain, swelling of extremities, and excruciating lower back pain, before you decide to get pregnant, you should lose at least 10-20% of your body weight. Better yet, strive to be within the normal BMI or, more correctly, the appropriate body fat percentage for your age. In addition to this, if you eat a proper diet, keep active and reduce stress and anxiety, both you and your child will be in great health and energy throughout your pregnancy. Your child will be of normal size and will not suffer the medical complications that being overweight can bring. Labor, delivery, and postpartum will be a pleasant and memorable experience. It will be all that a new mom could hope for.

**Too Many Carbohydrates**

Following the USDA guidelines, your dietician will probably recommend (on the average) about 2,200-2,500 calories per day, as already stated. This will most likely be divided among three meals and two snacks. Your dietician will probably recommend a diet that is low in fat (20-25 percent of calories), protein at about 10 to 20 percent of calories (from meat, poultry, fish, and legumes), and about 55 to 65 percent of calories from carbohydrates (such as bread, rice, cereal, pasta, potatoes, vegetables, and fruits).

A close evaluation of this diet will help you to understand the problem that you might face if you eat like this either when pregnant or not. A typical diet of 2,500 calories will consist of roughly 344-406 grams of carbohydrates that you consume daily. Knowing that eating habits do not necessary change drastically when one becomes pregnant, I will assume that most of the carbohydrates in your diet will be refined and high glycemic carbohydrates (such as white pasta, white rice, and white bread), starchy vegetables (such as potatoes and corn), and high glycemic fruits (overripe banana, raisins, and watermelon). These are the usual suspects that raise insulin levels, which may in turn increase inflammation.

Theoretically, this amount of carbohydrate will raise blood sugar levels by as much as 1,218 mg/dl (the normal blood sugar is 70-130 mg/dl. One gram of carbohydrate raises blood sugar by 3 points – according to the American Diabetic Association). This amount of blood sugar can over task the pancreas, causing blood sugar and insulin levels to become dangerously high and unhealthy for both you and your baby. You could become sick from this and have severe craving, restlessness, and food binges. This may be responsible for the increased appetite most pregnant women experience in their second and third trimesters.

All pregnancies, even those that are healthy, involve a state of hyperglycemia (high blood sugar) most of the time. Apparently, this is a normal process through which glucose provides most of the fuel that the growing fetus uses. As a result, there is a continuous transfer of sugar from mother to fetus. However, when there is sugar overload in the maternal blood, it could trigger the fetus' pancreas to produce extra insulin, causing excessive growth. It also raises the possibility that this could lead to the onset of low-grade chronic inflammation that may manifest itself in early childhood or later.

High blood sugar and insulin are detrimental to an unborn child, especially during the very early gestational period. This is when serious birth defects occur – before a woman even realizes that she is pregnant. So, even if she is willing to change bad eating habits during pregnancy, it may be too late.

*I know that it sounds like there is nothing a mom can do and puts her in a losing battle even before she has begun the process. I hope you don't feel that way. Doctors and nurses are trained to help you and your child through your pregnancy. However, the best thing that you can do for your baby and yourself is to take the time to make sure you are as healthy as you can be. Both you and your child will benefit from this extra care you give yourself before your life turns to baby.*

## More Nutrients and Antioxidants and Fewer Calories

Most authorities will agree that you don't have to eat many calories or foods when you are pregnant in order to have a healthy baby. But you do need to eat the right foods – foods that are high in nutrients and low in calories, such as non-starchy vegetables, fruits, legumes, whole grains, lean proteins, and healthy fats. Ideally, you should eat food according to your level of physical activity and special medical conditions. You should also take your prenatal vitamins and mineral supplements prescribed by your obstetrician. Your doctor knows what is best for you.

Your prenatal vitamins are specifically designed for you and your developing loved one. Vitamins provide adequate folic acid and other vital nutrients for the healthy growth and development of your child. For example, you could become anemic (low blood) and feel severely tired and pale in color if you fail to take your prenatal vitamins containing iron (iron is used to build hemoglobin, which circulates oxygen throughout your body and to your child). The blood that circulates from you to the child carries all the nutrients and oxygen your baby needs. It also removes toxic waste products from the baby to you. If the blood circulation is low, your baby may not be able to adequately remove waste materials or get enough nutrients to develop healthy.

Another important ingredient in your multivitamins is folic acid. It is a B-vitamin that can help prevent birth defects of the brain and spinal cord (called neural tube defects or NTDs). Folic acid works only if you take it before pregnancy and in the first few weeks of pregnancy.

The first few weeks of pregnancy are critical because that is when the fetus' brain and spinal cord are developing. Failure to have an adequate amount of folic acid during this period can cause neural tube defect, such as spina bifida (the vertebrae do not close completely and the spinal cord can protrude through the space). These are just few of the reasons you should take your vitamins regularly.

What if you can't take vitamins at all (some women can't tolerate them)? They have severe nausea that causes them to throw up any time they swallow vitamins. If you find yourself in this situation, eat more non-starchy dark leafy vegetables, low glycemic fruits, whole grains, and beans that are rich in nutrients. Folic acid, for instance, is found in Brussel sprouts, black beans, oatmeal, asparagus, wheat germ, and oranges.

Pregnancy is a state of heightened metabolic activities and both you and your unborn child are highly vulnerable at this period. Undernourishment or inadequate nutrients in this prenatal environment could lead to metabolic and cardiovascular disorders when your baby is born or even decades later. This is perhaps the most important period in shaping your child's destiny. Give your child a good start in life.

## Proper Brain Food A Necessity

### The Developing Brain Needs Omega-3 Fatty Acids

Not eating fish or having enough Omega-3 fatty acids in your diet can adversely affect your baby's brain development. The severity of the problem can range from behavioral to learning difficulties and depression. This is one major reason why eating healthy when you are pregnant is important and should be a primary focus.

The early development and shaping of your baby's brain before he or she is born depends on the availability of the proper types of fat. The brain's gray matter is about 60 percent fat, of which roughly one-third is DHA – the Omega-3 fatty acids that we saw in Chapter 3. DHA is used by the brain to build its basic structure and, hence, is vital for normal brain development, as well as for mental well being (see Chapter 12 for the selection of fish that are not contaminated with environmental toxins (such as mercury).

The baby's only source of DHA during pregnancy is you, the mother. The developing fetus gets adequate supply of these essential fatty acids when you eat fish, flaxseeds, flaxseed oil, dark green leafy vegetables, and nuts like walnuts. It is so important that the developing fetus will go to any length to get it from you. For example, if you are not eating enough fish or getting Omega-3 fatty acids from other dietary sources, the baby will get it directly from your own stores (such as the gray matter of the brain). This could deplete your own DHA and could set the stage for postpartum depression and other serious emotional disorders. Some studies have shown that the rates of postpartum depression are 50 times greater in countries where women don't eat fish.

The brain of a child that is severely deficient in Omega-3 fatty acids is poorly developed. This damage could persist through childhood and adult life. In a landmark study, Japanese researchers raised the possibility "that a relative Omega-3 deficiency may be affecting the behavioral pattern of a proportion of the young generations in industrialized countries."

This unfortunate and ugly circumstance can be prevented. You could give your child a better fighting chance if during your pregnancy you eat foods that are rich in Omega-3 fatty acids (more fish, dark green leafy vegetables, flaxseed oil, flaxseeds, butternuts, chestnuts, and walnuts). You should also cut back on animal fats and processed foods that are high in unhealthy fats. You can also use supplements if your dietary sources are not enough to meet your daily requirement (fish oil capsules, 1000 mg 3 times a day, or flaxseed oil 1 tbsp 1-2 times a day). Consult with your physician before using any supplements during pregnancy and lactation.

### Omega-3 (DHA) and Depression

DHA is so critical for the maintenance of brain function that some researchers think it may help to prevent degenerative brain diseases such as dementia and Alzheimer's disease. A low level of DHA is believed to be a significant risk factor for these diseases. The levels of DHA in the brains of people who are depressed are lower than those found in healthy people.

In some studies, fish oil supplements helped to relieve symptoms of depression and mood swings. Another group of people that have low levels of DHA are alcoholics. Alcohol is known to deplete the level of Omega-3 fatty acids in the brain. If you are pregnant, eat healthy and do not drink alcoholic beverages. Amongst the many adverse effects to your child may be permanent scarring of the brain.

### Pregnancy: A Highly Vulnerable Period

Pregnancy is a highly vulnerable period because of increased production of biological molecules, including DNA, RNA, proteins, enzymes, fats, cell membranes and cell organelles (brain, heart, liver, etc). All of these are sensitive to free-radical attacks, making lethal mutations more likely than any other period in your baby's life cycle. This probability is higher when your diet is deficient in antioxidants that help to neutralize free radicals. A diet high in refined carbohydrates, Omega-6 dominant vegetable oils and processed foods, including unhealthy fast foods, increases free radicals and inflammation that may play a role in the development of insulin resistance, obesity, diabetes, and heart disease in both you and your child years or decades later.

Within the last 30 years there has been a steady rise in the incidence of obesity and chronic diseases in our nation. The average size of babies born in the United States is increasing steadily. This is not good! The incidence of obesity among young children has also risen dramatically within the last 20 years. One-third of American children today are obese. It is no coincidence that this parallels the rise of type 2 diabetes, which now affects more than 500,000 children in the United States alone. Worldwide, the incidence of type 2 diabetes has risen and this seems to be associated with the diet typical of westernized societies.

But the increase in obesity and diabetes may have deeper roots. It may reflect the poor prenatal environment, which may be highly inflammatory and could set the stage for major health problems earlier or later in life. Both you and your child are susceptible to free radicals and inflammation if you eat poorly during your pregnancy.

Excessive calories can harm you and your child. Bad food choices delivering empty calories may displace healthier, nutrient-dense foods, causing excessive fat storage and weight gain in both you and your fetus. For example, saturated fats found in meat, cheese, whole dairy, and butter may interfere with the activity of cell membranes. They can cause stiffening and kinking of cell membranes, thereby diminishing their function in allowing the passage of nutrients into the cell and the removal of toxic wastes out of the cell. The cell malfunctions or dies if this role is not carried out properly.

Saturated fats also raise the levels of cholesterol, particularly LDL (bad), which could be oxidized by free radicals, leading to higher lipid peroxide levels. It is this process that makes LDL stick to walls of arteries and eventually form plaque. Processed and fast foods are rich sources of trans fats, which could block the enzymatic conversion of the anti-inflammatory Omega-3 fatty acids.

Eating a proper diet, being active and mentally relaxed when you are pregnant may reduce your risk of diabetes, toxemia, high blood pressure, and excessive weight gain and retention. A sedentary lifestyle in addition to eating badly and subdued by stress could be the worst nightmare for a pregnant woman.

It is never too late to eat healthy and to become active (*it is never too late to make a positive change*). I urge you to give this serious consideration, as it will make the difference between a healthy baby and a sick one or a brilliant child and a slow one.

We are fortunate that most of the dangers that I have briefly touched on here are either preventable or reversible if we intervene early enough. There is no doubt we cannot wait until the onset of disease or obesity before we intervene. Also, you need to take the option of planning ahead before you get pregnant: losing excess pounds or body fat, making better food choices, and keeping physically fit and healthy. It is also important to eliminate smoking, reduce coffee and alcohol, and eat in line with your level of activity.

Medical professionals trying to improve prenatal care will be more than appreciative if you take an active role in your own care. The prenatal environment may hold the key to changing the course of obesity, diabetes, and other chronic health problems that are draining resources and crippling lives. You have a vital role to play in this. After all, it is about you and your loved one.

*You must never diet or reduce your calories when pregnant. But you must eat to fullness and focus on increasing nutrients and antioxidants in every meal. Above all, keep physically active and reduce stress.*

# Chapter 7

# The Food Template: The Cornerstone

In this chapter, I will discuss the cornerstone of the UDP Weight Loss and Wellness Program, *The Food Template*. I will also compare the major differences between my recommendations and the USDA food pyramid. The food pyramid has been updated recently but many people are still confused. Many of us have grown up using this eating method and I think it will be useful to see how it compares to the UDP Plan.

**Our Food is Low in Vital Nutrients and Antioxidants**

Most of our food supply in America is grown in soil that is low in nutrients and contains chemical additives. As a result, today's foods are not only depleted of trace minerals, antioxidants, and phytonutrients, but they also contain toxic chemicals and pesticides that may increase inflammation and one's risk of cancer and chronic degenerative diseases.

Studies have shown that diet accounts for more than 35 percent of cancers. This is outrageous! As noted in previous chapters, the widespread consumption of refined flour has been associated with diabetes, heart disease, an increase in cancer rates, and an accelerated growth of tumors. Also, the common practice of using margarines and refined oils that are high in trans fats and inflammatory Omega-6 fats promotes cancer growth. Now that we know where many cancers and chronic diseases originate, it is time to take control of our health.

The easiest way to counteract the increasing levels of chemicals and the low levels of antioxidants in our food supply is to eat more whole foods that are low in calories but high in nutrients. Whole foods of plant origin (non-starchy vegetables, fresh fruits, legumes, soy, mushrooms, and seaweed) provide our bodies with a synergistic array of nutrients, antioxidants, vitamins, trace minerals, and powerful phytonutrients. Antioxidants (carotenoids, flavonoids, and crucifers) help us to counteract the free radicals that increase inflammation.

Flavonoids provide powerful antioxidant activity, cellular health, growth, and repair throughout the body. Common foods loaded with flavonoids are kale, green tea, red and black grapes, oranges, and grapefruit.

Carotenoids from carrots, tomatoes, spinach, broccoli, kale, collards, sweet potatoes, squash, cantaloupe, and peaches enhance cardiovascular health and battle LDL (bad cholesterol) oxidation – a process that leads to inflammation of the blood vessels and hardening of the arteries (arteriosclerosis). Carotenoids help to promote healthy vision and a healthy immune system so that our bodies can defend themselves against biological and chemical agents that are harmful.

Crucifers (broccoli, bok choy, Brussel sprouts, turnips, kohlrabi, radishes, and mustard greens) enhance and support enzyme activities that promote normal and healthy cell growth and repair.

**We Need More Non-Starchy Vegetables and Fruits in Our Diets**

Eating cruciferous vegetables, such as broccoli and cabbage, reduces the risk of getting breast cancer, prostate cancer, and colorectal cancer. Studies at UCLA Medical Center showed that men and women who ate about 4 cups of broccoli a week were 50% less likely to develop colorectal cancer than those who never consume broccoli. As little as ½ cup of broccoli sprouts two or more times a week can be protective and in fact seems to be more beneficial than eating the full grown vegetable. Researchers think that the sulforaphane, which is present in the broccoli sprout before the vegetable matures, may be the primary cancer-fighting agent.

No single food group provides all the flavonoids, carotenoids, and crucifers that we need to ward off diseases and enjoy a better quality of life. That's why it is important that we eat a broad spectrum of foods that includes dark leafy green, yellow, and red vegetables and all kinds of fresh fruits.

*To lose weight, as well as reduce health risk, you need to eat 1 to 2 servings (1-2 cups raw or ½ -1 cup cooked) of leafy green vegetables and other non-starchy vegetables before your major meals. To these vegetables, you will add healthy essential fats, vinegar, or lemon juice. This is the core foundation of the Food Template. This foundation of nutrients, antioxidants, anti-inflammatory foods, fiber and essential fats will be followed by other foods that provide mostly protein, carbohydrates, and a modest amount of non-essential (but, nevertheless, healthy) fats.*

Eating your vegetables before major meals may help you to eat fewer calories – but the real key is the hosts of nutrient and antioxidants you are getting. These can help to curb craving, release blood sugar slowly, and keep insulin levels from spiking. This is exactly what the body needs to burn fat efficiently.

The idea of eating vegetables in the morning may not appeal to some people, but there are those who can swear that it makes all the difference between starting the day with great energy, focus, and the ability to control stress more effectively.

A comparison of some of the breakfasts people eat will help to further illustrate the point. Some people start their day with a hefty bowl of refined cereal (sugar), milk (sugar and fat), a banana (sugar), and toast with butter (sugar and fat). Some people prefer a breakfast that is laden with both carbohydrates and fat, such as a bagel with cream cheese and a large cup of coffee with sugar and cream. These types of breakfasts are energy drainers and are definitely not the right foods with which to start your day. In simple terms, these breakfasts are grossly imbalanced.

In contrast, you could start your day with breakfasts that are balanced in carbohydrates, protein, and healthy fats. Your experience in terms of energy and concentration will be quite different from those who had carbohydrate- or fat-loaded breakfasts. An example of a balanced breakfast that would jumpstart your metabolism contains a variety of foods that are rich in powerful nutrients and antioxidants, whole vitamins and minerals: a vegetable omelet or scrambled eggs with spinach, red peppers, onions, and mushrooms with some lean protein (such as smoked salmon or Canadian bacon) with slices of tomato on a toasted small whole grain English muffin or multigrain bread.

Some people even go a step further and incorporate a powerhouse of nutrients and antioxidants in their breakfasts. For example, one of my favorite patients, a very busy corporate executive, enjoys a breakfast that would raise the eyebrows of most Americans who are accustomed to the more traditional breakfasts. Sharon's typical breakfast consists of ¼ raw squash/zucchini, 3 asparagus spears, 1 cup spinach, ½ cup broccoli florets, ½ red tomatoes, ½ cup romaine lettuce, 4 tbsp 2% cottage cheese, ½ medium apple, 2 fresh orange slices, 1 tsp canola oil, 3-multigrain crackers, 2 oz smoked salmon, and 2 tsp Clearly Fiber in a cup of green tea.

Sharon shared her enthusiasm with me one day in which she credited her newfound energy, concentration, and strength to handle daily stress on starting her days with solid breakfasts loaded with nutrients:

*"I feel so rejuvenated and awake and I had no idea that this was ever possible that you could feel so different and happy just by eating grocery foods." Smiling and glowing with inner confidence and radiance, she continued, "I have always accepted the fact that growing older and getting wrinkled, losing skin tone, and becoming flabby was all right. But I was dead wrong. We can all age gracefully and still be strong and fit at any age. That's the joy I have found in my middle age and it all starts with a simple breakfast that I never would have endorsed few years ago. Now, I don't go without it, even when I travel overseas on business trips."*

Apparently, not everyone will feel satisfied eating the type of breakfast that Sharon likes. It's uniquely Sharon's and was developed solely for her. At UDP, we work with each person to develop his or her own individualized program and meal plans. There are no generic plans – instead, we encourage your input in the designing of your program and continually work with you to modify it to your satisfaction.

As for Sharon, she is extremely health-conscious and was looking for alternatives to the cholesterol lowering medications she had being taken for years. Needless to say, her cholesterol on medication was over 300 and now it's around 180 without medications (see the complete meal plan for Sharon in Chapter 16 and her testimonial in Chapter 18).

The main reason for going through these elaborate explanations is to convince you that you should consider the idea of incorporating nutrient–rich, plant-based foods in your standard meals. You will be amazed with the degree of energy and vitality you will have.

I hope that the major differences between the four breakfasts I discussed above are now obvious to you – the real differences are that some of them are more nutritionally balanced than the others.

Again, adding vegetables to your breakfast is just one method to help stabilize blood-sugar spikes and the sugar rush that often follows a high-carbohydrate meal. Later in the book, I will discuss other practical methods.

At UDP, we do not omit or restrict carbohydrates or starches – even the bad ones. However, we do not believe that carbohydrates should dominate meals. To emphasize this idea, we treat carbohydrates and starchy vegetables and fruits as side dishes that one should learn to eat in line with activity level. This is a very simple and highly effective technique that will allow you to enjoy carbohydrates without the fear of eating too much (thereby triggering a strong insulin response) or eating too few and risking being hypoglycemic (symptoms associated with low blood sugar, such as headaches and dizziness).

As you will see later, neither the low glycemic carbohydrates nor the low glycemic load carbohydrates are foolproof. Of all the foods you will eat or are exposed to, carbohydrates are the only ones that induce a significant insulin response. Therefore, it is very important that you pay close attention to your portion sizes of this "instant" energy providing macronutrient. Of course, you should equally pay close attention to your portion sizes of protein and fat too. Even though these will not invoke a strong insulin response, they provide calories that can be converted into fat.

The template model was designed to make it easy for you to stay the course and to eat healthily without dieting. Following the template will help you to easily control your food portion size, reduce unneeded extra calories, eat what your body can burn, and, most importantly, feel satisfied while at the same time getting an adequate amount of nutrients and antioxidants.

You will be able to tell if you are doing the right things and the program is working for you in just a few weeks. First, the horrible cravings are resolved in just a few days as you provide your brain and body with vital nutrients instead of empty calories. Second, your energy level will dramatically increase and you may begin to feel the way you felt a decade or two ago. Third, your sleep pattern will improve and your mood will be pleasant and high and people close to you will notice your personality change. Fourth, your skin will become radiant and well toned. Fifth, the contour of your face and body shape will begin to change and it will make you appear much younger than your chronological age. You will realize most of these changes even before there is a significant change in your weight.

If you do not notice or feel a reasonable degree of progress right away, it may be that you are not eating an adequate amount of non-starchy vegetables, essential fatty acids, or protein. You may also be eating more carbohydrates or fats than your body can actually burn. One simple means to zero in on the problem is to keep a food and activity journal.

In most cases, it will point to a very common problem: too much food and not enough activity to burn off the calories before they turn to fat. That is why tailoring your food intake, particularly carbohydrates, to your level of activity makes sense. It is not dieting. It is simply a vehicle that enables you to provide your body with adequate nutrients without over flooding it with unusable extra calories. In other words, you learn to listen to your body in a way that you are more aware of its need and not just using it as a dumping ground of calories and debris.

If you have made the necessary adjustments – including boosting your activity level to match your food intake – and there is still no significant progress, you will need to customize your eating plan. This process is described in Chapters 14 and 15.

The UDP Program is based on a solid foundation (or template) of whole foods of plant origin and essential fatty acids – not grains or starchy carbohydrates, such as those recommended by the USDA food pyramid.

*Eating about five to seven servings of non-starchy leafy vegetables and low glycemic fruits daily will guarantee an adequate supply of the nutrients and antioxidants that are indispensable to weight loss and good health. Any of the following equals one serving: 1 cup raw leafy vegetables or ½ cup cooked leafy vegetables, ½ cup raw or cooked non-leafy vegetables, ½ cup cooked beans, 1 piece of fruit, ½ cup fresh fruit, ¼ cup dried fruit, and ¾ cup unsweetened fresh fruit juice. The key is to eat these nutrient-loaded whole foods before your main course. In essence, you are building a barrier of defense that will help to ward off dangerous free radicals in foods.*

Those of us who are not accustomed to eating vegetables and fruits might think it is difficult to have at least five servings a day. It is actually very simple. All it takes is a little planning. For example, to get seven servings of vegetables and fruits requires eating only half a grapefruit or 1 medium apple for breakfast or a mid-morning snack, 1 cup cooked or 3 cups raw vegetables for lunch, half a grapefruit or 1 medium apple or peach or ½ cup berries for an afternoon snack, and 1 cup cooked or 2 cups raw vegetables for dinner.

**Vitamin and Mineral Supplements Are Inferior to Whole Foods**

Vitamin and mineral supplements in synthetic forms are inferior to the vitamins, nutrients, and trace minerals found in whole foods from a clean environment. Vitamins and nutrients are better absorbed in their natural form and, that's why I recommend natural whole foods over supplements. However, if you are not getting enough dark green leafy vegetables, fresh fruits, beans, lentils, seaweeds, mushrooms, essential fatty acids, fish, and lean meat in your diet, you should supplement your diet with high-grade vitamins, minerals, or other nutrients (see: Building on a Solid Foundation later in this chapter). For example, fish is a major source of the beneficial Omega-3 fatty acids, whereas meat is a major source of B-vitamins that are needed for energy transformation.

**The Composition of the Food Template**

The Food Template consists of foods that are high in nutrients but low in calories, carbohydrates, and fats. The list of these foods is long and it is included in your shopping list. They include cooked or raw non-starchy vegetables, low-glycemic fruits, tomatoes, mushrooms, onions, garlic, carrots, zucchini, yellow squash, egg whites, whole egg, ground flaxseeds, wheat germ, nuts, avocado, flaxseed oil, fish oils, bean sprouts, algae, seaweed, lemon juice, vinegar, and legumes (beans, peas, lentils, and soy). Also included are vegetable soups without potatoes, corn, creams, or pasta. Other items included are sources of soluble fiber, such as oat bran (1-2 tbsp), wheat bran (1-2 tbsp), and fiber supplements (*Benefiber* and *Clearly Fiber*) for those not getting adequate soluble fiber.

The Food Template is not your typical American salad that consists of iceberg lettuce, tomato slices, and a hefty dose of salad dressing. Neither is it potato salad (cubed high glycemic potatoes, boiled eggs, celery, and mayonnaise). These are the same ingredients people like with their luncheon meat sandwiches and hamburgers.

Americans love their white potatoes and other starchy vegetables and sweet fruits, knowing very well that they can raise blood sugar and insulin levels and cause fat storage. The risk of adding extra fat and pounds far outweighs their health benefits if you eat large portions of these starchy foods. By comparison, the non-starchy vegetables and low starch fruits provide powerful combinations of antioxidants, fiber, and phytonutrients without the extra high glycemic starches that may trigger inflammation.

Vegetables come in various shapes and colors. You are probably getting more nutrient-dense vegetables if you select the leafy dark green vegetables, such as romaine lettuce, arugula, butter head lettuce, red leaf lettuce, spinach, broccoli, cauliflower, kale, cabbage, and collard greens. When you eat a combination of these, you can be assured that you are getting a powerful dose of antioxidants, phytonutrients, vitamins, and minerals (Vitamin A, beta-carotene, B2, B6, Folic acid, vitamin C, potassium, magnesium, and iron) that can help fight heart disease, cancer, and also help burn fat more efficiently.

As a rule, the more colorful and varied vegetables and plant-based foods you include in your Food Template, the more diverse and higher the quality of nutrients you will be getting. One sure way of getting enough vegetables and plant-based foods is to make a conscious effort to include them as the foundation of your meals. Losing weight and keeping it off is very simple if you get accustomed to eating a diet that is low in calories and high in nutrients. The Food Template is designed to help you achieve this goal without struggling. Once mastered, it eliminates the need to diet, count calories, or starve.

## What Is Not Recommended in the Food Template

Foods that are high in starch – even those that are low glycemic or whole grains – are excluded from the food template. Whole grains, such as barley, whole-wheat pasta and brown rice, even though they are low glycemic, are starchy (carbohydrate loaded) and may cause weight gain if you are physically inactive. Fruits, such as plantains, bananas, papaya, mango, raisins, and pineapples (which are all high glycemic) are also excluded. They release their sugar too quickly, flooding the body with too much energy.

Another reason to exclude grains and starchy foods from the template is because most of us eat too much of the wrong kinds (see the Harvard studies in Chapter 4). That is one reason so many of us are overweight. Carbohydrates, such as white bread, muffins, doughnuts, bagels, pizza, and white pasta are highly refined grains that are high in fats and sugar. Their fiber content is very low. Nutrients are concentrated in the fiber, which also has a filling effect that prompts us to eat less food. You might recall that foods that are high in fiber promote weight loss by helping the body to burn stored fats more efficiently and also help to slow the conversion of carbohydrates to blood sugar. This, in turn, helps to protect us against Syndrome X, insulin resistance, heart disease, and diabetes.

## Planning Is Key

Planning and preparation is the key to incorporating non-starchy vegetables and low glycemic fruits into your diet. They are not bland and tasteless if you know how to prepare them – and you don't have to be a chef. Vegetables can be prepared raw, baked, grilled, steamed, incorporated in light vegetable soups or stir-fried with a small amount of extra virgin olive oil or canola oil. Flavors can be enhanced with spices, herbs, and low salt seasonings. If you have a very busy lifestyle, you can prepare a large batch of vegetable soups or salad greens that you can refrigerate until needed. Taste and flavor are enhanced over time. Fruits can be eaten as is or incorporated into smoothies or fruit cocktails that can be eaten before meals or as snacks. Adding vinegar or lemon juice enhances their nutritional quality. They both help with food digestion and also delay stomach emptying.

**Low-Calorie, High Nutrition Diets**

All of the diets that scientists have studied and found to be healthy have one common denominator: they are low in calories and high in nutrients and antioxidants. Dr. Roy Walford of UCLA Medical School and his former graduate student, Dr. Rick Weihdruch, along with other researchers, found that when monkeys and mice were put on low-calorie, high-nutrient diets, they had lower blood sugar, insulin, and cholesterol levels, lower blood pressure, and a much stronger immune system. They also aged slower and lived longer. In contrast, laboratory animals that ate the typical Western diets not only lost their health, but they also aged more rapidly. These findings hold true for humans as well.

In 1991, Dr. Walford and his researchers in the Biosphere 2 Project were trying to see if they could survive entirely on the small ecosystems growing inside a three-acre greenhouse when they realized that they were low on food production. They unexpectedly found themselves on low-calorie, high-nutrient diets, similar to the one prescribed for the lab animals. Surprisingly, the team discovered that they too had experienced some health benefits similar to those observed in the laboratory animals.

In fact, for the last 30 years of his life, Dr. Walford himself ate a low-calorie, high-nutrient diet consisting of mostly vegetables, fruits, fish, and lean meat. At a height of 5'9" his weight was around 130 pounds.

What was truly remarkable was that he only ate about 1,600 calories a day compared to one of 2,000-2,800 calories that most men his age eat. He credited his longevity and good health to his diet and physical activity. He was in relatively good mental and physical health until his death last year – of Lou Gehrig's Disease (a condition that may not respond to dietary manipulations), a few months before his eightieth birthday.

Some of the other well-known, low-calorie, high-nutrient diets are the traditional Okinawa diet and the traditional Crete/Mediterranean diet. These are not diets of starvation or deprivation. The individuals eat to satiety (fullness) and are not hungry between meals. The key lies in their choice of foods: non-starchy vegetables, fresh fruits, fish, beans, lentils, and lean meat. Even though these types of foods are low in calories, they are quite high in essential nutrients that are needed for efficient metabolism of food and proper functioning of the digestive system, brain, lungs, kidneys, heart, and muscles.

They also provide the entire body with a host of powerful compounds that help to battle and neutralize harmful free radicals that trigger inflammation and cause diseases, including obesity. It is for this reason that low-calorie, high-nutrient diets are so successful in promoting real weight loss and health. These diets may probably work by forcing the body to release its fat reserve for energy – so that you lose weight gradually until you reach your ideal weight. Unlike calorie restricted diets that are lacking in nutrients, muscle mass is preserved, resulting in a more efficient and higher metabolism.

**Why It Is Important to Reduce Calories**

Our body generates energy from food through a process that removes electrons one step at a time until they are oxidized. The entire process creates a chemical energy called ATP. Scientists call this process oxidation (which literally means the burning of food with the help of oxygen) and it is essential to life. When you do aerobic exercise, you are basically using the same system to burn fat or release energy locked in food and body fat.

**Oxygen Kills**

Sometimes oxygen and other small molecules become electron deficient or "hungry". These unpaired electrons form free-radical molecules (also called oxygen radicals) that are highly unstable and chemically reactive (causing oxidative stress). The free-radical molecules can attack DNA and cause damage that, unless repaired, may lead to a defective DNA strand that makes a non-functional protein, hormone, or enzyme. Besides DNA, other biological molecules are susceptible to attack, including RNA, proteins, enzymes, and lipids (fats).

**LDL (Bad) Cholesterol Is Bad Only When It Is Oxidized**

The good news is that LDL (bad) cholesterol is not harmful to your body until it becomes oxidized and sticks to the walls of blood vessels. This is what causes inflammation and leads to the hardening of the arteries. Otherwise, most LDL circulates through your blood vessels and into organs and tissues where it serves as an energy source or is used for the production of compounds, such as testosterone and estrogen. The bad news is that highly refined carbohydrates and simple sugars cause the formation of free radicals that oxidize LDL, which then transforms it from good cholesterol to bad cholesterol (or sticky cholesterol).

**Our Cell Membranes Are Protective Barriers**

One of the areas of the body that is most susceptible to free-radical damage is the cell membrane that surrounds and protects all cells. The membrane regulates the passage of materials and nutrients into and out of the cell. The membrane is a double layer of proteins and fats, including the essential fatty acids (Omega-6 and Omega-3) that I discussed briefly in earlier chapters. The presence of these fatty acids contributes to the flexibility and fluidity of biological membranes. The cell membrane is essential to life and damage to it can set the stage for diseases and even death of the cell. This topic has been thoroughly covered by Dr. Nicholas Perricone in his book, *The Perricone Prescription*.

The reason the cell membrane is so susceptible to free-radical damage is that it has one of the largest surface areas of the body and free-radical molecules readily react with the fatty acids imbedded in its wall. This interaction may set off a chain reaction that triggers inflammation, leading to chronic degenerative diseases (such as premature aging, obesity, diabetes, heart disease, and cancer).

### The Destruction of the Cell Membrane Can Lead to Syndrome X

In the previous chapter, I discussed Syndrome X and diabetes at length. A disruption of the cell membrane could impair glucose transport into muscle and cells, leading to insulin resistance syndrome (Syndrome X) and eventually to diabetes and heart disease.

Pregnant women need to be especially careful because, if they are not getting adequate essential fatty acids from their diet, it could hinder the growth and development of their child's brain and other organs even after birth. The fetus completely depends on the flow of nutrients and removal of waste products through a healthy cell membrane that is fluid because of a rich supply of essential fatty acids. In pregnancies where the levels of essential fatty acids are low, it is not hard to imagine how the integrity of the cell membrane of the fetus can be easily compromised, allowing waste products and toxic chemicals to accumulate inside the cell. This eventually could cause damage to cells and hinder the development of vital organs, such as the brain and heart (refer back to Chapter 6).

### The More Food You Eat, the More Free Radicals There Are

The more food you eat, the more free radicals your body produces. Free radicals are an unavoidable by-product of the energy processing machinery. Eating less food, particularly the empty calorie, high-fat and refined foods, helps you stay healthier and live longer because fewer free radicals are produced. When your food is high in antioxidants, your body can defend itself effectively against free radicals, which increase your chance of developing Syndrome X, diabetes, heart disease, cancer, obesity, and other chronic degenerative diseases. In addition, you are more likely to burn body fat and lose weight. This is probably one of the reasons the traditional Okinawa diet, the traditional Mediterranean diet, and other low calorie/high nutrient diets promote health and longevity. The UDP program is no exception.

## Antioxidants: The Body's Defense

To prevent cell damage by free-radical molecules, the body uses natural defenses that capture and neutralize reactive electrons. These defenses are antioxidants. They include enzyme systems, such as glutathione peroxidase, catalase, and superoxide dismutase. Other antioxidants are found in foods and are Vitamins A, C, E, selenium, zinc, beta-carotene, and Coenzymes Q10.

A constant battle is being waged between free radicals and antioxidants in the body. As one ages, the body's ability to produce natural antioxidants decreases. Therefore, eating foods that contain appropriate plant antioxidants and phytonutrients is necessary to protect the body against free radicals and oxidative stress that can damage or destroy cells. If cells are harmed and they have no means to quickly repair the damage, it could lead to the earliest stages of disease. In this way, antioxidants and phytonutrients are indispensable in the fight against free radicals – by not only blocking them, but helping with the repair process as well.

**Whole Foods Are Better**

Whole or unprocessed foods provide a synergistic array of antioxidants and nutrients (carotenoids, flavonoids, crucifers, vitamins, minerals, fiber, etc.) that help the body neutralize free radicals and protect fats and proteins embedded in cell membranes. These foods provide the best protection against free radicals that trigger inflammation.

Many of the foods that we eat today are depleted of vital antioxidants, vitamins, minerals, fiber, and phytonutrients. Research shows that antioxidant levels in food have decreased significantly in the last three decades. Low levels of antioxidants are ineffective in protecting the body from the increasing levels of free radicals from toxic chemicals in foods and those generated in the body from eating large amounts of highly refined and processed foods. And, as I stated earlier, our food supply is produced with higher levels of pesticides and other harmful chemicals compared to decades ago.

**Foods Rich in Antioxidants Promote Health and Increase Life Expectancy**

The older generations of Okinawa people enjoy a longer life expectancy with substantially lower rates of heart disease, stroke, and cancers, such as breast, colon, or prostate cancer than Americans or those living in Westernized mainland Japan. Interestingly, when the Okinawa people migrate to the mainland, eat, and live like westerners – they too experience a higher rate of heart disease and cancer and a shorter lifespan.

The secret to their longevity and good health is believed to be their plant-based diet centered on non-starchy leafy green vegetables, fresh fruits, beans, soy, and whole grains. Their diet provides adequate amounts of antioxidants, trace minerals, vitamins, fiber, and phytonutrients that help to neutralize free radicals before they inflict serious damage to vital cells and organs. In short, their diet is anti-inflammatory.

The Okinawa diet calls for about seven servings of vegetables and fruits daily. In contrast, the average American has about three to four servings daily. Instead of leafy green antioxidant rich vegetables, the American staple is iceberg lettuce, corn, and potatoes. The Okinawa diet's main sources of protein are fish, soy foods, beans, and other plant-based proteins. In contrast, the American diet's main sources of protein are red meat, cheese, and dairy foods – all of which are fatty, high-caloric foods that are fattening and largely pro-inflammatory.

**The New Okinawa Experience**

Unfortunately, the younger generations of Okinawa people are deviating away from their traditional way of eating just like the Pima Indians of the Southwestern deserts of the United

States. After the Second World War, Okinawa came under the jurisdiction of the United States – up until 1972. Naturally, the natives adopted the Americanized diet consisting of large amounts of Omega-6 dominant vegetable oils, such as corn oil. The natives also shifted from a healthy diet dominant in fish and seafood and whole grains to one dominant in meat and highly refined grains. The combination of Omega-6 dominant vegetable oils, meat, and refined grains created the kind of drastic shift in the ratio of Omega-6 to Omega-3 that is typical to the ratio found in Westernized countries. This shift resulted in a rise in degenerative diseases never seen before in Okinawa (diabetes, heart disease, stroke, arthritis, cancer, etc.).

By 1990, the longevity of the Okinawa people was reported to be fifth among Japanese from the 47 prefectures of Japan. These results represent a drastic decline from the number one position the Okinawa have enjoyed in Japan and, indeed, the top position in the entire world. Perhaps we can learn a lesson from the Okinawa experience.

### Mounting an Adequate Defense

As I have pointed out, some of the foods that we eat are sources of toxic compounds that can hurt us. The more vegetables, fruits, and plant-based foods we eat, the better we are able to fight back. Conversely, high calorie fatty foods and carbohydrate-loaded foods like refined breakfast cereals, white pasta, white bread, white potatoes, big steaks, creamy dressings, and sugary desserts weaken our defenses and make us vulnerable.

The natural biological process that converts food into energy is the same process that causes the formation of dangerous free radicals that trigger inflammation and set the stage for chronic diseases, premature aging, and death. It seems like there is nothing we can do about it but that is not the case. We can fight back by reducing the amount of food and calories we consume, as this would reduce the amounts of free radicals that are produced during food digestion and metabolism. Most importantly, we could eat selectively and choose foods with lots of antioxidants to help neutralize the free radicals produced from digestion and metabolism of food. And, finally, even though vitamins are inferior to whole foods, it is still a good idea to take vitamin and mineral supplements, such as vitamins A, E, and C.

Mounting an adequate defense against free radicals is the main objective of the food template and also the reason for encouraging you to eat abundant amount of non-starchy leafy green vegetables and other colored vegetables before your meals. You should also increase your level of antioxidants by eating more leafy dark green vegetables any time you make poor choices. It is a good insurance policy!

## Benefits of the Food Template

### Boosts Energy and Well-Being

The food template may provide protection against the ravages of destructible free radicals that drain energy and inhibit the production of vital compounds. It may also indirectly provide a sense of security and well-being that you will notice immediately as a result of the dramatic increase in energy. The high dose of nutrients helps the body function at an optimum level.

Most of us do not make the effort to include healthy foods in our diets on a regular basis. To make matters worse, we often eat foods that taste great but offer very little in terms of nutrients and antioxidants. This is a practice that is easy to accept because most people do not associate food with health and disease. But hopefully that will change as people become more aware of the health benefits of vegetables and fruits. They are not only good for people trying to lose weight, but also for those interested in boosting their energy and improving their health and longevity as well. My own personal experience and those of my patients have provided enough evidence that the concept of the Food Template forces us not only to think more seriously about our food choices, but to consider having these healthy, non-starchy, plant-based foods as a cornerstone of every meal.

The low-calorie, high-nutrient diet is not at all your typical low-calorie diet, which is actually a starvation diet that is unhealthy and not recommended. The conventional low-calorie diets are often deficient in vital nutrients. One might experience an impressive weight loss in a short period of time and that's why these diets are so attractive. However, the aggressive weight loss is usually due to loss of muscle instead of fat. As a result, the body is saggy and clothes do not fit well. In fact, the individual may appear malnourished instead of healthy. These types of diets are also difficult to maintain over long periods of time and, in many cases, may even lead to more weight gain and health risks.

**May Slow Down Food Digestion and Absorption**

The Food Template may help to slow down the digestion and absorption of food, especially if you include vegetables with soluble fiber (such as broccoli, okra, navy beans, lima beans, cactus, and chana dal lentil). As a result, blood sugar and insulin levels rise more slowly. The lower insulin levels help the body to burn fat and, ultimately, lose body fat instead of muscle. By comparison, high blood sugar and insulin levels promote fat storage, weight gain, and resistance to weight loss in addition to causing inflammation.

*Cholesterol also improves when your blood sugar and insulin levels are low. The opposite is true when your blood sugar and insulin levels rise. Diabetics are also able to reduce insulin dosage and have better control of their blood sugar. You should always eat non-starchy leafy dark green vegetables or fruits (the foundation of the Food Template) before your meals in order to provide a "safety net" that protects you against blood sugar and insulin surges.*

**You Have Better Control Over Your Calories**

To lose weight, you need to consume fewer calories and burn more calories than you consume. This is why eating meals that are low in calories help you lose weight – provided that they are high in nutrients. For example, if you reduce your portion of pasta from 2 cups to 1 cup, you will lower your calories and insulin response. However, this is most effective if you also had adequate vegetables before eating the pasta. It is important to point out that you would probably not get the same protective benefit if you ate the pasta and vegetables together.

In my own experience, I am never full and satisfied eating the vegetables and pasta together. But it's quite the opposite if I ate the vegetables first and then followed with the same amount of pasta or another carbohydrate source of equal portion (I described this way of eating as "eating in courses" and it is described fully in Chapter 14).

*There is ample antidotal evidence to support the fact that it's the order in which the food is presented to the body that is the most important aspect of curbing our appetite and craving and not necessarily the reduction of calories alone.*

Eating in sequence will give you a sensation of fullness and satisfaction that helps to put a brake on how much food you eat. In essence, you will feel great on fewer calories because the food is high in nutrients, antioxidants, and fiber that take time to digest. So, you will not be hungry between meals. You can also control your cravings and hunger pangs better because of the low levels of insulin in your bloodstream. You recall that insulin is an appetite stimulator that makes you crave sugary and junk foods, as well as eat recklessly.

**Possible Explanations**

A possible explanation why eating non-starchy leafy dark green vegetables (such as broccoli florets, spinach, and collard greens) before meals helps to curb appetite and overeating may involve stretch receptors in the stomach walls. Loading with vegetables or light vegetable soups causes stomach distention, which stretches nerve receptors on the walls of the stomach. Nerve impulses are quickly conducted to the brain center that controls craving, hunger and satiety. As a result, you eat less food and feel quite satisfied on smaller amounts of food.

This is not a problem as long as your meals contain adequate nutrients and antioxidants. As you continue to eat smaller meals, your entire stomach sac and digestive bowel adapt and become a smaller sac over time. This can be seen as loss of mid-section abdominal fat as well as belly fat because the intestine, subcutaneous fat layer and the omentum shrink considerably (the omentum is a fold of fat that connects the stomach with the liver and other abdominal organs. It is usually large in an obese person and smaller in a slim person).

A similar change is probably seen in people who had gastric bypass, stomach banding or other procedures that reduce the stomach volume. You can appreciate that a much smaller stomach is more likely to be stretched by smaller amounts of food compared to a larger stomach.

Apparently, both procedures work, but only the practice of loading up on vegetables before meals are safe and without surgical risks. Most importantly, eating more vegetables delivers a powerhouse of nutrients and antioxidants that can help promote healthy weight loss and optimum health that is superior to all others. In contrast, surgical patients still have to learn to eat healthy and modulate their lifestyle or they inevitably fail.

**Decrease the Risk of Cancer and Other Health Problems**

Research shows that vegetables and fruits are the richest sources of antioxidants – notably vitamins A, C, E, and the mineral selenium. As you already know, antioxidants help prevent oxidative cell damage – which is the underlying cause of chronic degenerative diseases, including obesity.

A recent study of Greek women showed that women who had 4-5 servings (2-2 ½ cups cooked or 4-5 cups raw) per day of vegetables had a 46 percent reduction of breast cancer risk compared with women who had less than 2 servings (1 cup cooked or 2 cups raw) per day. Similar findings were found with fruits. According to the American Institute for Cancer Research, a plant-based diet that is high in antioxidants and phytonutrients can reduce the risk of cancer by as much as 30 to 40 percent.

## A Diet High in Fiber

A plant-based, high-fiber diet decreases fat digestion and reduces the amount of fat (including cholesterol) that is absorbed by the body. It also helps to stabilize blood sugar, preventing the swings in blood-sugar levels that are problematic for people with insulin resistance syndrome and diabetes. I have already discussed some of the important health benefits of fiber in Chapter 3. For example, the soluble fiber found in oatmeal, oat bran, fruit, legumes, barley, cactus, okra, and dietary supplements (such as *Benefiber* and *Clearly Fiber*) can bind and eliminate cholesterol with the stool.

## The Isoflavone-Health Connection

Soy is the powerhouse of phytonutrients and antioxidants that supports and strengthens the cardiovascular and immune systems, bones, muscles, prostate gland, kidneys, and gastrointestinal tract. Soy is rich in calcium, B-vitamins and zinc and is low in saturated fat. Soy is a major factor in the lower rate of breast and prostate cancer found in Asian people.

The health benefits of soy are derived from a class of compounds called isoflavones (such as genistein and daidzein). They are found in soybeans (also known as edamame) and legumes. However, the highest concentrations are in soy, such as soy cheese, soy hot dogs, tempeh, textured soy protein, tofu, soy flour, miso, soy nuts, and soymilk.

Soy isoflavones have been shown to help prevent the formation of arterial plaque, which reduces the risk of stroke and cardiovascular disease. They have antioxidant properties, which may help prevent the oxidation of LDL (bad) cholesterol into the form that accumulates as plaque in the arteries. They may also help to reduce cholesterol.

Soy isoflavones may help reduce human breast cancer by blocking the growth of estrogen-stimulated breast cancer. They may also inhibit prostate cancer by blocking cell growth. They are useful in the fight against osteoporosis. They can stimulate bone formation and prevent bone resorption (breakdown of bone). Soy isoflavones can help to relieve pre-menopausal and menopausal symptoms, such as hot flashes, night sweats, sleep disturbances, and other symptoms as well. A third compound found in soybeans (saponins) can help reduce the metastasis or spread of colon cancer. It can also reduce cholesterol.

Soy isoflavones can make you feel full and satisfied without the risks of increasing saturated fats, cholesterol, or blood sugar. Soy is low-glycemic and can prevent blood sugar and insulin levels from rising too much. The better you manage your sugar and insulin levels, the lower your cravings for carbohydrates and sugary foods will be. In addition, you will be better able to lower your cholesterol and blood-glucose levels and thereby reduce the risk of diabetes and heart disease.

Recent studies presented to the American Diabetic Association suggest that soy isoflavones lower blood sugar as much as some well known prescription drugs that are used to control diabetes – and without the side effects! In the study, women who ate or sprinkled their food daily with 30 grams of soy protein powder containing about 132 mg of soy isoflavones for three months had lower blood sugar and cholesterol levels than women who did not have soy protein. The women who had soy also had improved insulin resistance (Syndrome X), meaning that they decreased their risk of developing diabetes.

Soy isoflavones oppose insulin action and can help increase lean muscle mass and body metabolism. The more muscle mass you have, the more calories and body fat you burn for energy and the easier it is to lose weight or maintain your ideal weight. This is particularly important for people in their thirties and older – whose muscle mass is replaced by fat at a rate of one quarter pound per year. It is equally important for people with health problems or weight issues that prevent them from exercising effectively during the early stages of weight loss. The replacement of muscle with fat can slow down your metabolic rate, causing more fat storage. One way to prevent this process is to eat soy protein on a regular basis and exercise regularly.

**The Amount of Soy Isoflavones You Need**

Isoflavones work in concert with soy protein and the best way to consume isoflavones is in the form of whole foods instead of pills. Only the food form contains all the nutrients that are necessary for optimum health and protection. If you are not yet familiar with soy, you can incorporate various soy products gradually (see recipes). For example, use tofu instead of meat, eggs, or cheese in simple delicious dishes. Make delicious smoothies using soymilk and textured soy protein. Soybeans are flavorful and they are high in protein and low in fat. They are great in soups, side dishes, and snacks.

The FDA suggests a minimum of 25 grams of soy protein daily as part of a diet low in saturated fat and cholesterol as an effective means of reducing the risk of coronary artery disease. Asians consume a huge amount of soy without any known adverse effects. Most experts agree that consuming about three servings (25-30 grams soy protein) a day is sufficient to provide most of the health benefits of soy. A serving is the equivalent of the following: 8 ounces of soymilk; 1 tbsp of soy protein powder; 2 by 2 inch square of tofu (½ inch thick); 1 cup raw soybeans or edamame; or ½ cup toasted soybeans. The health benefits are due largely to the isoflavones. To give you an idea, about ½ cup of tofu has 25 to 35 mg isoflavones; 1 cup of soymilk contains about 30 to 40 mg isoflavones; 1 scoop soy protein powder contains about 50 mg isoflavones.

## Building on a Solid Foundation

### The USDA Food Pyramid

The U.S. Department of Agriculture (USDA) recommends carbohydrates or grains as the foundation of our diet, followed by produce (vegetables and fruits), protein, dairy products and fats, oils, and sweets with the warning to "eat sparingly". It appears to be a healthy recommendation, but it is not supported by current research.

### The Problem

Dr. Walter Willet and his colleagues at the Harvard School of Public Health showed that the USDA dietary plan does not promote health. It promotes a diet rich in grains and starches and low in good fats and sugar. To the contrary, the Harvard researchers found that the Harvard-designed diet (which is high in vegetables and fruits and healthy fats) outperforms the food pyramid. It appears that the USDA model emphasizes calories at the expense of nutrients.

*A high-carbohydrate diet may be appropriate for athletes and other very active individuals or those blessed with a fast metabolism that can burn up the calories before they convert to fat in the body. In contrast, when individuals who are physically inactive or have a slow metabolism eat a meal high in carbohydrates, it is very likely that they will end up storing fat and gaining weight, including triggering high levels of insulin and inflammatory compounds.*

This is so worrisome that some researchers believe that the USDA recommendation could increase the risk of heart attack in some individuals who have insulin resistance or Syndrome X. You may recall that one in three Americans has this condition and may not even be aware of it. As mentioned previously, studies done at Stanford University also showed that high-carbohydrate diets recommended for diabetics might hurt them instead of helping them. The message that will be repeated over and over again in this book is that one should eat carbohydrates according to his or her level of physical activity instead of going on a low or high carbohydrate diet.

### Why Carbohydrates Should Not Be At the Base

One strong argument for cutting back on carbohydrates (according to Professor Paul LaChance and Dr. David Heber) is that most Americans eat too much of the wrong kinds of carbohydrates, mostly the simple and highly refined ones. Most refined carbohydrates are also high in fat and sugar and can make you gain weight as well as raise cholesterol levels. In addition, refined carbohydrates are deficient in fiber and other vital nutrients that help to control appetite. Lucky for us, most of the vital nutrients located in whole grains are very similar to those found in vegetables and fruits and, therefore, they can easily be substituted in the food template.

Another argument for cutting back is that we are not as active as we were two or three decades ago. We drive everywhere and walk or exercise very little compared to Europeans and Asians. Professor John Pucher of Rutgers University believes this is one reason why Americans are far more obese than Europeans or Asians (approximately 25-30 percent of Americans are obese, compared to only 7 percent of Europeans).

Americans eat too many calories and burn less by way of physical activity, such as walking. This by no means suggests that every American is sedentary and eats too much. Such a view will be consistent with a one-size-fits-all approach, which is misleading. On the other hand, it does help to explain why people who are active should eat more food and carbohydrates, as suggested by the USDA; those who are moderately active should eat fewer carbohydrates; and those who are sedentary should even eat fewer.

## The UDP Food Pyramid: What Should Be At the Base

### Providers of Nutrients and Cellular Protection

Foods that are appropriate for the foundation of healthy meals provides low-calorie, high-nutrients (antioxidants, phytonutrients, fiber, minerals, vitamins, and essential fatty acids) that have healing properties and also promote the burning of body fat. Furthermore, these are foods we can afford to eat abundantly because they are low in carbohydrates, sugars, and fat.

For your convenience, some are listed here again: vegetables low in starch, low-glycemic fruits, soy foods, beans (very small amount), mushrooms, algae, seaweed, bean sprouts, green snap, green peas, split peas, yellow snap, lentils, soybeans, peas, wheat germ, wheat bran, oat bran, ground cinnamon, sauerkraut, beets, radishes, carrots, zucchini, eggplants, pumpkins, summer squash, winter hubbard squash, nuts (1 tbsp chopped or sliced), lemon, vinegar, ground flaxseeds, and the essential fatty acids. Also included are: vitamins and mineral supplements, green or black tea, and water. Of course, we should not forget physical activity, adequate rest, sleep, and maintaining a low stress level – all are essential building blocks of health and weight loss.

Essential fatty acids (Omega-6 and Omega-3) are critical for health and – since our bodies do not make them – they must be included in our diet in a ratio of 2:1 or 1:1. One way to ensure that you get adequate Omega-6 and Omega-3 is to add them as supplements or whole foods to your vegetables, fruit cocktails, cereals, smoothies, sorbet, or beans. Actually the best way to get the Omega-3 fatty acids is to eat fatty fish, such as salmon, mackerel, and tuna at least four times a week. But if fish or seafood is not in your meal plan, your secondary sources of this very important nutrient are flaxseeds, flaxseed oil, walnuts, and dark green leafy vegetables. Some people may need fish oil or flaxseed oil supplements. You can easily add Omega-6 fatty acids to your template by using cold-pressed canola oil or 1-3 tsp of corn or safflower oil.

Soy foods, lentils, and beans help our bodies fight heart disease and cancer and are therefore included at the base because of their nutritional value. They also help us to lose weight. Though beans are moderately high in starch, they are also one of the highest sources of fiber and their starch does not convert to sugar quickly. However, keep your portion size small (about ¼ cup or 1-3 tablespoons) when including beans as part of your template, or consider them as a primary carbohydrate source in your meal.

Fruits are a major source of carbohydrates and natural sugars in our diet but they are also loaded with nutrients that are required for health and weight loss. However, most fruits will fall under the category of carbohydrate and sugar providers on the second level of the pyramid. The ones that I recommend for your template are low glycemic with less than 15 grams of carbohydrate per serving (such as blueberries, blackberries, raspberries, strawberries, gooseberries, cherries, cranberries, grapefruit slices, tangerines, grapes, kiwi, orange slices, honeydew, passion fruit, fresh apricots, fresh figs, plum, avocado slices, and peaches. Cantaloupe, pineapple, papaya, and watermelon are high glycemic (as pointed out before) but you can include a small amount in your template (such as ½-1 cup of watermelon and ¼ cup or a few thin slices of cantaloupe).

Low glycemic fruits that are high in carbohydrates and sugars can be incorporated into your template provided you use portions that are small and the carbohydrate concentration is less than 15 grams. For example, ½ a medium apple delivers about 10-15 grams of carbohydrate and will be suitable for your template.

Also included at the base are vitamins and mineral supplements, water and green tea, adequate rest and sleep, a low stress environment, and exercise. Exercise of any kind as a regular way of life is beneficial and can help improve weight loss. Water is very much an essential nutrient without which biological and chemical reactions, including our metabolism and ability to fight disease and lose weight, is severely compromised. About six to eight cups of water a day keeps energy levels and metabolism high.

## Cortisol Stress Connection

In Chapter 1, you saw how chronic stress is bad for your health and can cause weight gain, including the piling up of stubborn belly fat. I will add a little bit more to that here. Cortisol is induced by all kinds of stress, including the day-to-day stress in our lives. Under normal conditions, the level of cortisol tends to return to baseline when the stress is over. However, elevated levels of cortisol may linger on for days under conditions of chronic stress (the body's response to stress is to release cortisol and adrenaline).

This is toxic to the body. It can cause the breakdown of muscle tissue, resulting in the release of large amounts of blood sugar into the blood stream. The rapid rise in blood sugar causes a spike in insulin levels, resulting in fat storage in the belly area and intense inflammation, which can increase risk of Syndrome X, diabetes, heart disease, stroke, arthritis, cancer, and even obesity.

Chronically elevated levels of cortisol can potentially destroy every organ system in the body. Our brain cells and nervous systems are particularly vulnerable to the toxic effects of cortisol. It can shrink and destroy our brain cells, the immune system, blood vessels, and muscle tissue. It can also cause premature aging and early death.

In pregnancy, the hormone could cross to the baby's environment and affect the fetus' brain, leading to mental and emotional problems, such as depression and learning difficulties in later years.

Normally, cortisol is released under stressful situations to help us escape from dangerous situations, increasing the chances of survival. This is called the "fight or flight" syndrome. This primitive automatic response probably worked well for people who lived thousands of years ago. They were able to escape from charging lions and bone crushing hyenas. But that was then and our own environment is uniquely different from the one I just described. However, we do have similar challengers and pressures, such as family discord, job pressures, financial problems, road rage, relationship problems, examinations and tests, and in general fear of failure (to name a few).

Confronting these problems on a daily basis can lead to chronic levels of cortisol, causing us to crave our favorite sugary foods, such as cookies, candies, sodas, chocolates, and ice cream. We crave under stress because it is a coping mechanism.

When we are under chronic stress, the levels of serotonin and dopamine (neurotransmitters in the brain) are significantly reduced. We need an adequate amount of serotonin and dopamine to make us happy, feel calm, secure, and content. Therefore, when our brains don't have enough of these chemicals, we become depressed, unhappy, and moody. As a result, we crave high-sugary foods to stimulate serotonin and dopamine production to help calm us and make us feel good. This also explains the reason we often feel so calm, relaxed, and sleepy after a heavy loaded carbohydrate meal at lunch.

But the feeling of 'euphoria' is usually short-lived and we are forced to continue eating even when we are not hungry. This behavior is called stress eating and I described ways to overcome it in Chapter 8.

Another aspect of chronically elevated cortisol levels is that it can cause a low body metabolism that even exercise may not adequately combat. Overstressed adrenal glands may also lead to lower thyroid function (hypothyroidism), which, in turn, lowers body metabolism, leading to more weight gain and fat storage.

Just like the way in which a depressed or 'burned out' pancreas leads to diabetes, exhausted adrenal glands may cause fatigue, depression, and sleep problems. The dark circles under the eyes are typical signs of worn out adrenal glands, chronic stress, and high cortisol levels.

A high level of cortisol naturally occurs as we age, but it is chronic stress that causes the greatest rise in cortisol levels, which floods the circulation system and organs causing loss of vital muscle, increase in body fat and a weakened immune system that is incapable of mounting an adequate defense.

The good news is that you can prevent toxic accumulation of cortisol by finding ways to deal with your stress appropriately instead of allowing it to build up in your system and affect your daily function. Maintaining a steady flow of energy by eating three balanced meals with snacks is also helpful. Learn to relax, and this could be highly beneficial in difficult situations.

Skipping meals and eating low-quality foods can trigger or lower your threshold to deal with stress in a positive way. Meditation and self-hypnosis can help you feel good, help breakdown destructive thoughts, and open the door to rejuvenation, self-awareness, and peace of mind. The technique is simple: choose a quiet place and repeat a meaningful word or short phrase silently as you exhale and inhale.

## We All Need Vitamins

Vitamins and trace minerals are essential catalysts to fire up your metabolism and other vital chemical reactions. Your body does not make them and you need to include them in your diet unless you are eating a balanced diet consistently. Using supplements is not a bad idea as long as they are of good grades and you are not overdosing on them.

Vitamins are not food and by no means replace whole food. Also, they do not make you eat more. Some people may experience an increase in appetite, but only because their body metabolism is geared up and burning calories and body fat. The net result is not a weight gain, but rather a melting of body fat. Vitamins and minerals are indispensable in the transformation of food into energy that is vital to life. In very simple terms, vitamins help to speed up biological and chemical reactions in your body, so that the brain cells, muscles, liver, kidneys, heart, and digestive systems work better. You probably don't need vitamin supplements if you eat a wide variety of foods most of the time. Unfortunately, most of us don't eat well at all. We often eat the same foods over and over again instead of diversifying. Worst of all, we eat too many highly processed and refined foods that have their vitamins and minerals stripped off.

Vitamins like beta-carotene (the carotenoids are converted to vitamin A), E, and C are powerful antioxidants that help to neutralize destructive free radicals that trigger inflammation and cause diseases, including cancer. The problem is choosing the right vitamins and minerals since the marketplace is flooded with so many different types – all-claiming to be good for us. For example, calcium carbonate is a form of calcium that is used as a dietary supplement that is used widely in inexpensive brands. But it is not well absorbed. In fact, the chalk used on blackboards is mostly calcium carbonate. Another example is *Tums*, which is also widely promoted as a source of calcium. Unfortunately, *Tums* is anti-acid and you need an acidic environment for the gut to absorb calcium, otherwise most of it ends up in the stool instead of the blood stream. On the other hand, calcium citrate is acidic and well absorbed.

I do not recommend taking vitamins and mineral supplements once a day (except prolonged release formulations), for the same reason, I would not advise you eat one meal for the entire day. Most vitamins and mineral supplements contain barely the minimum dose (RDA) needed for healthy normal individuals or to prevent deficiency diseases that are now rare in developed and Westernized societies. The therapeutic doses are much higher. For example, a clearer anti-inflammatory effect is observed at 800-1,200 IU daily of vitamin E. But most vitamins people buy in stores and pharmacies contain much less and, therefore, will be ineffective in reducing inflammation. To make matters worse, the amount of vitamin E in some popular once-a-day supplements is only 60 IU and that of vitamin C is 120 mg. These are well below the effective doses to combat major illness and more so if you are taking only one pill or capsule daily.

Another example is FOCUSFactor, which was brought to my attention by one of my patients. The pleasant sixty-year-old woman took FOCUSFactor for over a year to help improve her memory and concentration. She had learned about the supplement through a television advertisement that even promised a free one-month trial. She stopped taking her own regular multivitamins because she was assured that she didn't need them if she was on FOCUSFactor. That was a terrible mistake!

The promise of a better memory and focus appeals to most of us; but before you spend money on any nutritional supplements, first check the label for the quality and the amount of ingredients per serving. Just taking the bare minimum amount may not help your condition. For example, the nutritional labeling for the adult formula of FOCUSFactor is as follows: The serving size is 4 tablets and the servings per container is 30. The amounts per serving of antioxidants and nutrients that support brain function are listed and the italics are those found in some vitamin supplements that support proper nerve function and relaxation – vitamin C 250 mg (*500 mg twice a day of ester vitamin C*), vitamin E 30 IU (*400-800 IU*), vitamin A 4,000 IU (*5,000 IU*), vitamin B2 1.7 mg (*15-75 mg*), vitamin B6 15 mg (*50-100 mg*), vitamin B12 20 mcg (*50-100 mcg*), folic acid 400 mcg (*400 mcg*), selenium 50 mcg (*200 mcg*), and 15% DHA from fish oil (*200 mg DHA with 300 mg EPA three times daily* ).

I am not sure whether the ingredients and antioxidants in this supplement are adequate to support the claim of a better memory, focus, and concentration. You decide! Hopefully, what you have learned here will help you to be more investigative and to pay attention to labeling information. Below, I will show you the foods, vitamins and mineral supplements, and daily activities that will sharpen your memory, focus, and concentration.

**Foods for Brain Power**

First and foremost are the natural whole foods with high levels of antioxidants and nutrients that help to protect the brain and nerves from oxidative damage caused by free radicals and inflammation. You are probably familiar with the key players by now – the non-starchy dark green leafy vegetables, such as kale, broccoli, cabbage, cauliflower, spinach, Brussel sprouts, romaine lettuce, arugula lettuce, collards, and turnip greens. Fruits also contain high amounts of antioxidant properties, such as prunes, blueberries, blackberries, and strawberries. Others include citrus fruits (oranges, tangerines, and grapefruits) and the Beta-carotene found in yellow orange, green fruits, and carrots. The lycopenes also have antioxidant properties and are found in fruits, such as tomatoes, tomato sauce and tomato based products, pink grapefruit, pink guava, watermelon, and papaya. Green tea and mushrooms also have antioxidant properties.

When the antioxidant properties of vegetables and fruits were determined, prunes had more antioxidants than any of them, followed by raisins, blueberries, and blackberries. Next in line was kale, followed by strawberries and spinach. Spinach is believed to be the brain food needed to prevent memory loss and Alzheimer's disease. For example, in experiments in which women were given ten ounces of fresh raw spinach, their ORAC score (measures the ability of the blood, foods or any other substances to neutralize free radicals) was better than when they took 1,250 milligram of vitamin C. However, vitamin C was more effective than an eight-ounce serving of strawberries.

## Vitamins and Minerals With Antioxidant Activity

The primary ones are vitamin E, beta-carotene or vitamin A, vitamin C, and the metal selenium. Vitamin E is found in soybeans, seeds, nuts, and vegetable oils. Vitamin E is believed to reduce the risk of inflammation and heart disease. Most authorities recommend 400-800 IU daily for vitamin E and 500 mg twice a day of ester vitamin C. Both vitamins are antioxidants that improve memory, reduce wrinkles, and decrease risk of hardening of arteries (atherosclerosis).

Vitamin C is found in citrus fruits (oranges, tangerines, grapefruits, etc.), broccoli, green and red peppers, Brussel sprouts, tomatoes, cabbage, strawberries, and potatoes. Beta-carotene (which is converted to vitamin A) is found in orange, yellow fruits, and dark green leafy vegetables, such as carrots, spinach, kale, and sweet potatoes. Selenium is found in seafood, whole grains, and Brazil nuts.

The B-vitamins or B-complex (B1, B2, B5, B6, B12, Biotin and Folic acid) are very important in promoting healthy brain function. They are needed for the normal function of the brain and nerves. They are involved in the production of all brain chemicals and neurotransmitters (such as serotonin, dopamine, histamine, norepinephrine, taurine, and gamma-aminobutyric acid – also known as GABA). The B-vitamins also play a critical role in neutralizing harmful free radicals, insulating and protecting the brain and nerve cells, and enhancing memory. Check your multivitamin or B-complex vitamins to make sure you are getting adequate amounts. Otherwise, your brain and nervous system will not function normally (such as poor memory, difficulty learning and sleeping, poor concentration, and depression).

Diseases of the brain, such as depression, anxiety, fatigue, irritability, paranoia, learning difficulties, and insomnia are linked with B-vitamin deficiencies. The good news is that these diseases can be reversed or their stressor reduced if you take adequate amounts of B-vitamins or eat enough foods containing these vitamins. Another important contribution of the B-vitamins is that they are involved in the transformation of foods into energy. As a result, if you are not getting adequate amounts, you will be weak and low in energy.

## The Causes of B-Vitamin Deficiency

Some medications commonly prescribed for depression can cause B-vitamin deficiency and further aggravate the problem. Other common causes are alcohol, drugs, contraceptives, estrogen therapy, and diets high in highly refined carbohydrates, including processed foods and antibiotics used in farming and food production.

## Sources of B-Vitamins

The well-established sources are whole grains, wheat germ, whole grain pasta, rice, nuts, and lean meats. These vitamins are water-soluble and are excreted in the urine daily if your body fails to use them. Therefore, it is very important to take adequate amounts of B-vitamins daily.

## Omega-3 Fatty Acids Are the Quintessential Brain Food

The same Omega-3 fatty acids that promote a healthy heart and weight loss also help to build and maintain the billions of brain cells and nerves. Our brain tissue is largely composed of fats (the Omega-3 DHA). DHA is critical for maintaining brain function (memory, focus, concentration, thought processes, etc.) by promoting communication between brain cells and the nervous system.

As you already know, the Omega-3 fatty acids are anti-inflammatory and the primary sources of these nutrients is cold-water fish, such as salmon, tuna, mackerel, sardines, herring, and anchovies. Other sources of Omega-3 fatty acids are flaxseed oil, ground flaxseeds and canola oil. Extra virgin olive oil lacks Omega-3 fatty acids but it is also anti-inflammatory. This will be discussed in depth in Chapter 12.

## Other Compounds That Promote Brain Health

Alpha-lipoic acid is a potent antioxidant that can help to recycle other antioxidants, such as vitamin C, vitamin E, coenzyme Q10, and glutathione. It may help protect against atherosclerosis and slow the progression of diabetic complications. It is found in red meat, liver, and yeast.

Coenzyme Q10 is a powerful antioxidant that is beneficial to the heart and also takes part in energy production. It is found in organ meat, especially the heart. Chicken and beef contain small amounts.

Green tea contains catechins that have antioxidant activity. The most potent catechin is called Epigallocatechin-3-Gallate (EGCG) and may protect against cancer and atherosclerosis and have anti-inflammatory properties. It may also help burn body fat.

## Final Recommendations for Brain Food

My final recommendation for enhancing brain function, memory and concentration, is to follow the same principles for healthy weight loss, reduction of body fat, and optimum health outlined in this book. Eat meals high in non-starchy dark green leafy vegetables, fresh fruits, legumes, soy, mushrooms, seafood, and fish with high Omega-3 fatty acids, flaxseed oil and ground flaxseeds, nuts, lean meat, and whole grains. In addition, make physical activity a part of your daily routine.

Aerobic exercises increase the flow and delivery of oxygen and nutrients to brain cells and nerves. A reduction of blood flow to the brain cells can cause damage to brain cells, stroke, or loss of function, resulting in paralysis of the affected structures and extremities. If the brain goes for over five minutes without blood flow that carries oxygen and nutrients, brain death could occur. That's the rational for initiating early CPR in a person having a heart attack. The goal is to quickly restore blood flow and oxygen to the brain.

Smoking negatively affects the delivery of oxygen and nutrients to the brain and can promote loss of memory. On the other hand, reading regularly, doing puzzles, learning new languages, or games can help to keep the brain and mind sharp and young.

Remember that a single dose of vitamin and mineral supplements may not meet your health need. They may be convenient, but that is all you might get. Read the labels to make sure that the right amount of vitamins and minerals are what you are getting.

Toxicity and death from pure vitamins and minerals are rare. Most of these are due to the fat-soluble vitamins (A, E, D, and E). These can be stored in large amounts in fatty tissue. On the other hand, the water-soluble vitamins like C and B-vitamins are largely excreted through the urine when excessive amounts are ingested. The minerals are also water-soluble.

If you are really interested in quality, I suggest the nutrient rich super foods in powder form for maximum bioavailability. These formulations provide a full complement of vitamins, minerals, and digestive enzymes with amino acids to support brain and heart functions. They also contain powerful antioxidants, such as DMG, CoQ10, and Alpha lipoic acid to support immune function and energy levels. The super foods that I am familiar with are the Spectra Multi Age, Spectra Reds Powder and Spectra Greens (*DaVinci Laboratories* of Vermont), and Perfect Food (*Garden of Life*).

Like everything else, you have to do your homework and pay attention to the details on the nutritional label before you make up your mind to purchase any product. The scope of this book does not allow me to go in depth, but there are many good books out there that will help you – or you can ask your pharmacy for assistance. In Chapter 15, you will see the vitamins and supplements that I recommend. These vitamins and minerals can help to compliment a good diet and enhance the nutritional quality of food.

## The Second Level

### Providers of Primary Energy and Structural Support

Foods on the second level of the pyramid provide primary energy and structural support. These are the ones that we must closely tailor to our level of activity or risk flooding our body with excess calories that can be converted to fat. They include carbohydrates (whole grains, low-glycemic starches and starchy vegetables, and most fruits) and protein (fish, soy products, skinless chicken and turkey breasts, lean meat and low-fat cheeses, low-fat milk, low-fat yogurt, and other low-fat dairy products).

The carbohydrates emphasized are whole grains (multigrain breads, brown rice, long grain white rice, parboiled rice, *Uncle Ben's* converted white rice, whole-wheat pasta, Chinese vermicelli noodles, protein-enriched pastas, barley, bulgur, basmati rice, wild rice, and high fiber cereals), low glycemic starches and vegetables (sweet potatoes, yams, yellow sweet corn, squashes, beans, and new potatoes), and most fruits with carbohydrate content greater than 15 grams per serving (such as whole apples, mangos, pears, nectarines, pineapples, plums, prunes, unripe bananas, unripe plantains, cantaloupe, pomegranate, rutabagas, and papaya).

Consider beans and lentils (except for soybeans) to be a major source of carbohydrate if you eat more than ½ cup. One mistake that people often make is failure to account for the various foods that are contributing carbohydrate to a meal, such as fruits. For instance, recognizing that ½ cup of most cooked beans will provide about 20 grams carbohydrate, will caution you from adding another high carbohydrate source that will potentially raise blood sugar and insulin levels (such as 1 cup rice or pasta, each delivering about 40-50 grams carbohydrate).

On the other hand, ½-1 cup cooked beans will be perfectly suitable as a major source of carbohydrate for a person who is sedentary and eating 1,300 calories a day. Always keep in mind that even the non-starchy vegetables and fruits that I encourage you to eat do also contribute to the overall carbohydrate load. You will do fine if you keep in mind to eat not more than what your body can burn or use within a short period.

It is also important to know that beans are not a major source of protein as you might have been led to believe. Simply compare the carbohydrate to protein ratio listed on canned beans and you will agree. Therefore, if you are a vegetarian or are relying on beans as a primary protein source, you should include other protein sources that are not very high in carbohydrates. Otherwise, your diet could be extremely high in carbohydrates and relatively low in proteins. This could hinder weight loss.

Again, the key to preventing carbohydrate overload is to make sure you eat roughly what your body can burn and that has to do with whether you are physically active or not. Also, eat carbohydrates in an inverse relationship to protein. In other words, when the diet is low in carbohydrates, the protein portion should be increased slightly to compensate for energy deficit and visa versa. This will help to stabilize your muscle tissue. Also, eat carbohydrates with proteins, good fats, lemon juice, or vinegar to help prevent abnormal sugar spikes that could trigger excessive release of insulin.

As you grow older, your energy requirements will also drop. So naturally, you need to cut back on your total calories and carbohydrate intake. However, this may also require that you increase slightly protein consumption, preferably from fish, soy protein, beans, and other lean sources that are low in saturated fat and cholesterol – in order to save your muscle and bones and maintain an efficient metabolism.

## The Third Level

### Protectors and Providers of a Secondary Energy Source

The third level of the UDP food pyramid includes good fats (clean fuel) that the body uses as a secondary energy source and also to protect and keep the body healthy and fit. To be exact, we only need a small amount of these fats in our food supply because they are calorie dense. Using just small amounts in the food template, such as for light salad dressings is all right for those trying to lose weight.

These are our primary sources of fat (extra virgin olive oil, cold-pressed canola oil, red palm oil, and macadamia oil). These oils are rich in monounsaturated fats that are good for the heart. They also help to lower LDL (bad) cholesterol and raise HDL (good) cholesterol, factors that can lower the risk of heart attack and stroke. Monounsaturated fats, such as olive oil are also anti-inflammatory. However, canola oil, besides being high in monounsaturated fats, has the best ratio of Omega-6 to Omega-3 (2:1). Therefore, if you are trying to get a good ratio of Omega-6 to Omega-3, the best oil to use is canola oil and not olive oil. I will clarify in Chapter 12. Meanwhile, a good practice is to alternate or use combinations of canola and olive oils so that you get the best of both.

Use olive oil and canola oil as your standard cooking oils and the highly refined unsaturated vegetable oils, such as corn oil, peanut oil, soy oil, safflower oil, and other vegetable oils as secondary oils. Most of us get our fats from highly refined vegetable oils like corn oil and animal fats. The problem is that these vegetable oils have very high amounts of Omega-6 fats compared to Omega-3 fats and can easily shift the balance so that the diet is pro-inflammatory, as we saw for the newer generations of Okinawa natives.

This can drive your good cholesterol (HDL) down and increase risk of stroke and heart attack. A better way of cooking with vegetable oils is to combine them with either olive or canola oil (such as mixing 2 parts of olive oil with 1 part of peanut or corn oil). The fat in avocado fruit is also a source of healthy fat similar to the one found in olive and canola oil. But you only need to eat a small slice of this fruit or risk a heavy fat load. Avocado is used in Mexican dishes to make guacamole.

Similarly, nuts are rich in heart healthy fats, but most of them have a higher ratio of Omega-6 to Omega-3 (such as almonds, pecans, peanuts, cashews, and pistachios). Since Omega-6 fats can depress your HDL (good) cholesterol, you should limit nuts that are high in Omega-6 fats. On the other hand, walnuts and butternuts have higher amounts of Omega-3 and are preferred if you are trying to raise your HDL (good) cholesterol.

In general, you should not eat too many nuts at once because they are calorie dense. The standard serving size for a snack is one ounce and delivers close to 200 calories and about 19-21 grams of fat. This is more than the amount of fat you probably need for an entire meal. But ½ ounce or 1-2 tablespoons chopped nuts can be well tolerated and can be added to your template, cereals, and yogurt.

**Low-Fat Diets Are Not Healthy**

Contrary to popular belief, eating low-fat diets can force your body to manufacture fats that raise blood-cholesterol levels, which may actually increase health risk. Studies show that all fats are not created equal. The saturated fats found in animal products, the trans fats found in margarine, and processed foods do indeed raise your risk of heart disease, cancer, and other chronic degenerative diseases.

*Eating too much animal fat (fatty cuts of meat), dairy fat (butter, milk, and ice cream), and finely refined vegetable oils (corn oil) can indirectly raise insulin levels and promote fat storage as well as insulin resistance and inflammation – all of which can increase health risk. On the other hand, healthy fats, such as olive and canola oils and the fish Omega-3 fats, promote optimum health and weight loss.*

Some of us are afraid to eat fats, even the healthy ones. But what you need to know is that when you eliminate healthy fats from your diet, you will probably eat fat substitutes, which will make your body crave real fat. As a result you might be forced to eat larger portions of meat at the expense of nutrient rich vegetables, fruits, and legumes.

Eating a low-fat diet that is deficient in essential fatty acids does cause severe craving but also anxiety, depression, poor concentration, and can include loss of hair, nails, and dry-scaly skin. Low - fat diets can interfere with absorption of fat-soluble vitamins like vitamin A and E, resulting in serious deficiency. So, you should think about these things before going on a low-fat diet. In fact, most people on a low-fat diet end up gaining weight and raising their cholesterol to dangerous levels, while the HDL (good) cholesterol remains low. It's also very difficult to lose weight on a low-fat diet.

It's equally important to be modest with your portions of healthy fats. They are naturally high in calories but, when used in moderation, they can boost your metabolism and help burn calories and body fat. In Chapters 15 and 16, I will show you the right amounts of fats that you can have without risking gaining weight. For now, just remember to use healthy fats in order to neutralize the harmful effects of saturated fats any time you eat a meal that is high in bad fats (such as pork spare ribs).

## The Tip of the Food Pyramid

### Providers of Empty Calories, Bad Fats, Insulin, and Cortisol

At the tip of the UDP food pyramid are foods and compounds that may induce a strong insulin and cortisol response, raise cholesterol, and are largely fattening and pro-inflammatory. They also cause the breakdown of muscle tissue while promoting the storage of toxic fat in the belly area.

The foods and compounds in this group can actually harm our body, particularly if we are sedentary, smoke, and drink excessively. They include highly refined carbohydrates (such as white bread, highly refined breakfast cereals, short grain white rice, white flour tortillas, pizza, white pasta, bagels, donuts, waffles, and pancakes), simple sugars (such as sugary cakes, cookies, ice creams, sweetened juices and sodas, fruit punch and lemonade, candies, and fructose), starchy high-glycemic carbohydrates (such as white and red potatoes, rutabagas, fufu, and farina), high-glycemic fruits (such as overripe bananas and plantains, raisins, dried dates, and other dried fruits), and snack foods (such as corn chips, pretzels, potato chips, and popcorn).

Other cautionary foods to be aware of are red or fatty meats, poultry with skin, organ meat, whole milk, whole cheese, butter, premium ice cream, stick or hard margarine, fried fast foods, refried beans, baked beans, broad beans, palm kernel oil, coconut oil, coconut meat, processed meats high in salt and additives, processed foods high in trans fats (cookies, crackers, frozen entrees, and snack cakes), alcohol, and foods sweetened with fructose.

Foods listed in this group should be very low in your diet, especially if you are sedentary, obese, or have Syndrome X, diabetes, heart disease, cancer, high blood pressure, or arthritis. You will certainly improve your health if you limit these types of foods in your meal plans. But, if you can't do that, you should have them infrequently in combination with abundant healthier foods like fresh dark leafy green vegetables or fruits, such as blueberries and prunes, which are high in antioxidants. You should also keep your portion size small.

Diets high in red meat are believed to increase the risk of breast and colon cancer in susceptible individuals. Over-consumption of refined carbohydrates and simple sugars promotes inflammation and increases tryglycerides and risk of heart attack and breast cancer. Remember, foods high in trans fats lower good cholesterol and increase bad cholesterol. Vegetable oils like corn oil that are high in Omega-6 fats and low in Omega-3 fats promote inflammation and blood clots (a recipe for stroke and heart attack). Alcohol provides empty calories and uses up B-vitamins, even when the carbohydrate content is reduced. It is very hard to lose weight, even if you are eating healthy and drinking alcohol moderately on a regular basis (1-2 drinks a day).

In concluding this chapter, I will like to stress the point that some of the things that we are so concerned about are not even foods but, nevertheless, they have powerful influences on us. To refresh your memory, they include stress, alcohol, insulin, cortisol, smoking, and a sedentary lifestyle, as well as our state of mind. Our mind and thoughts are powerful source of energy that could also be cause of cellular degeneration and disease. All of these can exert strong negative influences on our brain, muscle, and virtually every organ in our body. They promote fat storage and weight gain and also prevent us from losing and keeping the weight off. Typically, they increase health risk, premature aging, and early death.

Now you can see how the food pyramid and the food template compare. And, as we go on, you will learn more and soon will be designing your own personal food template and healthy meal plan.

# Chapter 8

# Eat According to Your Energy Level

## We Eat Too Many Calories

### It's Easy to Eat Too Many Calories

In order to be successful in losing weight and keeping it off, you need to learn to eat just the right amount of food that your body needs in order to function properly. This is very difficult to do in a culture where food is cheap and readily available. However, I will show how to keep your portion in line with your level of activity without sacrificing nutrients and antioxidants. You will also learn tips and techniques how to maintain physical activity over the long-term. Exercise don't have to be strenuous activities to burn excess body fat and calories.

The formula seems simple enough. Yet, the number of people who are overweight or obese has been rising steadily for the past 20 to 30 years. This is in part because we are taking in too many calories – especially from the wrong kinds of food – and we are not active. For example, the USDA reports that Americans are now eating about 150 to 200 more calories a day than they were two decades ago. The average person consumes more than 2,000 calories a day, which can easily add 10 to 15 pounds per year.

I have often tried to impress upon my patients the importance of thinking of all foods as sources of calories. One of the fundamental errors I see frequently is that people tend to eat more if they believe the food they are eating is healthy. Making better food choices is only one piece of the solution. You also need to control your portion size. The bigger the portion, the more calories you are consuming, even if you are eating foods that are healthy. Understanding this concept has helped most of my patients change their relationship with food.

> Change your relationship with food. Think of food as providing calories that turn to fat unless you burn them off.

A sedentary lifestyle, one with minimal activity or an inconsistent exercise routine, can cause you to store fat even if you are eating fewer calories than you used to. Your caloric intake needs to reflect your activity level and energy demands on a meal-to-meal basis. Otherwise, your weight-loss effort will not be effective.

## How to Conquer Your Emotional Eating

Emotional or stress eating is a big factor in the consumption of too many extra calories. Traditional wisdom, which seems to rely on willpower, is proving to be inadequate in helping people to resolve this problem. I believe that understanding the science will empower you to conquer emotional eating. In previous chapters, I tried to show you why it is more rewarding to eat a proper meal that is low in calories but high in nutrients and antioxidants. Here, I will go a step further using an emotional eater, Patricia, to bring the point home.

Patricia is a 50-year-old woman who recently underwent treatment for breast cancer. At 253 pounds, she was more than 100 pounds overweight. She consumed about 3,000 calories a day and led a sedentary lifestyle.

No matter how much she ate, Patricia was always hungry a few hours later. This is a classic sign that she was eating the wrong kinds of food. It was also an indication of nutritional deficiency. Exercise was out of the question for Patricia because even walking was a heavy burden. Her energy was low and she suffered from severe fatigue.

Patricia had a wonderful and supportive network of family and friends as well as a successful business. Yet, she was not a happy person. Food controlled her life in a way that made her miserable. One serious mistake that Patricia made was, instead of taking action, she thought her eating was due to her emotions. Many experts would agree, but let's take a closer look at the underlying issues that may be hindering Patricia's progress. Only then can we truly say that emotional factors were her biggest enemy.

My approach was simply to help Patricia change her relationship with food, and eat an anti- inflammatory diet. Her new eating plan was focused on getting adequate nutrients and antioxidants, instead of calories during each meal. To her surprise, in just a few weeks, she felt completely satisfied eating about half the calories she had previously consumed. Her cravings disappeared along with her restlessness and she had more energy than she has had in a long time.

**In order to burn fat, you need nutrients, not calories!**

It is obvious that Patricia's problems were not due to lack of calories, but rather due to inadequate nutrients and antioxidants. And this is the reason she responded so well when her new diet was changed to one that emphasized nutrients and antioxidants instead of mere calories. The old diet lacked vital nutrients and antioxidants – these are necessary to help burn body fat and control cravings. For example, Omega-6 was 28 times the Omega-3 in her diet. This coupled with other bad fats and refined carbohydrates may have contributed to her breast cancer as well. Omega-6 fats are not only pro-inflammatory but they also promote cancer growth, whereas Omega-3 fats are anti-inflammatory and inhibit cancer growth. Omega-3 fatty acids also increase insulin sensitivity. This would also explain the reason why increasing the Omega-3 and reducing intake of Omega-6 and refined carbohydrates helped Patricia control her craving and binges.

Making better food choices and eating a proper meal rewarded Patricia with improved health and a better self-image. Her skin became radiant and toned and she looked and felt better. She was able to wear clothes that she hadn't worn for years. To top it all off, she lost 21 pounds (18 pounds was body fat) in two months.

**Is It Emotions or Something Else?**

Patricia's story shows us that it is quite possible to conquer our own emotional eating. The key is to eat a meal that consists of vital nutrients and antioxidants instead of just calories and never to go without food for a prolonged period of time.

**What Triggers You to Eat Compulsively?**

To answer this question, you should ask yourself, "Is it emotions or something else that prompts me to eat." Stress can drive you to overeat and drink, and that's the major reason to learn proper stress management. The root cause of some of these emotional eating can be traced back to deep psychological components (such as past issues and conflicts)—appropriate interventions by qualified professionals can help to resolve some of these issues. But suppose there was a simple, logical, biological explanation that would help you to understand the reasons for most of your emotional eating and binges? For instance, low levels of serotonin and dopamine in the brain can trigger craving, anxiety, overeating and mood swings. Perhaps, this will demystify cravings and provide you with a powerful weapon to fight back.

We all know by now that the culprits are the two notorious hormones cortisol and insulin. They trigger your appetite and make you hungry. But can you blame these hormones for your poor food choices that you make through the course of the day? Definitely not! First and foremost, you are responsible for the food choices you make. For example, if you eat French fries, you will feel hungry a few hours later. Likewise, popcorn, corn chips, or soda will drive you to eat a few hours later as well. On the other hand, 100% whole-wheat crackers or multigrain bread would probably cause a lesser drive to eat. The underlying factor that triggered your appetite is definitely not your emotions, but a severe deficiency in nutrients and energy.

**We Have Defenses**

Most of us are so convinced that we have no defenses against our emotions and stress. The good news is that we do have powerful defenses and allies that we can use at will. I definitely don't mean willpower. It doesn't work once you have allowed things to get out of control. For example no amount of willpower will save you from craving and binges if you consistently make poor food choices or skip meals, especially breakfast, as well as allow stress to control your actions.

Through years of countless observations, it is crystal clear to me now that the central reason why most people crave and have abnormal emotions and mood swings may be largely due to meals that are deficient in nutrients that are critical for production, utilization, and maintenance of energy. For example, the B-complex vitamins help to efficiently convert food into energy, improve digestion, help prevent blood sugar spikes associated with mood swings, food craving and production of serotonin and dopamine. The best sources of these vitamins are in foods that are high in nutrients, such as whole grains, lean meats, wheat germ and rice. Omissions of foods that provide these nutrients have serious repercussions that could range from depression to craving and overeating.

Consider also the fact that the nutrients in most refined and processed foods have been stripped off and all you get is empty calories. On the contrary, whole foods and minimally processed foods have most of their nutrients intact and can literally deliver more nutrients than calories. That is why they are able to quench your craving and binge eating and, most importantly, are able to help boost your body metabolism so that you can burn body fat more efficiently and increase your cellular energy. Besides eating nutrient-rich foods, taking appropriate amounts of good quality vitamins and minerals can help to restore energy and decrease stress that triggers cravings and over-indulgence. Below, I will discuss other causes that could trigger craving and overeating and also show you easy techniques that will give you the winning edge.

## Most Emotional Eaters Skip Meals or Fail to Eat on Time

Your energy level will be at its lowest point and you will be very vulnerable if you skip a meal, delay your meals, or fail to take your vitamins and mineral supplements. For example, you are more likely to be stressed and eat out of control if you skipped breakfast, have an inadequate lunch or fail to have a late afternoon snack to help keep your blood sugar and energy level stable. You will also be vulnerable if you eat simple sugars and refined carbohydrates that drive your blood sugar down and, in addition, highjack your vitamins and minerals. For this reason, you need to take your vitamin and mineral supplements on schedule.

One of my patients recently confessed to me that she had noticed a significant decrease in energy when she went without her vitamin and mineral supplements. She even went further to reveal that her symptoms of depression and anxiety were lesser when she took her vitamins than the prescribed anti-depressant. In her experience, that may be true – but it would make more sense to take the anti-depressant in combination with the vitamins and mineral supplements and also to eat foods high in nutrients and antioxidants. Keeping physically active also helps to curb abnormal emotional impulses and depression.

## Cortisol Drives Our Energy Level

The bloodstream level of cortisol rises steadily in the morning and peaks at noon and then declines to a very low level in the evening. The flow of energy and body metabolism through our body follows a similar pattern of highs and lows. That is why your energy level drops predictably during the mid-afternoon (between 3:30 and 4:30) or approximately 3 hours after your lunch. Your blood sugar plummets, causing mental fatigue, headache, anxiety, mood swings, depression, and ultimately a feeling of being out of control – which forces you to crave and binge (this subject has been covered extensively by Dr. Pamela Peeke in her book, *Fight Fat after Forty*).

Most people's usual response is to restore energy quickly by turning to sugary snacks, sodas and stimulants, like coffee. None of these are good choices. They raise blood sugar and energy quickly, but they also trigger a strong insulin response that sets a cascade of events into motion: low blood sugar, hunger pangs, severe craving, and perhaps even a deeper and more intense mood swing.

Chronic low stress levels causes cortisol levels to go up and serotonin levels to drop significantly, leading to an intense craving for carbohydrates and sugary foods, fatigue, crying more easily, depression, feelings of hopelessness, and loss of short-term memory. It's like being thrown into a swirling whirlpool in which it seems there is no way out.

But there is a way out. Simple lifestyle changes can be very helpful – such as cutting back on sweets and sugary foods (soft drinks, cookies, candies, and white bread). Other helpful practices are relaxation techniques, such as deep breathing, music, meditation, yoga, tai chi, self-hypnosis and massage. Regular exercise also helps, including learning good stress-management.

When you have a mid-afternoon crisis or low energy, the proper response to this afternoon lull would be to have minimally refined carbohydrates (such as whole grains or multigrain) balanced with protein or foods that do not trigger a strong insulin response. Better yet, it would help greatly to have a well-balanced breakfast, an adequate lunch, and an afternoon snack. This approach is more likely to stabilize blood sugar and energy and keep your stress level from raging out of control. This same technique can be applied to reduce other emotional stress that could trigger craving and compulsive eating.

> When we have enough nutrients and energy, we can better control our emotions so things don't get out of hand

The take-home message here is that food has a powerful influence on your emotions, mood, and personality. Some of these changes are so profound that they can be compared with some potent prescribed drugs. For example, some of my patients have come off anti-depressants or are able to respond well on reduced dosage by simply making better food choices and, of course, maintaining a reasonable level of physical activity.

> Food has a powerful effect on our physical and mental state

## Cravings May Be the Result of Nutrient Deficiency

I hope you now understand that nutrient deficiency in our diets can trigger intense craving and overeating and, of course, promote fat storage and weight gain – all of which increases health risk. There is one important secret that you have to know. Do not be overly concerned about calories as long as the meals are balanced and there are adequate nutrients and antioxidants. Also keep in mind that too much of any thing can be bad for your health, including foods we consider healthy. Now, let me reveal a small secret to you: Most of us have a huge reservoir of energy and calories stored in our fat cells that literally could sustain us for months.

The question is, why are our bodies not releasing this huge amount of energy and calories that are stored in our fat cells? Consider the possibility that our bodies are unable to tap into the huge pool of energy reserve whenever there is a deficiency of vital nutrients (such as vitamin B12, B6, Folic acid, calcium, chromium, magnesium, zinc, essential fatty acids, and fiber). The simple reason for this is that our bodies need nutrients in order to convert food into energy or burn body fat. Without adequate nutrients in the foods that we eat, our bodies literally starve, and under perform. This is what you do to correct the problem:

*Physical activity is important, but it's only practical if we tailor our food intake to our level of activity, and most importantly, eat meals that are abundant in nutrients and antioxidants, but low in calories. This will help to keep you full, satisfied and energized.*

*Once you adopt this strategy of getting more nutrients and antioxidants, and lesser calories, you will have discovered the secret of losing weight and body fat and improving your health beyond your wildest dreams.*

Now you should be empowered knowing that some aspect of cravings and compulsive eating may be primarily due to nutrient deficiency that you can correct. As you leave this section, I want you to remember that poor quality foods and unhealthy lifestyle habits (such as smoking, alcohol, skipping meals, sugary foods and refined carbohydrates, poor stress management and inactivity) can trigger abnormal emotions, drain energy and plunge you into a vicious cycle of hunger, eating, and emotional lows. In contrast, good quality foods that are high in nutrients and antioxidants satisfy and control cravings and provide emotional and mental stability, provided it's accompanied with a healthy lifestyle.

Before you eat another meal, make sure that you are getting enough nutrients and antioxidants and fewer calories. One more piece of advice: Chronic stress, bad foods and inactivity drive our energy down and make us vulnerable and unable to respond appropriately. On the contrary, good foods and activity drive our energy up, making us less vulnerable to stress and binges.

## Is Your Caloric Intake in Line With Your Activity Level?

We often underestimate the number of calories we are consuming each day because of unfamiliarity with serving sizes. A key to controlling portion sizes and calories is to become familiar with serving sizes. This is easily done since most people eat the same foods over and over again. For example, most people assume that a bowl of cereal is one serving, whereas it may actually contain two-to-three times the suggested serving size. One way to avoid this mistake is to check nutritional labels more often and to get into the habit of measuring foods.

The suggested serving size for most breakfast cereals is ½-1 cup and not a bowl. For a bagel, the suggested size is not the large bagels that may contain three to four serving sizes and add a whopping 300-400 calories. It is even worse with pasta or spaghetti. The suggested serving size for pasta and rice is ½ cup cooked but some of us eat two or more cups in a sitting. This is the equivalent of four or more servings and, of course, four times the calories.

For example, ½ cup cooked rice contains about 22 grams carbohydrate, where as 2 cups contain 86 grams carbohydrate. The amount of pasta the average person eats in one setting is alarming to say the least.

In restaurants, a plate of pasta may contain six or more servings. In some instances, you may inadvertently consume a whole day's calories in one sitting and not even be aware of it. This is the reason why eating out frequently can cause you to gain weight or resist weight loss. The all-you-can-eat mentality is certainly aggravating the obesity epidemic. It encourages people to eat more because they believe they are getting a bargain.

**Why Do We Eat so Much?**

Most people overeat without realizing it, even when they are trying to cut back. Professor Brian Wansink of the University of Illinois at Urbana-Champaign found that moviegoers consumed 44 percent more popcorn when they ate from large containers than when they ate from smaller containers. The American Institute for Cancer Research study found that 67 percent of Americans cleared everything on their plates regardless of the amount of food served. And *Self*-magazine few years ago compiled a chart that compared portion sizes at restaurants in America and Europe. It clearly showed that Americans consume more calories than Europeans because we eat larger portion sizes.

**Super Sizing in America**

| **United States** | **Europe** |
|---|---|
| Fast Food Fries, 7 oz, 610 calories<br>Croissant, 4 oz, 430 calories<br>Steak, 20 oz, 1360 calories | London: Fries, 5.5 oz, 485 calories<br>France: Croissant, 2 oz, 215 calories<br>England: Steak, 8 oz, 545 calories |

In the past decade, portion sizes in the United States have become even larger. Our plates, cups, and glasses are also larger. For example, the cups and glasses used in restaurants contain 12 to 16 ounces of liquid, not the standard 8 ounces.

Professor Wansink coined the phrase "portion-size distortion" to describe America's obsession with large portions. Most of us are not even aware that we are eating far too many calories from foods high in saturated fats and refined carbohydrates that our bodies easily store as fat. Part of the problem is that most people are not aware of how much they should eat to maintain their ideal weight. Another problem is that most of us eat too few non-starchy vegetables and fruits and too many calorie-dense meat, cheese, and refined grains. The refined grains can stimulate your appetite and cause you to overeat.

Most of us have never measured the amount of food we eat. We simply eat until our plates are clean. As a rule, we eat excessively because food is available and not because we are hungry, but this is not a behavior that we are born with. Scientists believe we learned how to eat this way from our parents. Also, it only seems to be exhibited in the human species.

You don't see obese animals in the wild. They always stop eating when they are full. A similar behavior is seen among young children who have not yet developed this bad habit.

Three-year-old children listen to their bodies and stop eating when they are full, even when served excessive amounts of food. In contrast, five-year-old children and adults eat because the food is available, regardless of their energy needs (according to researchers).

> **One of the key ways to control calories is to eat smaller portions, even if you think you need more food. The amount you actually need may be much less than you realize.**

## What Is a Serving Size?

### Serving Sizes Can Be Confusing

Most people do not have a clue as to how to interpret the serving size on food labels. The concept is really easy to understand and it can help you to eat just the amount of food that your body needs. In very simple terms, the serving size states how much of a particular food is recommended. This information is usually found on the nutritional label and it is much smaller than most people realize (See Chapter 3).

Another important thing to know is that the serving size listed on a food label is not necessarily the amount of food that is intended for you. It only tells you the amount of calories, carbohydrates, fats, cholesterol, proteins, fiber, and minerals found in that particular amount of food. You have to figure out the actual amount suitable for you. For example, the serving size for Quaker Oats is ½ cup dry (27 grams carbohydrates). This may be suitable for someone whose lifestyle is inactive or who has Syndrome X or diabetes, whereas someone with an active lifestyle will probably need 1 cup (54 grams). The following chart lists what 1 serving size equals according to the USDA:

| | |
|---|---|
| 1 slice of whole-grain bread | ¾ cup vegetable juice |
| ½ cup cooked rice or pasta | 1 medium apple |
| ½ cup mashed potatoes | ½ grapefruit or mango |
| 3-4 small crackers | ½ cup berries |
| 1 small pancake or waffle | 1 cup yogurt or milk |
| 2 medium-sized cookies | 1 oz cheese |
| ½ cup cooked vegetables | 1 chicken breast |
| 1 cup raw vegetables | 1 medium pork chop |
| 1 cup (4 leaves) lettuce | ¼ pound hamburger patty |
| 1 small baked potato | ½ cup grains/cereals |
| ½ cup beans, lentils, soybeans | 1 medium ear or ½ cup corn |
| ½ bagel | 1 tsp butter/margarine |
| 1 tbsp oils | 1 oz or 1 tbsp nuts/seeds |
| 1 or ½ cup fresh fruits | 3 oz fish/meat |
| 1 large egg | 2 egg whites |
| 1 tbsp peanut butter (creamy) | 2 tbsp peanut butter (chunky) |

## What Is the Appropriate Portion Size?

### Eat What Your Body Can Burn

The amount of food that is appropriate for you depends upon your energy needs – and your energy needs change from day to day. You need to understand this in order to adjust your food intake accordingly. This means that you may have to cut back on calories when you are inactive or your exercise routine is not up to standard. At the same time, you may have to eat slightly more food as you become more active or begin exercising on a regular basis. The important thing is to do this on a meal-to-meal basis and to make sure that your food intake is in line with your activity level most of the time.

For example, an active person (a person who burns roughly 500 or more calories daily) may require a 1-1½ cups portion of whole grain cereal (2-3 servings since generally ½ cup is equal to 1 serving) during periods of moderate to intense activity. But may have to cut back or eat less (½-1 cup: about 1-2 servings) during periods of less activity. Similarly, an individual who is sedentary most of the time may need an even smaller amount (½ cup ). In the illustrations given, the point is made even clearer that your food intake should be based on your level of activity and not so much on your weight. There is a direct correlation between muscle mass and metabolism. A sedentary, obese individual usually has more fat in comparison to muscle mass, hence a lower metabolism than a person who has a greater amount of muscle mass. The bottom line is that you will gain weight if you are sedentary, your exercise routine is inconsistent or you exercise intensely but consume food that contains more calories than your body really needs, even if it is healthy food.

*It is also important to make adjustments as you grow older and possibly less active. Portions should be smaller to accommodate this change in lifestyle. Most people make the mistake of eating the same amount of food that they ate 20 to 30 years ago, even though their metabolism has changed dramatically.*

However, simply cutting back on food portions without paying attention to your energy needs can be a problem, too. Portions that are too small and not appropriate for you can leave you feeling hungrier and craving the wrong foods. One way to prevent this is to pay close attention to your body's needs and you will eventually know the portions of different foods that are suitable for you (meaning you learn to listen to your body). In Chapters 14 and 15, you will learn easy methods to help you gauge the amount of food that is suitable for your level of activity.

Once you understand the importance of eating foods according to your energy needs and activity levels, it is very easy to realistically lose weight and keep it off for good. This behavior can be learned, just like the bad eating habits you previously learned. If you fail to do so, your weight will soar regardless of your age, gender, or physical activity level. The good news is that, if you succeed in mastering portion sizes, you will be rewarded with better health, an amazing appearance, and an energy level you never suspected you had in you.

# Chapter 9

# Carbohydrates, Inflammation, and Fat Storage

## Not All Carbohydrates Are Equal

When you eat a meal containing carbohydrates, starches, and sugars, they convert to blood glucose at different rates. Simple sugars and refined carbohydrates (sugars, sweets, cakes, desserts, juices, and white flour products) convert rapidly to blood sugar. In today's American society, we eat excessive amounts of refined carbohydrates that can drain ones energy and increase health risk. Refined carbohydrates can also trigger a rapid rise in blood sugar, leading to fat storage and inflammation.

Complex carbohydrates are a better choice. They contain nutrients like fiber, iron, calcium and B-vitamins that are lacking in refined foods. Whole foods like whole-wheat pasta, multigrain bread, brown rice, barley, unrefined oat bran cereals, sweet potatoes, and fruits (such as apples, cherries, and grapefruit) release their glucose slowly. As a result, they do not trigger an intense insulin spike that leads to fat storage and cellular inflammation. Nonetheless, it is still necessary to be aware of your intake based on your dietary needs and level of activity.

On the other hand, some complex carbohydrates like white potatoes, parsnip, white bread, corn, short-grain white rice, plantains, and sweetened breakfast cereals behave like highly refined carbohydrates. They also release blood sugar in the body quickly causing a surge of glucose, which, unless used up immediately by active muscle tissue, will be converted into fat.

Diets high in saturated fat, trans fat, and Omega-6 fatty acids, such as beef, lamb, pork, dark poultry meat, and full fat dairy products are also bad for you. Like refined carbohydrates, they trigger fat storage and inflammation. This is why eating a huge amount of refined carbohydrates with a large piece of beef can cause weight gain as well as increase health risk.

## Glycemic Index and Weight Loss

The glycemic index (GI) is a numerical way of predicting how quickly food turns into sugar in your body – the higher the number, the quicker the conversion and the greater the blood sugar rise and vice versa. There are two systems for measuring the blood sugar rise. One system uses glucose as a standard and the other system uses white bread. We are using the system based on glucose. When reading other books, you might encounter either of these systems.

The glucose system rates the breakdown of carbohydrates to blood sugar using a glucose reference (glucose = 100). The glycemic response can soar greatly higher in some instances. For example, the GI of maltose (beer sugar) is 105. A glycemic number below 55 indicates that the carbohydrate breaks down slowly (low energy carbohydrate) and is less likely to spike insulin levels, except when you eat too much. To help you lose weight and improve overall health, choose foods with a glycemic index below 55. Remember, the glycemic index does not tell you the total amount of carbohydrate present in a meal, nor is the amount of fat, so you must pay attention to your portion sizes. For example, eating two slices of bread increases the blood sugar nearly two times compared to one slice of bread.

> If your lifestyle is sedentary to only slightly active (burning fewer than 250 calories/day), you can prevent fat storage by choosing low energy carbohydrate foods with a glycemic index below 55.

A glycemic index above 55 indicates the carbohydrate breaks down quickly (high energy carbohydrate) and is likely to raise insulin levels. Foods with higher numbers (approaching 100) are not healthy for individuals who are physically inactive or have medical problems (such as obesity, Syndrome X, diabetes, heart disease, or high blood pressure). In general, the higher the glycemic index number, the greater the blood sugar response and the greater the health risks.

For example, pretzels have a GI of 83, whereas sourdough bread has a GI of 52. This means sourdough bread is better for your weight and health than pretzels. Foods with extremely low carbohydrate content, such as meat, fish, fat and proteins do not cause blood sugar spikes. Eating these foods with carbohydrates in a meal can help to reduce the blood sugar response.

If you are reading a book in which the glycemic index is based on white bread, you can easily convert the numbers to those based on glucose by dividing by 1.4. A list of carbohydrates with their glycemic value is shown below. For more detailed information regarding the glycemic index, consult www.mendosa.com/gi.htm or *The Glucose Revolution* by Jennie Brand-Miller, PhD.

Eating low energy foods (glycemic index blow 55) gives better satiety, improves insulin resistance, lowers blood lipids, and promotes fat loss and weight loss. The list of these foods is long. Fruits that are high in fiber includes apples, pears, plums, and grapefruits- they elicit a low to moderate sugar response. The list also includes a host of whole foods that are high in fiber, such as oats, beans and lentils.

It is very important to mention that simply relying on the glycemic index of foods does not ensure that you will burn body fat and lose weight. Even low glycemic foods can cause weight gain if you eat more than what your body is capable of burning in a short period of time.

High-energy foods (glycemic index greater than 55) can trigger varying degrees of high blood sugar and insulin responses that promote fat storage, insulin resistance, elevated blood lipids, weight gain, and inflammation. Most of these foods are low in fiber and may be excessively refined. You should limit foods, even complex carbohydrates, whose glycemic index is greater than 55. These foods may be appropriate for individuals who burn significant amount of energy, such as athletes and manual laborers, but they are definitely not the right choice for individuals who burn a minimal amount of calories and energy, such as sedentary individuals and those with major health problems.

> If you are not in shape to burn about 500 calories/day in strenuous physical activity, stay away from foods with a glycemic index greater than 55. These high-energy foods can trigger cravings, mood swings and cause abnormal fat storage and cellular inflammation.

### The Kind of Food You Eat Affects Your Body Metabolism

I often counsel patients not to blame their weight on their body metabolism, but rather their food choices and lifestyle. Some people have a fast metabolism and can eat all they want without gaining weight. You may not be one of them. But this should not stop you from doing the right things that will help to raise your body metabolism. Even a depressed metabolism can be boasted, and this section and the chapter on protein will explain the way to do it. In addition to making better food choices, engaging in regular physical activity (even walking briskly for 4 miles, 5-7 times a week) can help to raise body metabolism and increase the effectiveness at which your body burns fat.

The rate at which the food you eat is digested can speed up or slow down your body metabolism (your ability to burn calories and body fat). Low glycemic carbohydrates, such as high–fiber, complex carbohydrates (multigrain bread, brown rice, whole-wheat pasta, barley pasta, apples, and beans) require more energy to digest and therefore their sugar is released slowly into the blood stream. Similarly, the digestion of protein requires more energy (about 25% or more). Because of this, both low glycemic carbohydrates and lean proteins can help speed up your metabolism. This is known as the "thermogenic effect of food." It also explains why combining protein and fat when eating carbohydrate foods helps to balance the blood sugar levels and prevents the highs (hyperglycemia) and lows (hypoglycemia) from occurring. Fats, especially saturated fats found in meat, dairy, cheese, the refined or high glycemic carbohydrates, and white flours have the least thermogenic effect and can cause fat storage that can slow down your metabolism.

> Eating carbohydrate foods in combination with lean proteins and healthy fats helps to balance the blood sugar levels and prevent excessive insulin production in the body. This can help your body to burn fat more efficiently.

## Don't Be Fooled by the Numbers

We have established that simple sugars and refined carbohydrate foods raise blood sugar levels quickly and can cause fat storage and inflammation. But some complex carbohydrate foods are also guilty of this as well. White potatoes (GI 93), for instance, raise blood sugar levels higher than table sugar (GI 63) or white bread (GI 73).

Other foods like banana bread, blueberry muffins, peanuts, and potato chips raise blood sugar slowly only because they are high in fat – that's why you should be cautionary with them. They contain high levels of saturated fats, trans fat, and Omega-6 fats like those found in beef, pork, lamb, cheese, other full fat dairy products, and processed foods. The problem here is that these fats can raise blood cholesterol levels as well as raise compounds that promote inflammation. Despite the low glycemic index, these foods should be limited for health reasons.

In general, most foods with lots of fat, fiber, or protein will have a low glycemic index, regardless of whether they cause fat storage or inflammation. Take a look at the list below and you will understand why you should not take the glycemic index for face value. Use the glycemic index of foods simply as a guide and not as an absolute number.

Low Glycemic Index Foods to Limit or Use Sparingly

| | |
|---|---|
| Chocolate (49) | Peanuts (20) |
| Banana Bread (47) | Potato Crisps (54) |
| Blueberry Muffin (59) | Pound Cake (54) |
| Ice Cream, Low-Fat (50) | Sponge cake (46) |
| Mars M&M (32) | Yogurt, low-fat and sugar (32) |
| Mars Snickers Bar (40) | |

Other foods to look out for with a low glycemic index, but nonetheless are health hazards, are some of our favorite household staples, such as whole milk, full fat yogurt, ice cream, cheese, and many other dairy products. For example, some brands of yogurt that are fat free may have as many as 44 grams of sugar in an 8 oz cup serving. On the other hand, a better choice would be those brands of yogurt that are not sweetened with fructose and have less than 15 grams of sugar per serving or are plain without additives.

## Low Energy Carbohydrates Cause Lower Levels of Insulin Release

There are actually no "good" or "bad" carbohydrates but there are clear distinctions in the ways they affect us. For example, eating refined sugars and carbohydrates after an exhausting sports competition is highly rewarding and beneficial to the body. Energy is quickly restored to normal and, in this setting; the refined carbohydrate is definitely a better choice than whole grains, which would restore energy very slowly.

On the other hand, when a sedentary person eats a large portion of refined carbohydrates, most of the calories will be stored as fat instead of being burned for energy. Here, it is the food choice that is the problem, not the food. Remember, it is how we perceive and use carbohydrates that make them a problem, not the foods themselves.

*Each person has a different level of tolerance for carbohydrates. You will have no problem if you eat the right types of carbohydrates that are suitable for your body and also stay within the limit that your body can effectively burn. If you take in the amounts that are in line with your metabolism, more of your calories will be burned for energy and not stored as fat.*

However, for the purpose of our discussion here we will divide carbohydrates into two categories – good and bad. The "good" carbohydrates usually release their energy slowly in our body. Also, they are usually minimally processed, low glycemic and are high in fiber and whole grains. They are high in nutrients including calcium, B-vitamins, and iron. They provide long-term energy, keep you full longer between meals, and help you to maintain stable blood sugar and insulin levels. They can also help to promote weight loss more effectively than the bad carbohydrates, especially if you eat them in combination with lean proteins, healthy fats, or non-starchy vegetables. In addition, they can help to boost your body metabolism into a fat-burning machine. Other benefits include a healthier digestive system and improved concentration, skin tone, and mood.

As a result of better blood sugar and insulin control, eating low energy carbohydrates (foods with a GI below 55) can help you to lose abdominal fat quickly – which can reduce the risk of insulin resistance syndrome (Syndrome X), diabetes, heart disease, high blood pressure, and breast and colon cancers. Again, it is important to emphasize that simply eating low energy foods is not enough to ensure weight loss and improvement of health. You must also cut calories and eat portion sizes suitable for your level of physical activity. This will ensure that the change in your body composition involves losing body fat rather than muscle mass.

*The following charts will give you a guide to make better carbohydrate choices. Later in the chapter, I will also give you another guide to cautionary carbohydrate choices. Right now, take a look over this list and be sure to read the notes as well. Once you experiment with these best carbohydrate choices, you will never feel the need to eliminate carbohydrates from your diet again!*

## BEST CARBOHYDRATE FOOD CHOICES

Low glycemic food choices (GI below 55. Glucose GI is 100). They induce low levels of insulin and are therefore considered to be non-inflammatory and non-fattening. The non-starchy vegetables are rich in antioxidants and essential nutrients (vitamins and minerals) that are vital to the proper functioning of every cell and organelle, including the brain and muscle.
The non-starchy vegetables and fruits should be the foundation (food template) of each meal.

### NON-STARCHY VEGETABLES (<15)

Arugula
Artichoke
Asparagus
Bamboo shoots
Bean Sprouts
Beet
Bitter Balls
Broccoli
Brussel Sprouts
Cabbage, all varieties
Carrots, raw
Cassava greens
Cauliflower
Celery
Chard
Chinese cabbage
Chicory
Collard Greens
Cucumbers
Dandelion Greens
Dill pickles
Eggplant
Endive
Escarole
Ethnic greens
Fennel Bulb
Garlic
Green Beans
Green Snap
Green Peas
Green Snap Peas
Heart of Palm
Kale
Kohlrabi
Leeks
Lettuce, all varieties
Mushrooms (all varieties)
Mustard Greens
Okra
Onions
Parsley
Peppers, all varieties
Potato greens
Radishes
Sauerkraut
Scallions
Sea vegetables
Snow peas
Spaghetti Squash
Tomato juice
Tomatoes
Turnip greens
Vegetable Juice
Watercress
Wax Beans
Yellow Snap
Young summer squash (yellow)
Zucchini

Note: Eat 5-7 servings daily (2 ½-3 ½ cups cooked or 5-7 cups raw) or more depending on caloric level and activity. Start each major meal with non-starchy vegetables (without the fatty and salty dressing) or vegetable soup (without potatoes, cream or corn). You can eat an abundant amount of non-starchy vegetables. They are 95% water. Serving size is ½ cup cooked or 1 cup raw.

## BEST STARCHY VEGETABLES

Carrots, cooked, ½ cup (49)
Cassava, boiled (46)
Sweet Corn* on the cob, 1 (70)
Sweet Corn*, kernels, ½ cup (70)
Sweet corn*, canned, ½ cup (70)
Squash, Hubbard, 1 cup (<55)
Green peas, fresh, frozen, boiled ½ cup (48)
Legumes: see legumes below
New potatoes**, 5 small, 6 oz (62)
Sweet potatoes** ½ cup mashed, (54)
Yam, 3 oz (51)

*Modern corn, unlike the Native Indian corn, has less soluble fiber and is therefore a high-energy food.

Corn is very controversial and most people are confused as to whether or not they should eat corn. My view is that corn is a natural food that you can enjoy in moderation. Pay attention to the serving sizes listed above, including food labels.

**Sweet potatoes and new potatoes convert to blood sugar slowly whereas white potatoes convert very quickly. However, you should keep your portions small (sweet and new potatoes) to prevent blood sugar over load. For example, a medium 4 oz sweet potato has about 28 grams carbohydrate and a 3 oz new potato has about 7 grams carbohydrates.

By comparison, a 2-3 oz small white potato contains about 27 grams of high-energy carbohydrate.

You can bake potato wedges with the skin using of course the types of potatoes that do not convert to sugar rapidly, such as sweet potato and new potato and the root vegetable, yam.

Cassava is popular in West Africa, especially in Nigeria. Cassava can be boiled, roasted and fried (not recommended). Farina or garri is made from cassava from drying and grinding the peeled cassava root, which also preserve the cassava. The cassava flour is used to make a very popular dish called fufu.

Fufu is usually eaten in large portions and is heavily loaded with starch – probably highly glycemic due to the refining process that removes nutrients and fiber, unlike the parent cassava root. Fufu is also made from other starches, such as potatoes, eddoes, plantain, and yam. These highly processed foods could be contributing to the development of diabetes, obesity, and other chronic degenerative diseases in societies that over-indulge in them, including West African immigrants to America.

## BEST FRUITS AND FRUIT PRODUCTS

Tangerine, 1 (<55)
Apple juice, unsweetened, 1 cup (40)
Apricot jam, w/o sugar, 1 tbsp, (55)
Apple, 1 medium (38)
Apricots, fresh, 3 medium (57)
Banana, raw, 1 medium, (55)
Cherries, 10 large (22)
Grapefruit, ½ medium (25)
Grapes, green, 1 cup (46)
Plums, 1 medium (39)
Pear, 1 medium (38)
Kiwi, 1 medium (52)
Nectarine, 1 medium (<55)
Orange, navel, 1 medium (44)
Orange juice, unsweetened, 1 cup (46)
Peach, 1 medium (42)
Peach/canned/natural juice, ½ cup (30)
Peach/light syrup, ½ cup (52)
Pear/canned/pear juice, ½ cup (44)
Pineapple juice, w/o sugar 8 oz (46)
Grapefruit juice, unsweetened, 1 cup (48)
Fruit cocktail in natural juice, ½ cup (55)
Strawberries and berries, ½ cup (<15)

## BEST LEGUMES

Baby lima beans, frozen, ½ cup (33)
Beans, Romano, ½ cup (46)
Black beans, boiled, ½ cup (30)
Butter beans, boiled, ½ cup (31)
Canned green lentils, ½ cup (52)
Canned kidney beans, ½ cup (52)
Chana dal, cooked, ½ cup (8)
Chickpeas, cooked, ½ cup (33)
Chickpeas, can, drained, ½ cup (43)
Black-eyed peas, boiled, ½ cup (42)
Great Northern, boiled, ½ cup
Green lentils, boiled, ½ cup (30)
Hummus Tahini, 2 tbsp (<15)
Kidney beans, boiled, ½ cup (27)
Lima beans, boiled, ½ cup
Mung beans, boiled, ½ cup, (38)
Navy beans, boiled, ½ cup (38)
Pinto beans, boiled, ½ cup (39)
Pinto beans, canned, drained, ½ cup (46)
Red lentils, boiled, ½ cup (26)
Soybeans, boiled, ½ cup (18)
Tofu or soybean curd, 2" cube
Yellow split peas, boiled, ½ cup (32)

*Legumes (beans, lentils, soybeans, and soy products) have a moderately high carbohydrate content, but they break down slowly due to high fiber. Incorporate beans and lentils in soups, vegetable salads, and snacks in major meals. A serving of ½ cup cooked is usually adequate as a primary carbohydrate source or side dish. Use lesser amounts for your vegetable template (2-4 tablespoons).

Soybeans or edamame has low carbohydrate and high protein profile. Incorporate soybeans and chana dal as side dishes to help lower cholesterol and blood sugar. Navy beans, kidney beans and lima beans (½ cup cooked) are high in soluble fiber and can also help to lower cholesterol and blood sugar and boost body metabolism.

## BEST SOUPS

(These soups are all low in calories, carbohydrates, fat and sodium. It's ok to use them as needed)

LoSod Veg Soup, 4 oz
Fat free Hearty Lentil w/ Veg soup
Low sod tomato soup, 4 oz
LoSod Veg Chicken soup, 4 oz
Egg Drop soup, 4 oz
Fat Free Hearty Lentil w/ Veg Soup, 5 oz
*Progresso* Healthy Classic Lentil soup, 4 oz
*Progresso* Hlthy Classic Tomato Garden soup, 4 oz
Fat free Lentil and Carrot soup, 4 oz
Wanton soup, 4 oz

## GOOD SOURCES OF FIBER

Flax seeds, ground, 1-2 tbsp
Oat bran (both soluble and insoluble fiber), 1-2 tbsp
Rice bran, 1 tbsp
Unprocessed wheat bran (insoluble fiber), 1-2 tbsp
Wheat germ (fiber, vitamin E and folic acid), 1-2 tbsp
Whole grains (breads, cereals and grains)
Vegetables, fruits, legumes

*Additional sources of fiber if you are not getting enough from whole food: *Benefiber* or *Clearly Fiber*.

## BEST BREADS

100% Stoneground whole-wheat, (53)
100% whole-wheat bread (40)
Bagel 100% whole-wheat
Barley kernel bread
Buckwheat bread
Muesli bread, (54)
*EagleMills*BreadMix-Soy+Flaxseed, (50)

Mixed grain bread or multigrain bread (48)
Oat bran bread, (48)
Oat bran/whole-wheat flour pita, *Joseph's* (<55)
Oat bran/whole-wheat flour tortilla, *Joseph's* (<55)
Pumpernickel, whole grain, (51)
Sourdough bread, (52)
Soy protein pita bread (<55)
Whole-wheat hamburger bun

(See Chapter 3 for complete list)

## BEST CEREAL GRAINS

Bulgur, cooked, ½ cup (48)
Barley, pearled, boiled, ½ cup (25)
Basmati rice, cooked, ½ cup (50)
Brown rice, cooked, ½ cup (50)
Buckwheat groats, cooked, ½ cup (54)

Parboiled rice, cooked, ½ cup (48)
Rice Bran, 1 tbsp (19)
*Uncle Ben's* Converted rice, cooked, ½ cup (44)
Wild rice, cooked, ½ cup (35)
Wheat kernels, cooked, ½ cup (42)

Note: Instant rice breaks down to sugar quickly and trigger insulin spike and should be limited.

(See Chapter 3 for complete list)

## BEST BREAKFAST CEREALS

Barley, pearled, boiled, ½ cup, (25)
Buckwheat, cooked, ½ cup, (54)
Bulgur, cooked, 2/3 cup, (48)
*All Bran* w/ extra fiber, ½ cup, (51)
*Bran Buds* w/ Psyllium, ½ cup, (45)
*Kellogg's Special K*, 1 cup, (54)
*Kashi Good Friends*, Original, ¾ cup

*Kashi GOLEAN*, 1 cup (<55)
Muesli, toasted, 2/3 cup, (43)
*Organic Flax Plus*, Multibran Cereal, ¾ cup
Oatmeal, old fashion, cooked, ½ cup, (49)
*Quaker Oats*, Oat bran cereal, ½ cup, (50)
Rice bran, 1 tbsp, (19)
*Uncle Sam* Cereal, 1 cup (<55)

Note: The serving sizes listed are appropriate for an individual who is moderately active. You can eat more or less depending on your caloric need and activity level. For example, 1 cup of Kashi GOLEAN would be appropriate for a person with a moderate caloric need and activity level. On the other hand, a person whose caloric need is less and his/her activity level is low can get by with ½ cup. See complete list in Chapter 3.

## PASTA TO HAVE IN MODERATION

Capellini, cooked, ½ cup (45)
Fettuccine, cooked, ½ cup (32)
Linguine thick, cooked, ½ cup (46)
Macaroni, cooked, ½ cup (45)
Protein-enriched spaghetti, ½ cup (27)
Ravioli, meat-filled, ½ cup (39)
Spirali, durum, cooked, ½ cup (43)
Star Pastina, cooked, ½ cup (38)
Tortellini, cheese, cooked, 1 cup (50)
Vermicelli noodles, cooked, ½ cup (35)
Whole grain spaghetti, cooked, ½ cup (38)
Whole-wheat pasta, cooked, ½ cup (50)

Pasta is extremely tricky. You may have noticed the low glycemic index, but that alone can be misleading. Pasta is a very high carbohydrate food and in spite of the favorable digestion profile, it can cause significant fat storage if you eat larger portions. For example, one cup of cooked fettuccini contains 57 grams of carbohydrate and two cups gives 114 grams.

The best way to approach pasta is to measure out the appropriate cooked portion size, such as a half cup of cooked fettuccine before you start to eat. Your body can safely handle the carbohydrate content in a half cup of cooked fettuccine and most other pastas. You can always add some pasta later if you are not satisfied. Eating your meals in courses will help you to control your pasta portion (see Chapters 14 and 15). Most people often eat large portions of pasta because the amount eaten is never measured out.

Among the pastas, tortellini has one of the lowest carbohydrate content and you can take advantage of this and eat a bit more than you would if you were eating fettuccini or macaroni. For example, one cup of cooked tortellini has 26 grams of carbohydrate, which should be suitable for most people trying to lose weight. The Chinese vermicelli noodles are also a good choice (½-1 cup cooked contains about 20-40 grams carbohydrate). They are great in soups, stir-fries, vegetable dishes, and side dishes. They are commonly served in Asian restaurants.

Do not cook your pasta too long, otherwise, it breaks down quickly and releases a lot of sugar all at once. On the other hand, when cooked for a short period of time (about 5-6 minutes), the internal carbohydrate structure holds together instead of breaking apart, resulting in slow blood sugar and insulin rise. The pasta should be sticky and resistant when chewed. When shopping, look for other good pastas that may not be familiar to most people – barley pasta and buckwheat pasta.

Eat your pastas with low calorie, low-fat sauce, and abundant non-starchy leafy dark green vegetables and lean low-fat proteins. This will help to delay stomach emptying and lower the chance of carbohydrate overload. In general the pastas that are enriched with protein or are made with whole-wheat are better for people trying to lose weight or control calories and carbohydrates. Make sure the protein is over 15 grams per serving. As a rule, check the amount of carbohydrate, protein, and fiber before purchasing (see Chapter 3).

## BEST DAIRY FOODS

Chocolate flavored milk, 1 cup, (34)
Fat free milk, 1 cup (33)
Mozzarella string cheese, 1
Mozzarella cheese, 1oz
Mozzarella cheese, fat free, 1oz
Cheeses with reduced fat or fat free**
Cottage cheese, low-fat, ½ cup (5g carb, 4 g sugar, 14 g protein, 1g fat)
Ice milk, vanilla, ½ cup (50)
Pudding (*Hunt's*), low sugar, low-fat, ½ cup (43)
Skim milk, 1 cup (32)
Soymilk, 1 cup (31)
Whole milk*, 1 cup (27)
Yogurt (*Cabot*), plain low-fat, 4 oz
Yogurt (*Free*), 50cal,straw/banana, 4 oz
Yogurt (*Knudsen*), 70cal, non-fat, lemon, 6 oz
Yogurt (*Ultimate*), 90 plain, 4 oz, 4 g sugar
Yogurt (Yoplait), plain, 6 oz, 0 sugar
Yogurt (*Dannon*), low sugar, low-fat, 4 oz (<15)

*Whole fat dairy foods and products are a source of bad fat, even those with a low glycemic index.

** Fat free or reduced fat cheeses are healthier than regular cheeses: *Swiss cheese, Light American cheese, Light Cheddar, Low-fat Parmesan, etc.*

## BEST BEVERAGES

Apple juice, unsweetened, 1 cup (40)
Crystal clear pure water (<15)
Grapefruit juice, sugar-free, 1 cup (48)
Green tea, (antioxidants) <15
Juice Spritzer (half fruit juice and half sparkling water)
Lemon or flavored sparkling water (non caloric)
Orange juice, unsweetened, 1 cup (46)
Soymilk, 1 cup (31)
Tomato juice, low sodium (<15)
Vegetable juice, low sodium (V-8) <15 Water

## BEST BAKERY PRODUCTS

Angel food cake 1 slice, 1 oz (67)
Pound cake, 1 slice, 3 oz (54)
Sponge cake, 1 slice, 3 oz (54)

Note: These cakes are among the best in bakery products that have GI rating. They appear to break down to sugar moderately. In spite of this, you should limit the frequency and portion sizes whenever you eat these foods, especially at a party in which you might be drinking also. They are loaded with sugar and fat.

For example, Angel food cake, which has the highest GI in this group, has the lowest carbohydrate content of 17 grams per slice, with no fat. By comparison, Pound cake has a low glycemic index (54), but 1 slice has 42 grams carbohydrate and 15 grams fat. Sponge cake, on the other hand, has 32 grams carbohydrate and 4 grams fat per slice or 1/12 cake.

This is a perfect example of situations that you will encounter on a regular basis. The challenge is to know which one of these items to choose if you are in a situation where you are forced to have foods that you know are not so healthy.

You could choose to completely avoid the unhealthy foods, but that may not always be the right thing to do. So, the next best or politically correct thing to do is to have the one that would cause the least rise in blood sugar, the least fat, and eat only a small portion. This scenario will repeat itself over and over again in parties, holidays, weddings, birthdays, and all kinds of celebrations and gatherings. Stop to think about it before you plunge head on.

Overindulging is a serious mistake that can change your body composition in a very short time (such as losing muscle and gaining fat). People with diabetes will be forced to use more insulin or medications to control their blood sugar as a result of storing extra fat. Those with serious insulin resistance or sugar- sensitivity may lose their control and return to binging on sweets and sugary foods. This is the reason you should consider the consequences of eating these types of foods in the first place, especially if you are vulnerable to craving sweets and fats, or diabetic.

## SNACK FOODS TO ENJOY

Dark chocolate (22)
Lentil soup, canned, ½ cup (44)
Low-fat cottage cheese, ½ cup
Nonfat yogurt with low sugar*, 4 oz
Oatmeal, 1 cookie (55)
Peanuts, boiled, 20, 64 cal, 4g fat
Peanut butter, chunky***, 1 tsp
Peanut butter, creamy***, 1 tsp
Roasted Vegetable Crackers (*Carr's*)
Edamame, ½ cup
Nuts (walnuts, almonds, etc.) 1 tbsp
Mozzarella string cheese, low-fat (3.5g fat)
Pudding, ½ cup, sugar free, (43)
*Social Tea* biscuits, Nabisco, 4 cookies (55)
Split peas, yellow, boiled, ½ cup (32)
Tomato soup, canned**, low sod, ½ cup, (38)
Vegetables and Fruits (see meal plan)
Soy beans, boiled, ½ cup (18)
Multigrain crackers (*Carr's*)
Soybeans (*Mighty Mo Munchies*), organic, ¼ cup, (11g carb, <1g sugar, 10g protein, 4g fat)

* See dairy foods for more listings.

** See the soup selections for more listings.

***Peanuts and peanut butter are high in fats, including Omega-6, which is pro-inflammatory and can also lower HDL (good) cholesterol. People whose HDL are below 45 regardless of a normal total cholesterol are still at increased risk of stroke and heart attack and foods high in Omega-6 are not wise choices. Nuts, such as almonds, cashews, pistachios, pecans, and macadamia are all high in Omega-6 fatty acids. On the other hand, walnuts, butternuts, and chestnuts have a considerable amount of Omega-3 fatty acids that are not only anti-inflammatory, but can also help to raise HDL cholesterol, thereby decreasing the risk of stroke and heart attack.

1 tbsp peanut butter has about 95 calories, 8 grams fat, 2 grams saturated, fat, and only 4 grams protein. Dry roasted peanuts are loaded with calories and fat. For example, 20 dry roasted peanuts contain 117 calories and 10 grams fat and a count of 30 peanuts has 175 calories and 15 grams fat (the amount of fat in a complete meal).

Nuts are notoriously loaded with fats and, though these are healthier fats compared to beef and whole dairy, they can cause fat storage and weight gain if one eats the recommended serving sizes on a regular basis. . For example, 1 oz serving of almonds contains 15 grams fat, walnuts 19 grams fat, and pecan 20 grams fat. Therefore, snack on smaller amounts instead of the recommended serving sizes on food label. For example, 1 –2 tbsp of chopped walnuts delivers only 4-8 grams fat and almonds 3-6 grams fat and these smaller amounts are perfectly suitable for healthy snacking.

## BEST COOKIES/CRACKERS

Oatmeal, 1 cookie, (55)
Social Tea biscuits, *Nabisco*, 4 cookies, (55)
Multigrain Crackers (*Carr's*), 3
Whole-wheat Crackers (Carr's), 2
Roasted Vegetable Crackers (*Carr's*), 3

Note: Oatmeal and Social Tea have the lowest glycemic index in their group. Their carbohydrate content is less than 15 grams per serving. However, you still have to eat a small portion at a time and it's best to accompany them with a protein source, such as mozzarella string cheese, smoked salmon, or 1 tbsp peanut butter to prevent a rapid rise in blood sugar. The glycemic indexes of the three Carr's crackers have not being determined. However, their carbohydrate is less than 15 grams per serving. The multigrain and whole-wheat crackers also have some fiber and they are quite delicious---enjoy them (see the meal plan in Chapter 16).

## Bad Carbohydrates Cause Higher Levels of Insulin and Inflammation

As we discussed earlier, these types of carbohydrates are only bad when the wrong person (such as someone that is physically inactive has Syndrome X, diabetes, heart disease, arthritis, or other chronic degenerative diseases) uses them in excessive amounts. With few exceptions, they are more likely to be nutrient-deficient, refined, and cause spikes in blood sugar and insulin levels.

They are digested very quickly and hence provide instant fuel for muscle use and are not suitable for you if you are physically inactive. They can also cause a strong insulin response that can promote abdominal fat storage, bloating, bowel irregularity, and can even trigger inflammation throughout the body. Naturally, you should limit these types of carbohydrates if you are at risk for heart disease, diabetes, arthritis, and other chronic health problems, including obesity.

### High Insulin Levels Are Bad for You

Carbohydrate foods that are quickly digested (high glycemic foods) raise insulin levels. As you already know, insulin is vital to health but too much and prolonged elevation of insulin can be very dangerous (see Chapter 5). High blood insulin increases hunger and promotes fat storage and weight gain. The experience of feeling hungry a few hours after eating a huge meal of refined or high glycemic carbohydrates (potatoes, pizza, spaghetti, white bread, and sodas) is due to the excessive production of insulin in the body. And this response is not limited to only refined and high glycemic carbohydrates. As you saw previously, even some favorite complex carbohydrate foods like fruits and starchy vegetables are equally dangerous. In fact, they can cause more harm because we don't suspect them.

Insulin is known to cause several abnormal metabolic profiles, all of which increase the risk for cardiovascular disease, diabetes, high blood pressure, and some cancers. The detrimental effects of the prolonged elevation of insulin in the body are summarized below:

- Insulin resistance syndrome
- Craving and increased appetite
- Mood swings and fatigue
- Poor concentration and memory lapses
- Increased risk of developing type 2 diabetes
- High blood pressure
- Low HDL (good) cholesterol
- High LDL (bad) cholesterol
- High triglycerides
- Fat storage in the belly area (visceral or toxic fat)
- Weight gain and/or resistance to weight loss

Most of the foods listed under bad carbohydrates are those more likely to cause prolonged elevation of insulin levels and the risk associated with it. When consumed in excess amounts by people who are sedentary or not active enough, they can cause metabolic disarray that preferentially stores belly fat rather than promotes the burning of carbohydrate for fuel. This is an important fact to consider.

I do not advocate omitting these types of carbohydrates completely from your diet, but I advise that you use them sparingly if you're sedentary or have chronic medical problems. Also eat only small portion sizes at a time, including generous servings of non-starchy vegetables with a combination of other foods containing protein and/or fat to help slow the release of blood sugar and insulin. Now, I will give you the guide to the cautionary carbohydrate choices.

## CAUTIONARY CARBOHYDRATE FOOD CHOICES

These are high glycemic foods (GI above 55. Glucose GI is 100). They can induce high levels of insulin and promote fat storage and inflammation. If you are overweight or sedentary, eat only small portions at a time and also limit the amount of times you eat these foods.

### CAUTIONARY STARCHY VEGETABLES

Baked potato, 1 medium, 4 oz (93)
Butternut and Acorn squash
French fries, large, 4.3 oz (75)
Instant mashed potato, ½ cup (86)
Parsnip, diced, 1 cup (97)
Potato, mashed, ½ cup, 4 oz (70)
Potato, microwave, 1 medium, 4 oz (82)
Pumpkin, peeled, boiled, mashed, ½ cup (75)
Red skinned potato, 1 medium (88)
Rutabaga mashed, 1 cup (72)

## CAUTIONARY FRUITS AND FRUIT PRODUCTS

Apricots, fresh, 3 medium, 3.3 oz (57)
Banana, overripe, 1 medium (64)**
Cantaloupe, raw, ¼ small, 6.5 oz (65)*
Dates dried, 5, 1.4 oz (103)
Mango, 1 small, 5 oz (61)
Watermelon, 1 cup, 5 oz (72)*
Papaya, ½ medium, 5 oz (58)*
Peach, canned, heavy syrup, ½ cup, 4 oz (58)
Pineapple, fresh, 2 slices, 4 oz (66)*
Plantains, ripe med (57 g carb) >55**
Raisins, ¼ cup, 1 oz (64)
Dried fruits – high in sugar

*These are tropical fruits that are known for their sweetness. If their carbohydrate and sugar content is low and you eat only a small portion size they may not elicit a strong insulin response. Enjoy these seasonal fruits; just be sure to stay within the appropriate portion size. Accompany with lemon juice or vinegar to "tame" them.

**Bananas and plantains are high in carbohydrate and turn to sugar rapidly when they are overripe and can hinder weight loss. If you are concerned about potassium replacements, there are many other safer sources (asparagus, broccoli, celery, fresh apricots, yams, sweet potatoes, new potatoes, beans, lentils, and oranges)

* Raisins have a high carbohydrate and sugar content (¼ cup has 28 grams of high glycemic carbohydrate). And they are used in several cold breakfast cereals. They also have a very high Glycemic load (28).

## CAUTIONARY LEGUMES

Baked beans*, ½ cup, (49)
Broad beans, ½ cup (79)
*Loaded with sugar.
Fava beans, ½ cup, (81)

## CAUTIONARY SOUPS

(Items in this section are either high in salt (Na) or carbohydrates).

Black bean soup, ½ cup, 4.5 oz (64)
Green pea soup, canned, 1 cup, (66)
Pea soup, 1 cup (66), 56 g carb
*Campbell's RTS Veg Soup, 7oz, 730 mg Na*
Split pea soup, 8 oz (60)
*Campbell's* chicken noodle soup, 7 oz, 810mg Na
*Campbell's* tomato soup, 7 oz, 790 mg Na

## CAUTIONARY BREADS

Banana bread* 1 slice, 3 oz (47)
Melba toast, 6 pieces (70)
Banana, low-fat, Muffin, 1 (65)
Blueberry muffin, 1 muffin, 2 oz (59)
Gluten-free bread, 1 slice (90)
Hamburger bun, 1, (61)
French baguette 1 oz (95)
Kaiser roll, 1 (73)
Oat kernel bread, 1 slice (66)
Pita bread, white, 6 ½ inch loaf (57)**
Pita bread, whole-wheat, 6 ½ inch loaf, 2 oz (57)**
Dark rye, black bread, 1 slice, 1.7 oz (76)
Pizza, cheese and tomato, 2 slices, 8 oz (57)
Rye bread, 1 slice, 1 oz (65)
Whole-wheat bread**, 1 slice 1 oz (69)
Light deli (American) rye, 1 slice, (68)
Semolina bread (66)
White bread, 1 slice (70)

*Banana bread is high in carbohydrate, sugar, and fat. There are not many good and healthy choices in this group. If you are sedentary and physically inactive, this is not a place to shop. Likewise those with diabetes, heart disease, high blood pressure, Syndrome X, and the overweight.

**Whole-wheat bread is caramelized white bread and they both release their sugar at the same rate. This is also true for whole-wheat pita bread and white pita bread. On the other hand, 100% whole grain or wheat bread or 100% whole-wheat or multigrain pita bread or oat bran/whole-wheat pita (*Joseph's*) are the real things.

## CAUTIONARY PASTA

Brown rice pasta, cooked, ½ cup (81)
Durum spaghetti, cooked, ½ cup (56)
Gnocchi, cooked, 1 cup (68)
Rice vermicelli, cooked, 1 cup, 6 oz (58)
Macaroni and cheese, *Kraft*, 1 cup, 7 oz (64)
Pizza, cheese, and tomato, 2 slices, 8 oz (60)

Note: There are two major concerns with the high glycemic pastas. They are loaded with carbohydrates and also break down to sugar rapidly. For example, one cup of cooked gnocchi contains 71 grams of carbohydrate and this has the potential to raise your blood sugar by 213 mg/dl – literally over working your pancreas to exhaustion and eventual collapse if this continues over a prolonged period. This of course will lead to the development of type 2 diabetes.

Note: Pizza, cheese and tomato are among Americans leisure and convenient foods, but they are poorer choices if your goal is to burn body fat and lose weight. In fact, they may cause weight gain and fat accumulation. For example, two slices of pizza with cheese and tomato sauce contain 56 grams of high glycemic carbohydrate and 22 grams of fat. On the other hand, a vegetarian pizza without cheese is a better option. This is the kind of thought process that should be going through your head as you approach a restaurant or other convenient food providers. The frozen counterparts are often worse in terms of chemical additives and sodium, including trans fats.

## CAUTIONARY BREAKFAST CEREALS

Bran Chex, 1 oz (59)
Bran Flakes, *Post*, 2/3 cup (74)
*Cheerios*, *General Mills*, 1 cup (74)
*Cocoa Krispies*, *Kellogg's*, 1 cup (77)
*Raisin Bran*, *Kellogg's*, ¾ cup (73)
*Corn Chex*, *Nabisco*, 1cup, 1 oz (83)
Corn flakes, *Kellogg's*, 1 cup (84)
Cream of Wheat, ½ cup (71)
*Crispix*, *Kellogg's*, 1 cup (87)
Frosted flakes, *Kellogg's*, ¾ cup (55)
*Grapenuts*, *Post*, ¼ cup (67)
*Grapenuts Flakes*, *Post*, ¾ cup (80)
*Kellogg's Just Right* (59)
*Kellogg's Mini-Wheats* (whole-wheat), 1 cup (57)
*Life*, *Quaker*, ¾ cup (66)
*Muesli*, natural muesli, 2/3 cups (56)
*Puffed Wheat*, *Quaker*, 2 cups (67)
Corn bran, *Quaker Crunchy*, ¾ cup (75)
*Rice Chex*, *General Mills*, 1 ¼ cups (82)
Shredded Wheat, spoon size, 2/3 cup (58)
*Shredded Wheat*, *Post*, *1 cup* (67)
Smacks, *Kellogg's*, ¾ cup (56)
*Team Flakes*, *Nabisco*, ¾ cup (82)
*Total*, *General Mills*, ¾ (76)
*WeetaBix*, 2 biscuits (75)
*Kellogg's Smart Start*

Note: Most of the breakfast cereals in this group break down to sugar quickly raising blood glucose and insulin levels. They are quite suitable for very active people and athletes because they provide instant high energy that is needed for performance, such as running, jogging, cycling, etc. On the other hand, people who are sedentary or only slightly active should stay away from this group. Otherwise, they risk storing body fat and gaining weight. But it doesn't stop there. They also risk triggering high levels of inflammatory compounds (such as C-reactive protein and IL-6) that could lead to Syndrome X, diabetes, heart disease, premature aging, cancer and even morbid obesity. As a rule if you are sedentary or obese and you eat foods that are high glycemic, keep the portion small and do not eat them frequently. An occasional treat is not likely to cause harm.

## CAUTIONARY CEREAL GRAINS

Cornmeal, whole grain, ½ cup, (68)
Couscous*, cooked, ½ cup, 3 oz (65)
Instant rice**, cooked, 1 cup (87)
Jasmine rice, cooked, 1 cup (109)
Basmati rice, boiled, 1 cup (58)
Millet (72)
White rice, short grain, cooked, 1 cup, (70)
Rice cakes, plain, 3 cakes, 1 oz (72)
Short grain rice, white, cooked, 1 cup, (72)
Puffed rice, cooked, 1 cup (85)
Taco shells, 2 shells, 1 oz (68)
Tapioca pudding, boiled with whole milk, 1 cup, 10 oz (81)

*Couscous tastes great and makes a delicious meal, provided the portion size is kept small. Half a cup of cooked couscous contains 21 grams of carbohydrate. Eating this amount or a bit more with protein and lots of non-starchy vegetables will not cause major harm to your body. Jasmine rice is terrible! A cup of cooked jasmine rice has about 51 grams high glycemic carbohydrate. For comparison, a cup of basmati rice has about 44 grams, and brown rice and *Uncle Ben's* converted rice, about 37 grams carbohydrate that is low to moderately glycemic.

**Note that the instant rice grains are highly refined and have lost most of their nutrients and fiber. Therefore, they should be limited if you are trying to lose weight or improve your health.

Also note that the long rice grains are usually low glycemic, where as the short rice grains are high glycemic. In general, you can prevent abnormal carbohydrate over load if you treat carbohydrates and starches regardless of their sources as side dishes, instead of the foundation of your meals. You may be pleasantly surprised that when you switch to eating the UDP way, you will be satisfied eating about ½ -1 cup rice or pasta, whereas before you might have needed three or more times this amount.

## CAUTIONARY DAIRY PRODUCTS

American cheese, 1 oz (9 grams fat)
Ice cream, 10% fat, ½ cup (61)
Provolone cheese, 1 oz (8 grams fat)
Swiss cheese, 1 oz (8 grams fat)
Whole fat milk, 1 cup, 8 oz (27)
All full fat cheeses--limit

Note: In general, limit whole fat diary foods, cheese, and processed products. They are heavy in fats, especially saturated fats that raise cholesterol levels. Eating a slice of regular cheese daily in sandwiches and salads can increase health risk and also hinder weight loss due to the fact that over time the amount of fat taken becomes significant. Substitute whole fat foods, such as cheese with reduced fat varieties.

## CAUTIONARY BAKERY PRODUCTS

Danish, 1 (60)
Bagel*, 1 small, plain, 2.3 oz (72)
Banana bread**, 1 slice, 3 oz (47)
Blueberry muffin, 1, 2 oz (59)
Croissant***, medium, 1.2 oz (67)
Doughnut, 1 medium (77)
Oat bran muffin, 1, 2 oz (60)
Pancakes, 1 medium (>55)
Rice cake, plain, 3 cakes, 1 oz (82)
Waffles, plain, 4 inch square, 1 oz (76)

*One small, plain bagel has 38 grams high glycemic carbohydrate.

**Banana bread has 46 grams of high glycemic carbohydrate and 7 grams bad fat.

***A medium croissant (1.2 oz) contains 27 grams carbohydrate and 14 grams fat and 4 oz Dunkin Donut Plain Bagel has 330 cal, 68 grams carb and only 3 grams fiber..

## CAUTIONARY BEVERAGES

(Fruits and products canned in heavy syrup are often loaded with sugar).

Fruits and products canned in heavy syrup (limit)
Sportplus, 1 cup, 8 oz (73)
Gatorade, 1 cup, 8 oz (78)
Isostar, 1 cup, 8 oz (73)
Soft drink, 1 can (68)

Note: Soft drinks are a concentrated source of sugar and a major source of empty calories.

Note: Sport drinks, such as Gatorade, are suitable for athletes and people who are fairly active. In addition, Gatorade helps to normalize body electrolytes during exercise activities and also to replace lost electrolytes in situations like high fever, diarrhea, and heat exhaustion. On the other hand, soft drinks do not provide a useful medical benefit. Diet sodas are no exceptions. They have the potential to be abused and thus increasing the risk of raising the levels of free radicals in the body since they contain chemical additives – some of which cause biological actions that are not well established at present.

## CAUTIONARY COOKIES/CRACKERS

Rice cakes, plain, 3 cakes, (82)
Crispbread, 3 crackers, (81)
Graham crackers, 4 squares, (74)
Stoned wheat thins, 3 crackers, (67)
*Arrowroot*, 3 cookies, (69)
Saltines, 8 crackers, (74)
*Ryvita* tasty dark rye whole grain crispbread, 2 slices, (69)
Shortbread, 4 small cookies, (64)
*Kavli* whole grain cripbread, 4 wafers, (71)
Vanilla wafers, 7 cookies, (77)
Water cracker, *Carr's*, 3 king size crackers, (78)

Note: Cookies and crackers are a major source of sugar and fat, especially trans fat in the diet. Trans fat has being implicated in several health risks, including increase in breast cancer and raising LDL (bad) cholesterol, while at the same time lowering HDL (good) cholesterol. This trend increases the risk of stroke and heart attack especially in people who are already susceptible.

Cookies and crackers, along with sodas that often accompany them can stimulate the appetite and cause severe cravings as a result of spiking insulin levels, leading to increase in inflammation and fat storage. They are relatively deficient in vital nutrients and are packed with empty calories that crowd out nutrients that the body needs to function at optimum level.

The take home message is to use these items sparingly and to keep portions small or few. They are not the best choices for you if you are trying to lose weight or improve your health (such as increasing HDL or lowering LDL cholesterols). Take note that the whole-grain varieties are no exception either. Therefore, don't assume that a cookie or cracker meets healthy standards because it is listed as whole grain. This applies to breads also as already pointed out.

## CAUTIONARY SNACK FOODS

Chocolate bar, 1.5 oz (49)
Corn Chips, 1 oz (72)
Potato chips, 14 pieces, 1 oz (84)
Pretzels, 1 oz (83)
Dates, dried (103)
Jelly beans, 10 large, 1 oz (80)
Life Savers (70)
Mars Almond Bar, 1.8 oz (65)
Mars M&Ms Chocolate Candies peanut, 1.7 oz package (33)
Popcorn, light, microwave, 2 cups popped (55)
Kudos Granola bars (whole grain), 1bar (62)

Note: This group also contains highly refined carbohydrates and simple sugars that can stimulate your appetite as well as cause cravings and binges. Most are also high in fats, including trans fat.

Note: Two of the most consumed forms of corn in America are popcorn and corn flakes and the latter are widely used in breakfast cereals. However, a treat of plain light, microwave popcorn (2 cups popped has about 12 grams of carbohydrate) with or without a teaspoon of olive oil or soft margarine should cause no real harm if eaten occasionally. But a serving of 6 cups (36 grams carbohydrate) with lots of butter could be a health hazard if eaten frequently.

Note: Corn chips and potato chips should be limited. For example, corn chips: (1 oz chips has 16 grams carbohydrate and 10 grams bad fat). Similarly, 14 plain potato chips or 1 oz has 15 grams carbohydrate and 11 grams bad fat.

These snack foods are also used to accompany sandwiches and hamburger buns at lunch and you can appreciate the total amount of fat consumed over time as one eats these types of snacks on a regular basis. On a positive note, you can bake potato wedges with the skin using of course the types of potatoes that do not convert to sugar rapidly, such as sweet potato and new potato.

Note: Dark chocolate (> 70% cacao) is a good treat whereas milk chocolate can induce craving. Adding a little bit of Splenda or stevia with 1-2 tbsp 2% whole milk can transform dark chocolate into a sweet tasting chocolate that may even satisfy the palate of most sweet seekers.

## Keeping Blood Sugar and Insulin Down Can Boost Your Metabolism

Eating the right variety of foods, decreasing stress, and maintaining a regular physical activity level in line with your energy needs can help you to lose weight and keep it off for good with the added benefit of improving your overall heath.

You can increase your chances of succeeding by applying simple techniques and tricks that can help your body burn fat more efficiently. Even a sluggish metabolism can benefit from a boost and here is how you do it:

- Have vegetable soup, broth, or a glass of water with lemon or apple cider vinegar before each meal.
- Add vinegar or lemon juice to fruits and vegetables.
- Eat abundant non-starchy leafy vegetables (template) before lunch and dinner. Better yet, turn your vegetables into tasty and delicious soups.
- Learn better and simple methods for preparing foods that are satisfying and low in calories.
- Tailor your calories and carbohydrate consumption to your activity level (see Chapters 14 and 15).
- Eat high fiber whole fruits with skin over fruit juices for snacks.
- Include legumes frequently (½ cup cooked beans, peas, lentils, or soy).
- Eat smaller portion sizes of carbohydrates and starches even if they are low glycemic (*Meaning treat carbohydrates as a side dish; just as the Asians do*).
- Eat carbohydrates with lean proteins and good fats.
- Eat a variety of whole foods with high fiber to counteract a meal's high glycemic load.
- Use vinegar and lemon juice dressing. Limit full fat commercial dressings.
- Eat brown rice, wild rice, *Uncle Ben's* Converted rice, or barley instead of short grain white rice and instant rice. Keep portions small (½ -1 cup *side dish*).
- Choose whole-wheat or protein enriched pasta over refined white pasta. Keep portions small, about ½ -1 cup (*side dish*).
- Substitute sweet potatoes and new potatoes for white potatoes. Eat a small portion (*side dish*) with skin.
- Add oat bran, ground flaxseeds, and wheat germ to cereals and yogurt to increase fiber and nutrients.
- Choose high fiber breakfast cereals made with bran, barley, and oats. Limit highly processed cereals, such as corn flakes and puffed wheat. Decrease the portion recommended on the label if you are not active and stay within the serving size if you are. Take the time to measure out the correct portion size.
- Eat high fiber multigrain breads such as 100% whole-grain or 100% whole-wheat made with whole seeds, oats or oat bran.
- Treat starchy vegetables and fruits as sources of carbohydrate and energy and take into account their contribution to your daily meals (*side dish*).
- Limit sugary soft drinks and highly processed foods.
- Eat fewer carbohydrates, fats, and calories at dinner.
- To reduce fat: roast, broil, bake, sauté, or grill.

## To Eat or Not to Eat?

### The Glycemic Load (GL)

The glycemic index (GI) tells us how quickly a particular carbohydrate food turns into blood sugar (glucose) but it really doesn't tell us much about the carbohydrate content. We need to know both in order to make appropriate food choices that are healthy for us. One way to do this is to take into consideration a food's GI as well as the amount of carbohydrate content per serving (this is referred to as the glycemic load or GL). For example, a bagel has a GI of 72 and a GL of 25. A GL of 10 or less is considered low and favorable. On the other hand, a baked potato has a GI of 93 and a GL of 26, whereas premium ice cream has a GI of 61 and a GL of 4. Does this mean ice cream is healthier for you than potatoes? I think not. The fact is that potatoes have valuable nutrients, such as potassium, magnesium, phosphorous, and fiber, whereas, ice cream offers very little besides calcium.

The same question can be asked of other foods whose GI is high but their GL appears to be in the low to medium range. These foods include graham crackers, shortbread, vanilla wafers, potato chips, pretzels, apple pie, and Coca Cola (to name just a few). With few exceptions, most of these are high in sugar and artery-clogging trans fats. It is conceivable from these examples that even the glycemic load is not perfect.

The Glycemic load does not tell you the amount of fat in a food or its fat-storage capacity. Therefore, it can be misleading. For example, the glycemic load of peanuts and cashew nuts is 1 and 2, respectively, even though these are loaded with fat. The fat-storage potential of a food is important and can help us to select foods that are non- fattening and low in calories. It would be a major breakthrough to have a system that addresses the qualitative aspect of both carbohydrates and fats in foods, since these are key players in energy production and fat storage.

### Some Useful Application of the Glycemic Load

The GL appears to work better with natural starches and sugars and less with foods that are highly refined, processed, or contains high fat. My best advice is use common sense. Check food labels for carbohydrate, sugar, and fat content. Limit refined foods regardless of their GI or GL.

Foods, such as beets, cooked carrots, watermelon, pumpkin, squash, and cantaloupe have a moderate to high glycemic index, but their carbohydrate content is very small. Therefore, if you eat only a small amount, it will probably have minimal negative effects. For example, watermelon (GI of 70) has 10 grams of carbohydrates in a 1 cup serving; cantaloupe (GI of 65) has 7 grams of carbohydrates in a ½ cup serving; beets have 6 grams carbohydrates in a ½ cup and cooked carrots (GI of 85) have 6 grams carbohydrates in a ½ cup serving.

For watermelon or cooked carrots to have a serious impact on your blood sugar, you will probably have to eat a substantial amount (over a pound or so). By comparison, a medium banana has a GI of 55-65 and a carbohydrate content of about 32 grams. Eating a banana (overripe banana) will have a much more powerful glycemic response than any of the other foods considered. Others that you have to be aware of are pineapple, prunes, papaya, pear, mango, fresh kernel corn, and canned corn – all can induce a strong insulin response just like bananas. On the other hand, corn fresh on the cob may induce a weak insulin response.

It is reasonable to assume that, if you eat only a small amount of any carbohydrate food with a high glycemic index, but whose carbohydrate content is low (15 grams or less per serving), the chance is that the blood sugar rise will not be as strong. It is important to know that, as with anything else, there are exceptions to the rule. This argument may not hold true for some carbohydrates such as, honey, fructose, *Gatorade*, and beer.

For example, beer has a GI of 110 and a carbohydrate content of 5 grams per serving. The problem with beer, alcoholic drinks, and other highly refined foods is their lack of nutrients, especially B-vitamins, which are important in the metabolism of carbohydrates. The depletion of these vitamins can lead to a sluggish metabolism and other serious medical conditions. In addition, beer and other alcoholic drinks contain lots of calories. The low carbohydrate beers may have as low as 3-6 grams of carbohydrate, but as many as 97 calories per twelve ounce serving. Drinking three to four of these can easily add up to the calories of an entire meal. Worst of all, these are non-nutritious calories that simply occupy space and crowd out vital nutrients.

Besides alcohol, you should also limit carbohydrate foods with low starch or sugar content that are highly refined or processed (such as hamburger buns, popcorn, soft-drinks, candy, chocolate, or ice cream), regardless of their glycemic index or glycemic load. However, it is perfectly all right to occasionally have these foods in small portions as long as there are other foods to help neutralize their effect – lemon juice, vinegar, proteins, and/or healthy fats. Dark chocolate is a good treat if you add Splenda or Stevia to enhance taste (smoothies and sorbets).

A short list of selected foods with their glycemic index and glycemic load is given below for comparison. It is accepted that foods with glycemic loads below 10 or less will not induce a strong insulin response but, as you have seen, that is not always the case. You can find a complete list at the University of Sydney website, Glycemicndex.com or in Dr. Willet's book, *Eat, Drink, and Be Happy*.

| | |
|---|---|
| All-Bran cereal (9) | Air-popped popcorn (4) |
| Banana, overripe (12) | Apples (6) |
| Banana, under-ripe (6) | Basmati rice, boiled (22) |
| Cornflakes (21) | Brown rice, boiled (18) |
| Dates, dried (42) | Carrots (10) |
| Doughnut (17) | Cassava, boiled (12) |
| Jasmine rice, boiled (46) | French fries (22) |
| Kidney beans, boiled (7) | Pancake (39) |
| Raisins (28) | Peanuts (1) |
| Saltines (25) | Potato, baked (26) |
| Spaghetti, white, boiled 10-15 min (18) | Sweet potatoes (17) |
| Spaghetti, whole-wheat, al dente (14) | White rice, boiled (23) |

## Carbohydrate Foods Used to Treat Diabetic Crisis

The standard of care when your blood sugar drops too low is to eat refined or high glycemic carbohydrates that will cause an instant rise in blood sugar. A brief review of some of the foods that physicians recommend for diabetics when their blood sugar drops too low (hypoglycemia) will help a great deal to shed light about the seriousness of overindulging on refined carbohydrates and high glycemic foods. Some are even common household names like oranges and grapes.

Doctors usually recommend sugar, orange juice, corn syrup, regular soda, and honey when blood sugar drops to dangerous levels. Does it surprise you that their carbohydrate content is only about 10-15 grams per serving? Yet, they can still raise your blood sugar by 30-45 points very quickly. For example, a glass of orange juice (8 oz) can rapidly raise blood sugar by 90 points.

This is the reason you should not have your breakfast cereal with toast and follow it with orange juice or a banana – carbohydrate overload could spike insulin levels. The second point is to have the fruits, such as orange with proteins or fats to help slow down their digestion – even a small amount can trigger a strong insulin response. A much more comprehensive list of foods used to treat diabetic crisis is given below.

You will agree with me that while these foods are appropriate for saving lives (such as during a life-threatening diabetic crisis), they are not the best choices for the average person who is physically inactive (most people are physically inactive!). Foods, such as sodas, sweetened fruit juices, honey, and ice cream are concentrated sources of energy that usually deliver more sugar and calories than our body can handle.

| **Foods Used to Treat Diabetic Crisis (hypoglycemia)** | |
|---|---|
| 2-5 glucose tablets | 6 Jellybeans |
| 5-7 Lifesavers | 4 oz orange juice |
| 6-8 oz skim or 1% milk | 10 Gumdrops |
| 2 Tbsp raisins | ½ can regular soda |
| 2 tsp sugar | 2 tsp honey |
| 2 tsp corn syrup | 1 tube cake mate decorator gel |

## Why Are Low Carbohydrate Diets Dangerous?

### Low-Carbohydrate Diets

It is not unusual these days to have a relative or friend on extremely low carbohydrate diets. These people are driven by the need to lose weight instantly and have therefore adopted extreme measures to eliminate all carbohydrates from their diet, such as bread, pasta, rice, fruits, and potatoes. This is not a practice that I recommend by any means.

The basic function of glucose is to provide fuel to the brain and muscle cells. We saw in previous chapters that when carbohydrate food is eaten, insulin helps the blood sugar to penetrate the muscles and cells, assuring the functioning of all organs. To ensure a steady supply of blood glucose, a small amount is stored as glycogen in the liver and muscles. The bulk is stored as fat if it is not immediately used up. If too little carbohydrate is consumed, the amount of glucose reserved as glycogen is small. Therefore, it is quickly depleted when needed (between meals or during physical activity) causing the blood sugar level to fall to abnormally low levels. This is called hypoglycemia and it is an abnormal condition that can literally put your body in a state of shock.

## Why Maryann Fainted on a Low-Carb Diet

Maryann, a 52-year-old, successful, self-employed businesswoman struggled with weight all her life. She had tried every diet program imaginable. She had struggled to lose 60 pounds over a twelve-month period dieting and she still had about 80 pounds to lose when I met her. She did it by eliminating bread, potatoes, pasta, and other starches and sugars. She came to see me because she had reached a plateau and saw no progress in six months. She was also worried about her health.

Maryann's medical and social history was a textbook case: she had high blood pressure, arthritis, thyroid disease, insomnia, frequent headaches, fatigue, anxiety, irritability, constipation, and she often craved sweets and carbohydrates. She had recently fainted at work and in another episode she was at home. She had a thorough medical workup at a prestigious medical institution that offered no explanations as to why she had fainted. But, in her mind, she blamed it on extreme stress and a lack of sleep and proper rest.

Maryann had faithfully followed a low carb diet that omitted most carbohydrates, including whole grains. She ate a very high protein, high fat, and low carbohydrate diet daily. It was also high in calories (about 2,300-2,500), cholesterol and fat (1,240 mg cholesterol, 96 grams total fat and 27 grams saturated fat). Her meals had very little fiber, including the all important soluble fiber.

Maryann's symptoms were quite predictable and are the consequences of inadequate carbohydrates and fiber in the diet. The symptoms can range from mild to life-threatening conditions: headaches, fatigue, weakness, irritability, anxiety, nervousness, depression, sweating, aggressiveness, lack of concentration, nausea, insomnia, dizziness, fainting, and even death.

You might have had similar experiences, even though they may not be as life-threatening as those suffered by Maryann. It could happen to you if you skipped meals or followed a diet program that was deficient in good carbohydrates. It could also happen to you if you took too much insulin.

## Don't Be Afraid to Eat Carbohydrates

Carbohydrates are essential for life. They are a powerful energy source that keeps our brain focused, sharpens our cognitive skills, and keeps our energy level high. The key is to balance the carbohydrates you eat with your level of physical activity because these are energy foods. Also, eat mostly whole-grains that are rich in fiber, antioxidants, and phytonutrients. Whole-grains, low glycemic fruits and legumes can help to stabilize blood sugar and prevent hypoglycemia. This will prevent an overload of blood sugar that can trigger an excessive insulin release and hypoglycemia.

## With Carbohydrates, Too High Is Just as Dangerous

### High-Carbohydrate Diets May Not Be Healthy

Low blood sugar (hypoglycemia) can also occur when too much insulin is released following a high carbohydrate meal consisting of huge amounts of refined or high glycemic carbohydrates. This could happen even with good carbohydrates.

You can probably recall eating a big meal loaded with carbohydrates (white bread, potatoes, bagel, rice, pasta, or corn, etc.) and, less than 3 hours later you, suddenly felt lethargic and hungry again. If you had checked your blood sugar then, as most diabetics do so often, it would probably have showed a low blood sugar (hypoglycemia).

Surprisingly, some people whose blood sugar is chronically elevated may even have symptoms at a relatively "normal" range of blood sugar. On the other hand, there are diabetics who can tolerate chronically low blood sugars because they have developed some adaptive mechanism over time.

It usually takes no time for your blood sugar level to rise rapidly when you eat a diet that is high in refined or high glycemic carbohydrates like white bread, bagels, pizza, or white pasta. This can cause a rush of energy that is only short lived.

Elevated levels of blood sugar can trigger the release of excessive amounts of insulin, which, in turn, quickly clears the sugar from the bloodstream. Insulin prevents the toxic accumulation of glucose but it may also cause the blood glucose level to drop too low. The net result is a situation that is very similar to those eating a very low carbohydrate diet that may not be in line with their level of activity.

Eating the wrong carbohydrates can also trigger your appetite and force you to eat when you may not even be hungry. In a worst case scenario, you might find yourself trapped in a vicious cycle of high energy followed by sudden low energy that can lead to intense cravings, constant hunger, depression, and even behavior that is typical of addicts.

Interestingly, alcohol can cause similar high and low cycles. Remember, alcohol is a highly refined carbohydrate that is deficient in nutrients and fiber just like white flour and white bread. An excessive intake of alcohol will initially give you the feeling of a rapid rise in energy and mood only to be followed shortly by a drop in energy and feeling of irritability as the blood alcohol and sugar levels drop. Often, the usual response is to have another drink in an attempt to restore energy quickly.

*For some people, alcohol is a powerful drug that simply provides temporary relief. Refined carbohydrates and simple sugars (such as sodas, sweetened juices, white bread, and candies) may provide the same function – except the consumer may not realize it. Both behaviors are due largely to chronically abnormal blood sugar levels and the depletion of B-vitamins.*

## Refined and Sugary Foods Can Sabotage Your Best Efforts

In the next few paragraphs, I will describe the experience of one my favorite patients and I hope you will learn from it. Shirley is a pleasant, 63-year old woman who lost control at a birthday party. She went to the party hungry and soon she was indulging in cookies, chocolate, cake, and sugary foods (including alcohol). When she returned home and realized what she had done, she felt depressed and disappointed with herself. But that was not her only problem.

When she got on the scale in the office, she was even more depressed. Her body fat percentage had increased by three percent in a single week. Interestingly, she maintained the same weight she had the previous week. How could this happen?

The simple explanation is that four pounds of muscle mass was lost and replaced by an equal amount of fat. Therefore, the net weight loss was zero. But it wasn't good because her progress was going in a negative direction. She had lost muscle instead of fat. The lesson learned is that it is easy to shift the balance between burning body fat and storing it, especially when alcohol is involved. Worst of all, this is done at the expense of muscle tissue.

One important thing that Shirley could have done to salvage the situation after binging on simple sugars and alcohol was to make sure she exercised twice as hard and ate healthy. But she didn't during that entire week because she was angry with herself. Another important fact that you should be aware off is that, after a high carbohydrate meal, especially if it is highly refined, it could take several days of vigorous exercise to burn it off.

Perhaps this type of behavior is the most common reason why most people drop out of weight loss programs. Remember that your progress and hard work could be wiped out in just a single weekend of binges, especially if alcohol was also involved.

Luckily for Shirley, she regrouped and was back on track the following week (making healthy food choices and exercising). There were other parties and celebrations that she afterwards attended, but she was in control and did not give in to the temptations of over-indulgence in bad foods. You will be challenged too and I hope you will do the right thing.

## Too Many Carbohydrates Linked to Breast Cancer

Recent studies by Dr. Walter Willet and colleagues in Mexico linked eating too many carbohydrates (corn, corn products, bread, and soft drinks) to breast cancer. The good news is that eating whole grain and high fiber carbohydrates that are minimally processed in the right amount that is in line with our level of physical activity may, in fact, help our body fight off cancer. As you already know, highly refined carbohydrates raise blood sugar and insulin levels rapidly, causing the formation of free radicals that trigger inflammation. They also appear to stimulate cells to divide rapidly and raise levels of estrogen in the bloodstream, which may promote breast cancer growth. The risk for cancer is even greater when the source of fat is meats, processed foods and dairy products that are heavy in saturated fat and trans fat.

The amount of carbohydrates that you should eat per meal should depend entirely upon your level of physical activity and must be adjusted on a meal-to-meal basis. For example, if you are sedentary, you should eat mostly low-energy carbohydrates that are high in fiber (minimally processed whole grains) and the amount you eat should reflect your current activity level. You can better appreciate this process if you think of what you normally do with your checking account, savings account, or credit cards. Some of us are poor money managers. Nevertheless, we can all agree that we fair well when we cut our budget down to what we can afford to pay for without putting us into a negative balance. We can also afford to buy more when the financial situation is good and less so when the reverse is true.

The high fiber, low glycemic carbohydrates are burned slowly in a very efficient process that delivers just the right amount of blood sugar that may not flood our body. This is why they are perfectly suitable for people who are not burning adequate calories and carbohydrates via exercise.

A sedentary person, an obese person or someone with major health problems who repeatedly eats high-energy carbohydrates like white potatoes and refined pizza as their staple is risking his or her health in a very real way. Eating these types of foods in large amounts, in combination with high fat foods (including fried foods) can cause fattening and inflammation – two of the greatest enemies against weight loss and optimum health.

In general, people who are moderately active (such as those burning around 500 or more calories a day during physical activity or manual labor) can afford to eat high-energy carbohydrate meals and get away with it. This is because their muscle is active enough to burn up the carbohydrates and calories before they get converted into fat.

The UDP program urges you to limit the frequent use of high-energy carbohydrates that drain energy, trigger inflammation, and cause fat storage if you are sedentary and at risk for major health problems. Instead, I encourage you to eat low-energy, high fiber carbohydrates that promote gradual but sustainable energy between meals. They are satisfying and can help to promote healthy weight loss and well-being.

Carbohydrates should be an important part of our daily meals and snacks, but choosing the right types of carbohydrate that are in line with our body metabolism is even more important. As already pointed out, the whole-grains and minimally refined types are more suitable for you if you are sedentary or barely moving. They may even help to boost your metabolism and help burn body fat provided you stay within the range your body can tolerate (such as 1-2 servings or 15-35 grams of carbohydrates per meal for sedentary individuals). Later in this book, I will show how you can arrive at the carbohydrate range or serving that is right for your activity level.

## Simple Sugars Cause Inflammation

### Too Much Sugar Is Bad for Your Health

Most sugars we use are pure chemical products that are problematic because of the proportion of it that is hidden in foods, such as preservatives, beverages, snacks, desserts, dressings, and condiments. The irony is that the body needs glucose as a primary source of energy but not sugar (sugar is a combination of glucose and fructose). Sugar (white, brown, powdered, and liquid sugar) along with other carbohydrates and starches found in grains, fruits, beans, honey, and unrefined foods are converted to glucose. That is why it is so easy to overload on glucose. For example, an 8 oz glass of grape juice or 1 cup of yogurt may contain 44 grams of sugar; the equivalent of about 3 slices of bread or 11 teaspoons of sugar. Juices served in restaurants may even contain more sugar. Recently, *McDonald's* introduced a healthy *Fruit and Walnut Salad* but it has 44 grams of carbohydrate and 32 grams of sugar (the equivalent of about 8 teaspoons of sugar). In addition, the salad has 13 grams fat and it is not even the main meal.

A small amount of sugar (about 1-2 tsp or 10 grams or less per serving) is probably not bad for your health. Excessive sugar consumption causes elevation of insulin and triglycerides – factors that can increase the risk of heart disease. *What is most frightening is the rampant use of sugar among children, young adults, and adults who have developed a tolerance for this chemical.*

Secondary effects of excessive sugar consumption include hypoglycemia, slow metabolism, and digestive problems. Just like other refined carbohydrates, too much sugar in the diet leads to B-vitamin deficiency, especially vitamin B1. The B-vitamins are needed to absorb and digest carbohydrates. A deficiency of B-vitamins can cause fatigue, muscle ache, depression, poor concentration, and loss of memory and perception.

## Sugar Causes More Than Dental and Oral Diseases

Excessive consumption of sugar has also been linked to dental and oral diseases, which are widespread in westernized countries today. For example, periodontal disease (gum disease) involves inflammation caused by plaque along the gum line and is now the second leading cause of heart disease (behind smoking). When plaque invades under the gum, the immune system attacks the plaque and other tissues leading to the erosion of the jawbone and deep cavities in the gum. The levels of C-reactive protein (CRP) increase substantially and may explain why people with severe gum disease tend to have heart disease.

Sugar causes inflammation (as has been discussed previously). To refresh your memory, high levels of blood sugar create free radicals that oxidize fats, particularly LDL (bad) cholesterol. As you know, the oxidation of LDL causes plaque formation in the arteries. The body interprets plaque deposits as an injury to the blood vessel walls. This causes white cells or inflammatory cells to attack the plaque, resulting in blood clots and heart attacks. This is why a diet that is high in refined carbohydrates or simple sugars can increase your risk for heart disease, especially if you are sedentary, smoke, or have high blood pressure or diabetes. People with diabetes have a higher risk of dying from heart attacks – probably due to their high blood sugar, which causes LDL to oxidize.

It is best to use granulated or cubed sugar cautiously, especially if you are at risk (sedentary, obesity, diabetes, heart disease, arthritis, etc.). Also limit foods high in concentrated sugar and their products (they contain calories but no nutrients), such as honey, sweetened juices, sodas, sweets, desserts, and other refined carbohydrates. To do this, you will need to check food labels carefully for added sugars, such as corn syrup, fructose, maltose, or dextrose. You can also replace granulated sugar with sugar substitutes, such as Splenda and Stevia.

## Sugar Substitutes

### Are They Safe?

There are many sugar substitutes on the market today but only two (Splenda and Stevia) stand above the rest. Splenda (also called Sucralose) is about 600 times sweeter than table sugar and is used in beverages, fruit juices, chewing gum, baked goods, and desserts. It is made from table sugar and tastes just like it. However, it does not significantly affect blood sugar or insulin levels and it does not add significant calories because it is not digested in the body. It is suitable for people with diabetes.

Stevia is a natural sweetener that is about 200-300 times sweeter than table sugar and has no calories. It is derived from a South American shrub and the natives have used it for hundreds of years without any known side effects. It, too, is suitable for diabetics and does not cause cavities in teeth. Stevia is popular in Japan but, in the United States, the FDA has not approved its use as a food additive yet. It can be found in most supermarkets and health food stores.

### Do Not Abuse

Be careful not to get addicted or to abuse these products. Because they are presumed safe, some people may be tempted to use a large quantity of Splenda or Stevia – and this is a mistake. A single packet at a time is usually sufficient. The data on long-term usage is not yet available. When margarine was first introduced to the public, no one suspected that trans fat could be so harmful to the body. Trans fat or partially hydrogenated oils from vegetable oils were made by simply moving the hydrogen molecule from the "cis" position to the " trans" position: a simple structural change that resulted in major health risk. No body knows for sure that a similar thing will happen with splenda following structural modification. Only time will tell. On the other hand, sugar or sucrose is the natural sugar from cane sugar and it is relatively safe in small amounts, such as 1-2 tsp (4-8 grams) per serving.

### Are Sugar Alcohols Safe?

Sugar alcohols are mentioned here briefly because you will see them listed in many low-carb products, such as protein bars and yogurts. They are fake sugars that include mannitol, maltose, sorbitol, lactitol, and Hydrolysed Starch Hydrolysates (HSH). They provide fewer calories and carbs than sugar and are not completely absorbed in the intestine. As a result, they produce a smaller rise in blood sugar and insulin. But so does fructose, which was once thought to be safe.

Most experts recommend using sugar alcohol with caution. They have a bad reputation of holding onto water and causing gas, bloating, and diarrhea. Overeating these products can trigger unpleasant symptoms and side effects. Some people may even experience a blood sugar rush from eating just a small amount. For example, protein bars sweetened with sugar alcohol may have lower carb grams, as opposed to regular bars, but they may trigger sweet cravings and carb binges.

# Chapter 10

# Fruits, Vegetables, and Your Weight

## Fruits Contain Carbohydrates and Sugar Too

In previous chapters, I emphasized the indispensable contribution of fruits to our health as sources of antioxidants and phytonutrients. Fruits are extremely important in our diet – but there is something important you must know before you start loading up or developing your template. Fruits contain carbohydrates, such as starch, glucose, sucrose (sugar), and fructose. They are also high in fiber, which helps to decrease the absorption of these sugars. As a result, they are not easily stored as fats in the body – with few exceptions (e.g. overripe bananas, raisins, plantains, tropical fruits, etc.).

Unfortunately, most of us have access to a wide variety of fruits, but we often choose the ones that are sweet (such as overripe bananas and sweet oranges). Without question, the most important message to take home from this chapter is that fruits are a major source of carbohydrates and sugar (natural sugar) that should be accounted for in your overall meal plan. Otherwise, you could easily overload on carbohydrates without realizing it. Serving sizes and equivalent calories are listed below:

| **FRUITS** | |
|---|---|
| **(60 calories in one serving)** | |
| **Fruit** | **Amount** |
| Apple | 1 small |
| Apricot, fresh | 4 whole |
| Banana | 1 small or ½ large |
| Blueberries | 3/4 cup |
| Cantaloupe | 1 cup cubed |
| Cherries | 1 cup |
| Dates | 3 |
| Grapefruit | 1 small or ½ large |
| Grapes | ½ cup or 10 |
| Honeydew Melon | 1 cup cubed |
| Kiwi | 1 large |
| Mango | ½ cup diced |

| | |
|---|---|
| Mixed Fruit | ½ cup |
| Nectarine | 1 |
| Orange | 1 medium |
| Orange Juice | ½ cup |
| Peach | 1 large |
| Pineapple | ½ cup cubed |
| Pear | 1 small |
| Plums | 2 |
| Prunes | 3 |
| Raisins | 2 tablespoons |
| Raspberries | 1 cup |
| Strawberries | 1 ½ cups whole |
| Tangerine | 1 |

The seriousness of underestimating the impact of fruits as contributors of carbohydrates came as a total surprise to me during a casual conversation with a physician friend. She honestly confessed, "I never thought about fruits and carbohydrates in the same sense. I always thought fruits were one thing and carbohydrates were another. When I think about carbohydrates, I think of bread, potatoes, pasta, and rice."

Unfortunately, many people share this view and, as a result, fruits are overlooked in the overall meal plan more often than not. As part of a healthy meal plan, you should strive to eat at least two fruits a day (they are good snack items). When eating fruits, be sure to include some source of protein, such as low-fat cheese like mozzarella string cheese, low-fat cottage cheese, egg whites, soy protein powder, low-fat peanut butter, nuts (a few walnuts, almonds, macadamias, peanuts, soy nuts, or hazelnuts), low-fat low-sugar yogurt, plain yogurt, a slice of grilled chicken, turkey, or smoked salmon. This will help to delay digestion and absorption of the fruit's sugar. Otherwise, within a few hours, you will be hungry and craving sugary foods.

### Limit Dried Fruits

Dried fruits are a concentrated source of sugar and fructose and should not replace fresh fruits. Water-packed canned fruits or light syrup are favored to those in heavy syrup, which contains large amounts of sugar or sweeteners like fructose. Whenever possible, eat the skin of the fruit because it is the richest part of the fruit in terms of fiber, nutrients, and vitamins. Eating the fruit with its skin can even help to lower the glycemic index and diminishes the absorption of sugars which will help burn body fat.

Below, I have included a list of fruits that you can enjoy. With few exceptions, their carbohydrates break down slowly, releasing glucose gradually. Aim for 1-2 fruits a day. They can easily be incorporated into your daily meal plan as snack items.

| FRUITS TO ENJOY FREQUENTLY | |
|---|---|
| Apples | Kiwi |
| Applesauce, unsweetened | Lemon/lime |
| Apricots, fresh | Oranges |
| Avocado | Peaches |
| Blackberries | Peaches/canned Pear/canned |
| Blueberries | Pears |
| Cherries | Plums |
| Figs, fresh | Raspberries |
| Fruit Cocktail/water | Strawberries |
| Fruit Cocktail/light syrup | Tangerine |
| Grapefruit | Tomatoes |
| Grapes | Guava |
| **Fruits to Enjoy Occasionally** | |
| Banana (not overripe) | Papaya |
| Cantaloupe | Pineapple, fresh chunk |
| Mango | Pineapple, waterpacked / Watermelon |
| Note: All these fruits release their sugar quickly and so do overripe bananas. | |
| **Cautionary Fruits** | |
| Dates, dried | Raisins |
| Dried Fruits | Raspberries, frozen/sweetened |
| Fruits packed in syrup | Strawberries, frozen/sweetened |
| Plantains | Very Ripe Bananas |

## Fruit Juices Are a Concentrated Source of Sugar and Fructose

### Be Careful With Juices

Fruit juices, including freshly squeezed juices, are not as good for the body as fresh fruits simply because they lack fiber. Drinking fruit juice, with the exception of lemon or lime juice, may even elevate your blood sugar levels. Commercial fruit juices, even those without added sugar, are lower in vitamins and fiber than fresh fruit juices. Most contain large amounts of fructose corn syrup, preservatives, artificial flavors, and colorings.

Unsweetened fruit juices are also a concentrated source of sugar that can hinder your weight loss progress, especially during the early phase. My opinion is to limit fruit juices (both sweetened or unsweetened) unless the carbohydrate or sugar content is low (below 10 grams per 8 oz); otherwise, it is very easy to overload on sugar. You saw previously that one-gram of carbohydrate will raise blood sugar by 3 mg/dl or 3 points. Thus an 8 oz orange juice containing 22 grams of carbohydrates will raise your blood sugar by (22 x 3) 66 mg/dl and an 8 oz grape juice will raise blood sugar by (44 x 3) 132 mg/dl.

Can you imagine the metabolic effects? Without proper physical activity, most of this energy will be stored as fat. However, you can overcome this problem by paying close attention to the carbohydrate and sugar content of the foods you eat. A healthy range of blood sugar is between 70 to 130 mg/dl. When your blood sugar drops below 70 mg/dl, you may begin to sweat and feel very anxious and agitated. In contrast, when your blood sugar shoots above 130 and higher for a long period of time, you might become restless, nervous, thirsty, and urinate frequently. Some people may even experience visual problems. Furthermore, it may increase risk of diabetes and heart disease.

You should not be afraid to eat fruits as long as you are eating them according to your level of physical activity and are accounting for them in your total meal plan. And remember, the whole fruit with the skin is a better choice than the juice.

That being said, I do recommend tomato juice and V-8 juice (low sodium) for your pantry. They are a better choice than sodas and fruit juices. Apple juice, grape juice, and orange juice all have a low glycemic index, but they are often high in sugar. Sugar breaks down to fructose and glucose. The more sugar there is in a juice, the more fructose – a toxic substance that is hazardous to health. Sports drinks like *Gatorade, Isostar,* and *Sportsplus* are high glycemic and designed to enhance athletic performance. Other options like sport shakes are a health hazard for physically inactive people. They may contain about 55-63 grams of sugar in a serving of eleven ounces (see other examples below).

**BEVERAGES**

| **Juice** | **Carbs/Sugar (Grams)** |
|---|---|
| Apple Juice (1 cup) | 29.5 |
| Apricot Nectar (1 cup) | 36.6 |
| Coke (12 fluid oz) | 39.0 |
| Cranapple (1 cup) | 41.0 |
| Cranberry Juice Cocktail (1 cup) | 41.7 |
| Cran-Cherry Juice (1 cup) | 39.0 |
| Hawaiian Fruit Punch (1 cup) | 30.0 |
| Gatorade, most flavors (1 cup) | 14.0 |
| Grapefruit Juice (1 cup) | 23.0 |
| Grape Juice (1 cup) | 42.0 |
| Lemon juice (1 tbsp) | 1.0 |
| Lemonade (1 cup) | 27.0 |

| | |
|---|---|
| Lime Juice (1 tbsp) | 1.0 |
| Mountain Dew (12 fluid oz) | 46.0 |
| Orange Minute Maid (12 fluid oz) | 47.0 |
| Orange *Slice* (12 fluid oz) | 51.0 |
| Orange Juice (1 cup) | 26.0 |
| Peach Nectar (1 cup) | 36.0 |
| Pear Nectar (1 cup) | 38.0 |
| Pineapple Juice (1 cup) | 34.0 |
| Prune Juice (1 cup) | 48.6 |
| Tea, Iced: | |
| Lipton (12 fluid oz) | 33.0 |
| Nestea (12 fluid oz) | 33.0 |
| Snapple (1 cup) | 25.0 |
| Fruit Flavored Teas (1 cup) | 26.0 |
| Tangerine Juice (1 cup) | 29.9 |
| Tomato Juice (1 cup) | 10.4 |
| V-8 (1 cup) | 10.0 |

## The Case Against Fructose (Fruit Sugar)

Fructose (also known as natural sugar) is a type of simple sugar found in fruits that does not elevate blood glucose levels like sugar. In spite of that, fructose poses a health hazard even more dangerous than sugar. It increases blood levels of cholesterol and triglycerides far more than sugar. As we already know, increased blood levels of sugar and triglycerides are associated with an increased risk of heart attack and stroke. This effect is even more pronounced in people who eat a diet that is high in saturated fat and cholesterol. Fructose is also implicated in contributing to Syndrome X and diabetes.

### Worse Than Sugar

For years, fructose has been thought to be a safe sugar for diabetics because it does not trigger a rapid rise in blood sugar. However, in January 2002 the American Diabetic Association stopped recommending fructose other than that which occurs naturally in fruits.

Since the 1970's food manufacturers have been using sugar from corn to make food sweeteners, which go under the names fructose, cornstarch, corn syrup, dextrose, dextrine, or high fructose corn syrup because it is much less expensive to produce. These corn sweeteners are nothing but a form of highly processed sugar that is used in everything – bread, pasta sauces, bacon, beer, breakfast cereals, ice cream, processed foods, and beverages. It is even used in health food products like protein energy bars, natural sodas, frozen desserts, jams, jellies, fat-free, low-fat, and sugar-free foods.

As with all refined foods, a small amount of fructose will probably not hurt you. But the problem is fructose in fruit juices and other products is like trans fat in cookies and processed foods. Most fructose comes "hidden" in processed foods, low-fat foods and sugar-free foods that you may not suspect. Fructose also sneaks into the diet as sucrose or table sugar, which breaks down during digestion into equal parts of glucose and fructose.

### Fructose in Fruits

Fructose is also found in fresh fruits. But you have nothing to worry about if you eat fresh fruit because fructose accounts for only a small percentage of the total weight of most fresh fruits. For example, fructose accounts for about only 5 to 8 percent of the weight of grapes, apples, bananas, pears and cherries. It only accounts for 2 to 3 percent of the weight of strawberries, blueberries, blackberries, grapefruits, and oranges. By comparison, honey contains 40 percent fructose.

Dried fruits and fruit juices are more concentrated sources of fructose than fresh fruits and should be restricted, particularly if you are at risk or have a health issue (such as Syndrome X, diabetes, heart disease, high cholesterol, high triglycerides, and other chronic degenerative diseases, even obesity). In general, processed foods are a greater health hazard than natural foods because their sugar or fructose is usually hidden. Furthermore, people tend to consume large quantities of these foods.

You can easily spot "hidden" fructose, if you get into the habit of reading food labels for high fructose corn syrup or corn syrup. It is a fairly common ingredient in fat-free, low-fat foods or sugar-free foods and this is one reason why these foods are not healthy.

## Vegetables Can Help You Lose Weight

I have already covered  the vegetables in previous chapters, so I hope to be very brief here. If you wish to succeed with your weight loss program, you must get accustomed to eating lots of non-starchy dark leafy vegetables (turn vegetables into soup). Eating just iceberg lettuce, cucumbers, green peas and tomatoes is barely enough to provide your body with the vital nutrients you need to help burn body fat as well neutralize harmful free radicals.

Besides eating more vegetables and fruits, you must also cut back the portion sizes of starchy carbohydrates (such as white potatoes, corn, and rice) that you eat. In Chapter 7, I encouraged you to start your meals with non-starchy vegetables and/or vegetable soups before your main course since this will help you cut down your overall caloric intake while, at the same time, filling your body with vital nutrients and antioxidants. Below are the serving sizes and calories of some common vegetables, but remember that you can eat more.

| VEGETABLES (25 calories in one serving) | |
|---|---|
| **Vegetable** | **Amount** |
| Asparagus | ½ cup cut in pieces |
| Broccoli | 1 cup florets |
| Brussel Sprouts | ½ cup cut in pieces |
| Carrots | ½ cup sliced or 1 medium |
| Cauliflower | 1 cup florets |
| Celery | 1 cup diced |
| Cherry Tomatoes | 8 |
| Cucumber | 1 cup sliced or 1 medium |
| Eggplant (cooked) | 1 cup |
| Grape Tomatoes | 8 |
| Green Beans | 3/4 cup |
| Green Bell Peppers | 1 cup sliced or 1 medium |
| Kale (cooked) | 2/3 cup |
| Lettuce | 2 cups shredded |
| Mushrooms | 1 cup whole |
| Onions | ½ cup sliced or 1 medium |
| Peas, Green | 1/3 cup |
| Spinach (cooked) | 1 cup |
| Spinach (raw) | 2 cups |
| Summer Squash | 3/4 cup sliced |
| Tomatillo | ½ cup diced |
| Tomato | 1 medium |
| Vegetable Juice | 4 ounces |

Non-starchy vegetables are low in calories and you cannot gain weight eating them. They are rich in nutrients and are high in minerals and antioxidants that have anti-cancer and cardiovascular activity. They help to keep blood sugar and insulin levels normal and they also suppress your appetite and food cravings. You can boost your metabolism and burn body fat if you get into the habit of eating abundant amounts of vegetable greens or dark leafy vegetables before your meals.

Spinach, kale, Bok choy and collard greens are example of common dark leafy non-starchy vegetables you can eat freely because they are generally low in calories, carbohydrates, and fats. The rest of the vegetables that you can eat freely are listed below and in your shopping list. Vegetables that are high in starch should be treated as you would rice, potatoes, and pasta, which are a major source of carbohydrate. Other starchy vegetables include corn, parsnip, rutabaga, and plantain. To get the full benefit in terms of nutrient and antioxidant power, aim for at least five to seven servings of vegetables a day (5-7 cups raw or 2 ½ -3 ½ cups cooked daily).

## Non-Starchy Vegetables to Enjoy

| | | |
|---|---|---|
| Alfalfa Seeds, Sprouted | Collards | Peppers, Sweet Green |
| Artichoke | Cucumber | Peppers, Sweet Red |
| Arugula | Dandelion Greens | Potato Greens |
| Asparagus | Endive | Pumpkin |
| Bamboo Shoots | Fennel, Bulb | Purslane |
| Bean Sprouts | Garlic | Raddicchio |
| Beans, Green | Hearts of Palm, Canned | Radishes |
| Beans, Snap | Jicama | Rhubarb |
| Beans, Yellow Snap | Kale | Sauerkraut |
| Beet Greens | Kohlrabi | Scallions |
| Bitter Balls | Lettuce, Butter Head | Spinach |
| Broccoli | Lettuce, Arugula | Spinach, Chinese |
| Brussel Sprouts | Lettuce, Romaine | Squash, Summer |
| Cabbage/Bok choy | Mushrooms | Tomatillos |
| Carrots, Raw | Mustard Greens | Tomato Juice |
| Cassava Greens | Nopales, Cooked | Tomatoes |
| Cauliflower | Okra | Turnip |
| Celeriac (Celery Root) | Parsley | Turnip Greens |
| Celery | Peppers, Jalapeno | Watercess |
| Chard, Swiss | Peppers, Serano | Zucchini |

**Starchy Vegetables to Enjoy in Moderation**

| | | |
|---|---|---|
| Beans | Lentils | Sweet Potatoes |
| Chana Dal | New Potatoes | Yams/Eddoes |

**Starchy Vegetables to Use Cautiously**

| | | |
|---|---|---|
| Baked Beans | Farina | Parsnip |
| Broad Beans | Fufu | Plantain |
| Cassava | Garri | Red Skinned Potatoes |
| Fried Beans | Grits | White Potatoes |
| Corn | | White Potatoes mashed |

# Chapter 11

# Protein Can Help Speed Body Metabolism

## Protein Grows Hair, Nails, and Muscle

Protein is found in animal and plant sources, such as fish, meat, beans, nuts, and seeds as well as soy and dairy products. Proteins are used in the building of skin, nails, hair, muscles, and bones. They are also used in the building of organs, such as the heart and liver.

Enzymes and hormones like insulin, testosterone, and estrogen are also included in this process. They come in many different forms and shapes and perform various functions that are necessary for life. The protein collagen is used to build skin, tendons, and bones. Crystalline is a lens protein that provides clear vision. Hair and nails are made of keratin and muscle is made of actin and myosin. The protein hemoglobin carries oxygen from the lungs to the rest of the body. Muscles contract when actin and myosin slide back and forth to give movement and motility. These contractions help move oxygen and nutrients throughout the body and help the lungs inhale and exhale.

Each protein is manufactured according to specific information coded on our DNA and RNA. Sometimes, a defective protein or wrong protein is made due to errors in the DNA as a result of damage inflicted by free radicals (which triggers inflammation). This is believed to be the root cause of most diseases including cancer and heart disease.

To make the right proteins, such as hemoglobin, you need adequate amounts of good quality proteins; otherwise, faulty and defective hemoglobin could be produced, causing problems with oxygen uptake and delivery. This is why you should concentrate on eating foods with good quality proteins, such as egg whites, beans, fish, and lean meat. Poor quality proteins are high in bad fats, which are readily stored and can also increase the risk of disease.

## Dieting or Fasting Breaks Down Muscle Tissue

During starvation or prolonged fasting, the body could “cannibalize” muscles and other vital protein tissues, including heart muscle. The muscle breakdown is more pronounced if you are on a diet that is low in carbohydrate and protein. Apparently, muscle protein and other tissues are broken down to release amino acids, which are readily converted to glucose in the liver (gluconeogenesis). This process provides energy when short-term carbohydrate stores are up in a few hours, if you are fasting or skipping meals.

This mechanism is important for survival because the body is capable of storing only a small amount of carbohydrate reserves in the muscles and liver. It is for this reason that eating frequent but small balanced meals consisting of unprocessed carbohydrates, proteins, and fat is healthier as opposed to prolonged starvation or eating fewer but larger meals, especially at dinnertime when body metabolism is lowest.

## Are You Losing Fat or Muscle?

When your diet is inadequate in protein or exercise, you may tend to lose weight quickly, but only to regain it rapidly. The apparent weight loss is mostly due to the breakdown of muscle tissue and loss of tissue water. Surprisingly, the total body fat goes up, but the bathroom scale might register a weight loss, giving the false impression that you are on track. The consequences of losing muscle while retaining or storing fat is enormous – the body's ability to burn fat and calories can be severely compromised. In general, a sluggish metabolism causes the body to store fat instead of burn it for fuel. And the higher your body fat in relationship to your muscle tissue, the more the calories that you consume is converted into fat, causing you to be weak and sluggish.

When weight loss plateaus in spite of regular exercise activity, it could be due to inadequate protein consumption. Increasing protein intake could correct this problem and put you back on the right track towards weight loss. In general, if adequate protein is not consumed during dieting, body metabolism, physical appearance, and overall health could be compromised. Hair and nail loss might be an indicator of inadequate protein consumption that you should be aware of.

## The Bathroom Scale Is Not Adequate

Your bathroom scale measures only your body weight. It does not distinguish between the pounds from fat and those from lean muscle. As a result, your scale is not telling you whether you are in a healthy weight range. This information is very important since it is so common to lose muscle and retain fat. The bathroom scale will not show any of these changes.

Losing muscle instead of excess body fat is probably the number one reason why people regain lost weight so quickly. The higher the amount of body fat, the higher the number of calories that are converted to fat. As a result, you feel weaker and have less energy. Measuring your body fat can help you manage your weight loss better. Whenever there is a shift toward muscle loss instead of fat loss, you can take appropriate steps to halt the trend.

Either the bathroom scale or the Body Mass Index (BMI) doesn't actually calculate body fat, so it is inaccurate for athletes, such as football players, body builders and anyone on a weight-training program, and for people who are muscular. It is also inaccurate for growing children, sedentary adults, and the very elderly. For these people, the best method is the body composition analysis, which actually calculates the body fat percentage. There are now reasonably priced body fat scales available that you can use to measure your body composition in the privacy of your own home (*Tanita* Body Composition Analysis or some other model).

## Know Your Body Fat Percentage

Before he entered the UDP program, Tony was 5'8", weighed 197 pounds, and had a body-fat level of 45%. After three months, his weight was 190 pounds but his body fat was down to 27%. His total fat loss was 37 pounds and he had gained 5 pounds of healthy, lean muscle. In addition to reducing his body fat, he also reduced his blood pressure and cholesterol because these are associated with excess body fat that is stored around the abdominal area. Conversely, Karen, who was 5'7" and weighed 214 pounds, had a body-fat level of 50% before entering the UDP program. After three months, she weighed 194 pounds with 48% body fat. It was clear that Karen's weight loss was due to muscle and water loss instead of fat ( this was mainly due to a lack of exercise or inactivity). She could not have known this if she was depending only upon her bathroom scale. Appropriate steps were taken to adjust her program and keep her weight loss moving in the right direction. Otherwise, she could have regained the weight very easily.

The weight reflected on the bathroom scale consists of both lean muscle mass and body fat. Lean muscle mass is the part of your body that is metabolically active and is responsible for burning calories and turning fat into energy. Therefore, the more lean mass you have, the more calories you burn and the leaner and firmer you will look, regardless of your weight.

What happens when your weight stays the same or even increases? Does that mean that you are not making progress? Actually, you could be making substantial progress, such as losing fat and gaining muscle, which is very healthy. Since muscle is bulkier than fat, you might look slimmer and trimmer and your clothes will fit better. You might also experience a surge of energy, stamina, and well-being, even though the scale may show either an increase in weight or no change at all. This is the fundamental reason why you should not rely solely on the ordinary bathroom scale. It does not tell you the whole story. Refer to the chart below to see if you are in the healthy fat range.

**Healthy Body Fat Range,
Standard Adult**

| Age: | 20-39 | 40-59 | 60-79 |
|---|---|---|---|
| Male: | 8-19% | 11-22% | 13-25% |
| Female: | 21-33% | 23-35% | 24-36% |

*Adapted for use from Gallagher et al, AJCN, Vol 72, Sept 2000*

## Where the Fat Is Located Is Very Important

For your health and well-being, it is important for you to know where most of your excess body fat is located. Excess body fat, especially in the abdominal area (apple-shaped figure), is not only cosmetically undesirable, but it is also linked to life threatening conditions including heart disease, stroke, type 2 diabetes, high blood pressure, and some cancers (breast and colon). Excessive belly fat is linked to high cholesterol and high sugar and insulin levels, which can trigger cellular inflammation throughout the body – the underlying cause of many diseases. It also depresses metabolism and causes more fat storage.

In contrast, fat around the hips and thighs (pear-shaped figure) – which is common in women – seems to present a lower risk of health problems. Therefore, accumulated fat in the abdominal area should provide a strong motivation to lose excess body fat, especially if there are other risk factors, such as smoking, alcohol usage, family history, and inactivity.

### Body Fat Increases With Age

Starting at age 30, we steadily lose muscle and gain fat – which, in turn, slows down our metabolic rate or our body's ability to burn calories. This is particularly true if we are sedentary and eating a typical American diet containing high amounts of fat and refined carbohydrates. Excessive body fat accelerates aging, drains energy, weakens the immune system, and may even affect bone density.

The good news is that eating a proper diet and engaging in regular physical activity can help to build or maintain lean muscle and reduce body fat to a healthy range, regardless of age. In fact, eating a proper diet and maintaining regular physical activity, combined with a healthy lifestyle (no smoking, minimal alcohol consumption, adequate sleep, and maintaining a low stress level), can slow the aging process and keep brain function intact.

### Eating Lean Protein Speeds Metabolism

In previous chapters, we learn that eating highly refined carbohydrates and even white potatoes that are complex carbohydrates can actually depress metabolism and cause fat storage. On the contrary, the opposite effect is seen with carbohydrate foods that are high in fiber, such as whole grains (they are slowly digested and absorbed). As a result, they help speed body metabolism and burn fat more efficiently. Proteins have similar effects on metabolism and you can take advantage of this fact.

In other words, eating adequate amounts of lean protein can help stimulate your metabolism even when you are sedentary or have a medical condition, such as hypothyroidism that could depress your metabolism. Protein affects your metabolism in a positive way because the body takes as much as 25% of its metabolic calories to digest and process a protein-rich meal. This is why eating a protein-rich meal raises metabolism by as much as 25%, in turn, allowing the body to burn more calories.

Calorie for calorie, fat calories will make people fatter than the same number of calories from carbohydrates or proteins because of the way the body metabolizes fat. It takes only about 3% of the body's energy to convert fat in food to body fats; whereas 17% of the energy is required to convert carbohydrate calories to body fat. This means that, when you consume an extra 100 fat calories (roughly the amount in a tablespoon of butter, margarine or oil), your body will store about 97 of the calories as fat. On the contrary, if you consume an extra 100 calories from protein, such as fish or chicken breast, only about 75 calories would be stored as fat.

## Conquering Craving and Hunger Drive

Proteins are usually large and complex molecules in 3-dimensional space and their digestion and metabolism requires more energy and takes considerable time. This is why eating a protein-enriched meal makes you full more quickly and less hungry between meals. Though protein foods are not high in fiber, they are typically low-glycemic and tend to curb cravings and appetite.

Protein-rich foods also help decrease stomach emptying, thereby preventing the rapid digestion of carbohydrates that causes sugar and insulin elevation. Therefore, when you eat carbohydrates with lean proteins, your blood sugar and insulin do not spike as much. Whereas eating carbohydrates alone, especially refined carbohydrates or foods made with white flour and even some complex carbohydrates (white potatoes and fruits), can drive the blood sugar up.

## Proteins Are Not All Equal

As stated above, eating meals and snacks with lean low-fat proteins may help increase body metabolism. However, the challenge is choosing the right protein sources that are low in artery-clogging saturated fats and trans fats. Fatty cuts of meat are definitely a poor choice of protein and should be eaten less. Excellent protein choices are lean and low in fat and contain more protein per ounce and fewer artery-clogging (bad) fats. They are also rich in nutrients, including B complex vitamins, iron, potassium, phosphorus, sulfur, and copper. These include fish, lean cuts of meats, legumes, seeds, and nuts. Legumes are exceptionally good because they contain some modest amounts of good quality proteins and fiber, both missing in animal and fish foods. Alternating or combining fish and meat with a variety of plant-based proteins (such as nuts, seeds, and legumes) can help establish a healthy balance that will keep metabolism in high gear.

Organic meats from free-range or wild game not only have less saturated fat and cholesterol but a higher percentage of healthy Omega-3 fatty acids. By comparison, conventionally raised meats and animals, including chickens fed grains, have flesh that are higher in saturated fats and Omega-6 fatty acids, with minimal Omega-3 fatty acids.

Recently, researchers in Northern Ireland were able to reduce the percentage of saturated fat in milk from 64% to about 50% while raising the percentage of unsaturated fat from 35% to 46%. The idea of improving the quality of meat and meat products by adapting similar techniques in the near future is quite exciting.

## Protein Sources High in Artery-Clogging Saturated Fat

High calorie, high fat protein foods are usually more flavorful but they are typically high in fats that can increase health risks – saturated fat, trans fats, cholesterol, Omega-6 fatty acids, and arachidonic acid. These are all inflammatory producing substances that not only raise blood cholesterol levels and lead to greater risk of heart disease and cancer, but cause fat storage and weight gain.

The usual culprits again are red meat, whole fat dairy (such as cheese) and poultry with skin, especially dark meat. Some of the worst, high fat protein sources are found in common foods that may be eaten regularly. A glance at the chart below of some favorite foods will indicate how easy it is to exceed the daily quota of fat. For reference purposes, people with a daily intake of 1,300 calories will need about 28-56 grams a day and those with a daily intake of 1,600 calories will need 42 to 70 grams of total fat per day.

| Meal | Fat Content |
|---|---|
| *McDonald's* Chicken Select Premium Breast Strips (10pc.) | 66 grams |
| *McDonald's* Deluxe Breakfast (5.6oz.) | 60 grams |
| *Burger King* Original Double Whopper/Cheese Sandwich (14oz.) | 69 grams |
| *Denny's* Hickory Cheeseburger (15oz.) | 71 grams |
| *Denny's* Bacon, Lettuce and Tomato (7oz.) | 38 grams |
| *Denny's* Clam Chowder (8oz.) | 42 grams |

Other commonly consumed fatty foods include processed meats, such as luncheon meats, frankfurters, and sausages. These are usually high in fats and often contain nitrates, which could be converted in the stomach to cancer-causing nitrosamines. You will not only succeed in losing weight, but you will also lower your cholesterol and tryglycerides if you limit these types of food in your meals. They are high in saturated fat that promotes fat storage and insulin resistance. Whenever you eat foods that are high in saturated fats, keep the portions small – you should apply this rule not only to meat, but also to whole dairy, cheese, and full-fat yogurt. The potential to store fat is greater in the evening when metabolism is slower; therefore, try to eat most meat and full fat cheese at lunch and reserve fish and other lean low-fat protein foods like chicken breast, beans, and soy products that are low in saturated fats for dinner. Also, limit consumption of processed foods that are high in salts and fat, especially in the evening, when the potential for the body to store fat is greatest.

### Drink Plenty of Water When Eating Protein Foods

You should eat protein, even those that are lean and nutrient-dense in moderation. This can be achieved by paying attention to serving sizes. Even though most of the proteins eaten end up in muscle tissue or are used to make new products like enzymes, extra calories in protein could find their way into fat, as in the case with carbohydrates. Your body needs healthy kidneys and adequate water intake in order to flush toxic protein by products, such as urea, which can be harmful to organs and cells.

## Making a Healthy Protein Choice

### Making Better Protein Choices

Most protein sources, such as fish have been covered in other chapters. Shrimp and other shellfish are mentioned here briefly. Their cholesterol content is high and squid, in particular, has more than twice the cholesterol content of meat, but the saturated fat portion is much lower.

| Food | Cholesterol (mg) | Saturated Fat (g) |
|---|---|---|
| Oysters (12 med.) | 115 | 1 |
| Baked Eel (3 oz.) | 137 | 3 |
| Shrimp (3 oz.) | 165 | 0 |
| Squid, fried (3 oz.) | 221 | 2 |

By comparison, a single medium-large size egg has about 213 mg of cholesterol, 5 grams of fat, 1.5 gram of saturated fat and 6 grams protein. Thus, a serving of two whole eggs would contain as much as 426-450 mg of cholesterol, which would exceed a whole day's recommendation. However, only about 30% of cholesterol in a diet contributes to the overall body cholesterol, when the body has enough substrates (saturated fats and excess carbohydrates) to synthesize it needs by the liver. In fact, most cholesterol synthesis in the liver comes from saturated fats and not from dietary cholesterol. Therefore, for those people who like shrimp and shellfish, moderation is urged. The exception is for those people whose cholesterol level is high in spite of all their efforts, including medications. Keeping cholesterol intake to no more than 300 mg daily (the equivalent of one whole egg) may result in a better cholesterol profile. The egg yolk contains all the fat and cholesterol and you could selectively reduce their contribution by omitting them in situations calling for more proteins, such as in omelets and scrambled eggs.

| **Protein Foods With Low Saturated Fat Content** |
|---|
| Best Sources of Protein |
| Legumes: Soy beans and soy based products, baked beans, kidney beans, chick peas, lentils, butterbeans, navy beans, black beans, white beans, chana dal, pinto beans, etc. |
| Fish: Salmon, trout, fresh tuna, tuna –canned in water or oil, haddock, sole, perch, bluefish, bass, shrimp, lobster, clams, scallops, muscles, squid, and other seafood |
| Eggs: Egg Whites or egg beaters |
| Poultry: Skinless chicken or turkey breast |

| Dairy: Nonfat yogurt, reduced fat cheese, skim milk, 1% milk, nonfat dry milk, and low-fat flavored yogurt (sugar less than 10 grams) |
|---|
| Meat: Lean cuts of beef, pork, lamb, and veal |

Egg protein (albumin), or egg white, is an excellent source of protein that is relatively inexpensive and is good in salads, soups, and other side dishes. One serving consists of three egg whites (12 grams protein, 0 grams fat, 0 mg cholesterol). The recommended serving for egg substitutes is ½ cup (12 grams protein, 0 grams fat, 0 mg cholesterol). Whole eggs from free-grazing chickens or those that have been fed flaxseed meal or vegetable based feeds have higher Omega-3 compared to those raised on grains (such as the Eggland's Best eggs). They also have lower cholesterol and saturated fat and are probably better for those people with cardiovascular disease. One whole egg a day or a few times a week, even from conventionally raised chickens is not likely to raise cholesterol levels. However, it is best to keep in mind that two medium whole eggs could contain as much as 426-450 mg of cholesterol and about 10-15 mg of fat. The American Heart Association recommends no more than 300 mg of cholesterol per day (the equivalent of a medium whole egg).

**Foods High in Saturated Fats and Trans Fat**

| **Protein Foods With High Saturated Fat and Trans Fat Content** |
|---|
| Protein Sources To Minimize |
| Fish: Frozen and breaded fish and fish sticks. Fish prepared in palm kernel, vegetable, peanut, or coconut oils. Fried fish in general. |
| Eggs: Whole eggs with yolk (eating more than 2/day) |
| Poultry: Turkey or chicken with skin; dark meat of poultry, such as thighs, legs, and wings; fried chicken and nuggets. |
| Dairy: Whole or homogenized milk, whole fat cheese. |
| Meats: Untrimmed red meats, heavily marbled cuts or roasts, or organs, such as liver, brain, and heart that are very high in saturated fats; spare ribs, cold cuts, sausage, salami, beef hot dogs, and bacon.<br>Foods high in trans fat: fast foods, stick margarine, cookies, and processed foods |

Foods that are high in saturated fats, trans fats, Omega-6 fats, cholesterol, and calories should be limited to only a few times a week and the portions should be kept small. To minimize fat and calories, the visible fats should be trimmed before and after cooking. Foods should be baked, broiled, roasted, grilled, or boiled instead of fried. They can also be sauteed or cooked in a small amount (1-2 tbsp) of canola or extra virgin olive oil. Nonstick sprays made with olive or canola oil should be used for browning or sautéing.

When preparing recipes containing protein that call for flour, coating mixes, or breadcrumbs, select whole grains, such as whole-wheat flour, oatmeal, oat bran, and whole cornmeal instead of refined white flour. Meat should be weighed after the bones and fat have been removed and again after cooking. A recommended serving size is four ounces before cooking and three ounces after. Meats, especially beef, should be limited to not more than 16 oz per week. This goal can be reached by alternating meat with chicken or fish three or four times per week.

### Plant Protein

Plant proteins are not only low in cholesterol and saturated fats, but they are quite high in fiber, particularly soluble and insoluble fibers, which can help to keep blood sugar and insulin levels from spiking. Legumes (canned or dried), such as kidney beans, navy beans, pinto beans, black beans, lima beans, peas, and lentils are all good choices. They can also substitute for starches because they are high in carbohydrates. Depending on the product, ½-1 cup is usually sufficient for most people, especially when another carbohydrate source is included.

Incorporating beans and lentils as a side dish can help to control your blood sugar and insulin levels. For best results, use legumes with high soluble fiber, such as navy beans, kidney beans and lima beans. Chana dal is a lentil that has one of the lowest glycemic indexes. It's well recognized for its potential to control blood sugar and may also lower cholesterol. A serving of ½ cup of this delicious tasting lentils with your meals is a worthwhile healthy treat. Textured vegetable proteins are tasty, crunchy and delicious for addition to snacks, vegetables, soups and breakfast cereals.

Other plant proteins include soybeans and soy-based products, such as soymilk, tofu, soy nuts, soy protein powders, soy butter, canned or frozen soy beans, dried raw soy beans, tempeh, miso, soy flour, soy burgers, hot dogs, and soy breakfast cereals. Nuts and seeds, including peanuts and peanut butter, are also sources of protein, but they should be used cautiously because they are high in fat (Omega-6 fats).

### Poultry Sources

Lean, skinless chicken, skinless turkey, skinless duck, and other wild game provide a good source of protein that is also lower in saturated fats than meat and meat products. Chicken and turkey breasts or white meat with the skin removed are the best choices. Darker meats of poultry, such as wings, thighs, and legs have more fat than white meat.

All visible fats on chicken, turkey, and duck should be removed before cooking since most of the fat is located in the skin. Cooking with the skin on can leave some fats in the liquid even if the skin is removed prior to serving. Broil, bake, grill, or sauté chicken in small amounts of olive or canola oil (1-2 tbsp) and limit deep-frying, as this can soak up a good portion of the fat in the meat. You can also add chunks of well-seasoned chicken breast into vegetable soups that you eat with your meals.

### Meat and Meat Products

These are high in protein but also higher in saturated fats, trans fat, and Omega-6 fat than any other protein sources. Red meats, like refined carbohydrates, should be kept to a minimum, especially during dinner when the possibility of fat storage is highest. Leaner cuts with reduced fats are better choices, but the portion size should be kept small. Most of the visible fats should be trimmed before cooking. Better choices are: top round steak, eye round steak, loin sirloin steak, and round tip roast.

Game meats, such as deer, rabbit, buffalo, ostrich, and elk are lean and provide a good source of protein. Their meat is healthier and contains less saturated fat than that of domesticated animals (cattle, chicken, goats, sheep, etc.), which are fed an artificial, grain based diet. Game meats also contain a better ratio of Omega-3 to Omega-6 fatty acids.

Lean cuts of pork and pork products are also a healthy source of protein. You can also use well-trimmed cuts of meat like Canadian bacon, loin chops, and roasts and tenderloin roasts and products (fresh, canned, cured, or boiled ham) that are better choices of lean protein. Other lean cuts of meat include veal and lamb, such as cutlets, shoulder blade steak, and shank. Typically, processed meat should be limited because they are laden with fat, salt, and additives. Some of the health risks of these are not well known (see fast food section in Chapter 13).

## Dairy Products May Have a Positive Effect on Weight Loss

### Milk and Dairy Products

Several reports in recent years have claimed positive health benefits, including weight reduction, with dairy products, such as milk and yogurt. The consumption of just two servings (2 cups) of dairy products a day may be linked to some reduction in fat and body weight, according to some studies. This may be due to the calcium and protein content found in dairy foods.

Milk and milk products are primary sources of calcium, which facilitates the growth and repair of bones and connective tissue, including muscle. Eating foods rich in calcium and nutrients (such as complete protein, riboflavin, thiamine, phosphorus, and vitamins B6 and B12) also helps prevent osteoporosis, cavities, stomach ulcers, and infection.

A cup of milk (skim or 1%) contains about 349 milligrams of calcium, whereas a cup of non-fat yogurt contains about 452 milligrams. The low-fat varieties are the best because they are low in saturated fats and suitable for people with high cholesterol or a history of heart disease, diabetes, and high blood pressure. Brands with reduced amounts of sugar (approximately 10 grams or less per serving) are preferred. Whole milk and cheese should be limited. They are linked to heart disease and breast cancer because of their high saturated fat content.

Today's milks are fortified with Vitamin D, which regulates calcium metabolism. Inadequate intake of Vitamin D causes bone softening and fractures, a common problem in menopausal women. Interestingly, people who have adequate exposure to sunlight can produce the active form of Vitamin D.

People with milk intolerance, who have symptoms, such as diarrhea, irritable bowel syndrome, asthma, and even rheumatoid arthritis, have alternatives – soymilk, goat milk, or non-lactated milk and milk products. Other sources of whole food calcium that are well-absorbed by the body includes beans, nuts, collard greens, and seaweed. Seaweeds like Wakame and Hijiki have over 1,000 mg of calcium per three ounce serving and are good in vegetable dishes, salads, and soups. They can be found in Oriental and health food stores.

**How Much Protein Is Adequate?**

The protein intake in the UDP program is about 20-35% of the total calories. For a sedentary woman eating 1,300 calories daily, that is 65 to 114 grams of protein (90 grams average per day). For a sedentary man eating 1,600 calories daily, about 80 to 140 grams of protein (110 grams average per day) will be appropriate.

Another method to determine the daily amount of protein consumed is this: divide your weight by 2.2 (2.2 lbs. equals 1 kilogram) and then multiply the result by 1.5. This gives roughly the number of grams of protein needed each day.

A useful guide that will help you keep your protein intake in the right range is this: eight grams of protein is approximately equal to an ounce of fish and lean meat, an ounce of tuna or cheese, a glass of milk or an egg, a half cup of cooked beans, or one tablespoon of peanut butter. Later, I will show how you can use this information to determine the amount of protein to be consumed per meal.

In general, a healthy meal should have adequate lean protein but low in red meat, processed meat products, and whole fat dairy. This can be easily achieved by alternating fish and poultry with lean meat, which, in turn, will help to keep saturated fat down and increase the sensitivity of muscle to insulin. For example, if steak is eaten at lunch, select fish, chicken, or turkey for dinner instead of another protein source that may be high in saturated fat. Alternating or mixing plant-based proteins with the primary protein source can also help to keep cholesterol down. Likewise, eating fish and meat with lots of non-starchy dark green leafy vegetables and a modest amount of whole grains will help you lose weight and keep it off, provided that you tailor your food intake to your level of physical activity (The UDP Mantra).

As protein intake is increased, saturated fat should be monitored carefully. For example, three ounces of loin sirloin steak contain 6 grams of total fat and 2 grams of saturated fat. Eating twice the serving size doubles both the total fat and the saturated fat and this could increase health risk and weight gain. Fatty meats and full fat dairy products are loaded with fats that increase the risks of weight gain and chronic health problems and should not be a major source of either fat or protein.

# Chapter 12

# Good Fats Promote Weight Loss and Health

## Our Bodies Need Good Fats

Our bodies need an adequate amount of good fats to maintain optimum body function as well as burn body fat. Most people on a 1,300 calorie meal plan will need about 2-4 tablespoons (28-56 grams) of healthy fats or oils a day, such as the monounsaturated fats found in olive oil, canola oil, macadamia oil, and the Omega-3 and Omega-6 fatty acids found in fish, flaxseed oil, dark green leafy vegetables, vegetable oil, and nuts. These fats in their right proportions promote weight loss and good health and help fight inflammation.

On the other hand, saturated fats in meat and dairy products and the trans fats found in hard margarine and processed foods do, indeed, raise the risk of heart disease and cancer. These food groups are pro-inflammatory and contain many calories.

A deficiency of fats, especially the essential fatty acids (Omega-6 and Omega-3), can lead to many serious health problems. Essential fatty acids are involved in vital life- functions throughout the body including energy production, growth, and emotional stability. They help provide protection against cellular damages from saturated fats and trans fats that are abundant in meat, dairy foods, and highly refined processed foods.

The deficiency of essential fatty acids can lead to inflammation, blood clots, blood clumping, abnormal cholesterol production, and the formation of cancerous cells. Other health conditions include high blood pressure, arthritis, asthma and allergies, depression, skin disorders (such as acne, eczema, and dermatitis), premenstrual syndrome, behavioral disorders, hyperactivity, learning disorders, diabetes, loss of hair and nails, dry skin, low metabolism, weakness, obesity, fibrocystic breast disease, and breast cancer.

Fat provides the basal metabolic energy that keeps us alive. Fat also keeps skin and tissues healthy and it helps with the absorption of vitamins that only dissolve in fat. If dietary fat is lowered too much, deficiencies in the essential vitamins A, K, D, and E will occur. This is what has probably happened to the American diet in the last thirty years.

## Fat Is Not the Enemy

The problem with the American diet is that fat intake comes mainly from animal and dairy products instead of fish, poultry and plants. A huge portion of body fat also comes from the conversion of refined and high-glycemic carbohydrates like white flour pasta, sweetened breakfast cereals, soft drinks, and sweetened fruit juices.

As body fat increases, so do blood sugar, insulin, and cholesterol. All of these contribute to cellular inflammation, which sets the stage for insulin resistance (Syndrome X), heart disease, stroke, high blood pressure, diabetes, and cancer – but low-fat diets are not the answer. They only stimulate the body to manufacture saturated fats that are converted to more cholesterol by the liver. Furthermore, most low-fat foods contain high amounts of refined sugars that promote inflammation. During the past thirty years, Americans have been consuming low-fat foods, but their waistlines have been getting bigger. This strongly suggests that the solution to the obesity problem is not a low-fat diet. Our bodies need healthy fats to carry out its numerous functions, some of which have already been discussed in this and previous chapters. You should not be afraid to eat moderate amounts of good fats.

### The Irrational Fear of Eating Fats

The irrational fear of gaining weight from eating fats is well understood. In America, people get a large portion of their fat from sources, such as meat, poultry with skin, whole and 2% milk, full-fat cheese, butter, margarine, premium ice cream, and Omega-6-dominant vegetable oils. As a result, Americans consume lots of artery-clogging saturated fats, dietary cholesterol and Omega-6 fatty acids. All of these increase the risk of inflammation, obesity, heart disease, diabetes and cancer. The good news is that eating less fatty meat, whole fat dairy, and processed foods can reverse this trend. Including more fatty fish, olive, canola, flaxseed and macadamia oils, seeds, nut, and non-starchy dark green leafy vegetables can also help reduce risk.

Omega-3 fatty acids and monounsaturated acids can stimulate metabolism and help you lose weight, fight disease, and enhance your mood. They can also cut cravings, reduce insomnia, irritability, depression, and premenstrual symptoms (PMS), prevent muscle and joint pain, strengthen nails and hair, and help fight cancer, heart disease, and diabetes.

Including moderate amounts of healthy fats like fish, extra virgin olive, canola, or flax oils in each meal can improve the nutritional quality of your diet. Eating fat does not make you fat if you eat healthy fats in moderate portions. Low-fat diets are not healthy and may even cause weight gain and poor health, triggering loss of hair and nails and dry skin. In fact, you need to eat moderate amounts of healthy fats to burn fat and lose weight. People in cultures where fat intake is based solely upon monounsaturated fats and Omega-3 fats enjoy a low incidence of obesity, heart disease, stroke, and other chronic health problems that are so common in America and other westernized societies.

## Fats That Make People Fat and Sick

### Saturated Fats Raise Body Fat and Decrease Metabolism

As discussed in previous chapters, there are three kinds of fats that raise the cholesterol level of the blood and increase the risk of heart disease, breast, and colon cancers: saturated fats, trans-fats, and, to some extent, fats from refined vegetable oils. A diet high in saturated fats and dietary cholesterol can significantly increase LDL (bad) cholesterol, which can stick to walls of the arteries, triggering inflammation and hardening that leads to heart disease and stroke. A diet high in saturated fats can also cause the body to store fat rather than burn it, as well as increase insulin resistance. Animal fats (meat, egg yolks and full fat cheeses, whole milk, full fat yogurt, and ice cream) and vegetable oils (corn and safflower oil) are also high in arachidonic acid and Omega-6 fatty acids, which can spur inflammation when consumed in excess, especially when the diet is deficient in Omega-3 fatty acids.

Your consumption of saturated fat should be less than 10% of the day's calories, which comes to about 14 grams in a 1,300–calories-per-day diet and about 18 grams in a 1,600-calories-per-day diet. Limiting animal and dairy fats can help keep your saturated fat down. When shopping, look for foods that are low in total fat (less than 5 grams per ounce except for fatty fish) as these are usually low in saturated fat. The portions of meat and full-fat dairy should be kept small in order to reduce the amounts of total fat and saturated fat that you consume.

Additional Omega-3 acids (flaxseed oil, flaxseeds or fish oil) can be taken to counteract saturated fats. These will provide the essential nutrients the body needs to perform at optimal level. As a result, you will burn body fat more efficiently and increase metabolism and energy production, becoming more alert and energetic. To get the most benefit, you should also limit the consumption of fried foods, butter, premium ice cream, whole milk, whole cheese, fatty cuts of meat, poultry with skin, and highly refined vegetable oils. Eating these foods along with foods high in Omega-3 fatty acids dilutes their metabolic benefits.

**Some Helpful Steps in Cutting Back Saturated Fats and Cholesterol**

- Keep meat portions small and low in fat, and limit to 2-3 times per week.
- Choose lean cuts of meat and chicken or turkey without the skin.
- Limit cooking with highly refined oils made from (corn, peanut, and coconut).
- Sprinkle 1-3 tbsp soy protein powder to yogurts, cottage cheese, and other foods
- Red palm oil is low in saturated fat and high in carotenes, natural vitamin A and tocotrienols, a form of vitamin E that are super-antioxidants, and more potent than vitamin E tocopherol supplements on the market. It contains high amounts of plant phytosterols that are used in margarines and spread to reduce cholesterol levels. It's free of trans fat and cholesterol and low in pro-inflammatory Omega-6 fatty acids. Its exceptional resistance to rancidity and excellent stability at high temperatures makes it suitable for cooking, baking, frying and spreads.
- Choose low or non-fat milk, cheese, yogurt, and ice cream with reduced sugar.
- Limit deep fried foods and fried snack foods (high in trans fat).
- Avoid or limit foods with trans-fats, such as hard margarine and shortening.
- Counteract the effects of bad fats by adding good fats to each meals and recipes.
- Use food labels to help select foods that are low total fat and saturated fats.
- Bake, broil, saute, grill, roast, or poach food rather than frying.

- Add 1-3 tsp flaxseed oil, ground flaxseed, or wheat germ to yogurt, vegetables, and cereals.

**Some Favorite Foods Are Loaded With Trans Fats**

The problem with controlling the intake of bad fats (saturated fats, trans fats, and cholesterol) is that we don't always know their sources (especially the trans fats). On food labels, the amounts of saturated fats and cholesterol are usually listed, but not the amounts of trans fats until recently (you will begin to see this on food label). Therefore, it is often difficult to tell if you are eating too many trans fats. One thing is clear, the more fast foods, processed, or packaged foods you eat, the more trans fats you may be consuming. The good news is that you can use the nutritional label to estimate the trans fat content of a product: Add the saturated fat, monounsaturated fats, and polyunsaturated fats. Subtract this number from the total fat number and the remainder is likely trans fat. Also, if the package ingredients list contains partially hydrogenated oil, the product may contain trans fat. Below are some common foods that most of us would not suspect to be high in trans fat.

**Some Common Foods That Are High in Trans Fats**

| | |
|---|---|
| Mrs. Smith's Apple Pie | Pound cake |
| Potato Chips | Popcorn |
| Burger King Dutch Apple Pie | Nabisco Original Wheat Thins |
| French fries | Sunshine Cheez-It Baked crackers |
| Swanson Potato Top Chicken Pot Pie | Corn chips |
| Donuts | Kellogg's Cracklin Oat Bran cereal |
| Cream filled cookies | Post's Select Great Grains |
| KFC Original Recipe chicken dinner | Chocolate chip cookies |
| Bisquick | Nondairy creamers |
| Cake mixes | Flavored coffee |
| Shortening | Whipped toppings |
| Bean Dips | Gravy Mixes |
| Salad dressings | Cheese cvrackers |
| Waffles | Stick margarine |
| Nabisco Animal Crackers | Potato chips |
| Quaker Chewy Low-fat Granola Bars | |
| G. Mills Cinnamon Toast Crunch Cereal | |

**Margarine or Butter – Which Is Better for You?**

Margarine is a butter substitute made by hardening vegetable oils, such as corn and safflower. Salts and artificial flavoring are added to make it taste like butter. The process of hardening oils (called partially hydrogenated) creates entirely new compounds called trans fats that are harmful to the body. As already stated, the trans fats in margarine do three things that can increase health risk significantly: they raise artery-clogging LDL (bad) cholesterol as well as triglyceride and, at the same time, they lower artery-cleansing HDL (good) cholesterol.

The saturated fats in butter, on the other hand, only raise LDL (bad) cholesterol without affecting the good cholesterol. In this respect, it appears butter is a healthier choice than margarine; however, certain types of margarines enriched with plant sterols have been shown to lower cholesterol and they include Benecol, Take Control, and Becel. They block the absorption of cholesterol from the gut.

Plant sterols are present naturally in small quantities in many vegetables, fruits, nuts, seeds, cereals, legumes, vegetable oils, and other plant sources. Similarly, plant stanols are found in even smaller amounts in many of the same food sources. For example, both plant sterols and stanols are found in vegetable oils. Both sterols and stanols are essential components of plant cell membranes and structurally resemble cholesterol.

Cholesterol, as the name suggests, is itself a sterol that is predominately found in animals. In humans, the liver synthesizes the bulk of cholesterol, but an additional amount may also come through dietary sources. Its presence in the body is essential for life, since it is a building block for steroid hormones, such as testosterone and estrogen, and for cell walls (refer to Chapter 3).

In recent years the new health claim is based on evidence that plant sterol or plant stanol esters may help to reduce the risk of Coronary heart disease (CHD). Coronary heart disease is one of the most common and serious forms of cardiovascular disease, and causes more deaths in the U.S. than any other disease (see Chapter 5). Risk factors for CHD include high total cholesterol levels and high levels of LDL (bad) cholesterol. Foods that may qualify for the health claim based on plant sterol ester content include spreads and salad dressings. Among the foods that may qualify for claims based on plant stanol ester content are spreads, salad dressings, snack bars, and dietary supplements in softgel form.

Foods supplemented with plant sterols or stanols may reduce cholesterol and lower heart disease risk (such as Benecol, Take Control, Smart Balance Omega Plus and Smart Balance Omega Natural Peanut Butter). But, food manufacturers can only make the health claim for plant stanol or sterol esters to reduce cholesterol levels, as well as the risk of heart disease, if they meet the FDA standard. This is what you should look for:

- Foods should contain at least 0.65 grams per serving of plant sterol esters, eaten twice a day with meals for a daily total intake of at least 1.3 grams, as part of a diet low in saturated fat and cholesterol.
- Also diets low in saturated fat and cholesterol that include at least 1.3 grams of plant sterol esters or 3.4 grams of plant stanol esters, consumed in 2 meals with other foods.

The margarine spread, Smart Balance Omega Plus has been in the market for sometime, but Smart Balance Omega Natural Peanut Butter spread is a recent arrival. They contain no trans fats or cholesterol. They are made with soy, palm, canola, and olive oils to produce a balance of monounsaturated fatty acids, polyunsaturated fatty acids, and saturated fats. The manufacturer claims that it helps reduce cholesterol levels as well as improves the ratio of good and bad cholesterol.

- Stick margarine has 2.8 grams of trans-fat per tablespoon and 2.1 grams of saturated fat.
- Tub margarine has 0.6 grams of trans-fat per tablespoon and 1.2 grams of saturated fat.
- Butter has 0.3 grams of trans-fat per tablespoon and 7.2 grams of saturated fat.

### Plans to Reduce Trans Fats

- First and foremost, identify the source: Read the list of ingredients. Look for listing of trans fat that is now required by law. A listing of partially hydrogenated vegetable oil or partially hydrogenated vegetable shortening near the top may indicate a high amount of trans fats in cases that do not list the actual amount of trans fat yet.
- However, a listing at the bottom may suggest a small amount of trans fat. Beginning this year, food labels will mandatory carry the amounts of trans fat per serving.
- Limit foods with trans fat – cookies, pies, shortenings, and processed foods.
- Choose soft or liquid margarines enriched with plant sterols (Benecol and Take Control) instead of hard or stick margarines, which tend to have more trans fats.
- Keep your portion size of suspected foods small. The bigger the portion size, the more likely the product will have high amounts of trans fat.

## Fats That Promote Health and Help Burn Body Fat

The healthy fats that promote health and help you lose weight are unsaturated fish oils and plant oils, such as cold-pressed canola and extra virgin olive oils and those from dark green leafy vegetables, nuts, seeds, and avocados. You should replace most of the saturated, trans-fats, and highly refined vegetable oils in your diet with these healthier fats. The monounsaturated fatty acid (MUFA) from canola and olive oil and nuts like almonds and macadamia can help to lower blood cholesterol and reduce the risk of heart attack, high blood pressure, and cancer.

Fats from flaxseed oil and fish oil that are rich in Omega-3 fatty acids have also been shown to help protect the heart and help control depression, mood, attention deficit disorder (ADD), arthritis, and high blood pressure. They help burn excess calories and also stimulate the body to burn fat. Eating enough good fats can speed up your metabolism and help burn body fat even faster. By contrast, saturated fats found in meats, whole dairy and fried foods actually slow metabolism down.

Some of us are born with a sluggish metabolism or go about our daily life being sedentary. Nevertheless, there is still hope that we too can experience the benefits of a fast metabolism. This is how you do it: simply replace the saturated fats in your meal with those that are unsaturated and are used by the body to increase metabolism and energy production. This means eat more fish- and plant-based foods (such as soy, beans, lentils, canola oil, olive oil, flaxseed oil, and flaxseeds) and less fatty meat, full fat dairy, and poultry with skin. If your caloric intake is 1,300 calories, you need about 1½-2 tablespoons daily of essential fatty acids (such as 2-3 teaspoons of fish or flaxseed oil and 2-3 teaspoons safflower oil or corn oil or soybean oil, or 2 tablespoons of canola oil).

To prevent fatty acid oxidation, you should also take a multivitamin with vitamin E or take extra vitamin E, 400 IU. One to two tablespoons of wheat germ may provide adequate amounts of vitamin E in whole foods that is well absorbed by the body. Your metabolism will run even faster if you increase your intake of flaxseed oil or fish oil.

## Omega-6 Dominant Vegetable Oils Are Inflammatory

Vegetable oils, unlike animal fats, are unsaturated, containing Omega-6 fatty acids and Omega-3 fatty acids in varying amounts. However, vegetable oils from corn, soybeans, peanuts, sunflowers, and safflowers contain high amounts of Omega-6 fats in comparison to Omega-3 fatty acids. Some are even completely devoid of Omega-3 fatty acids. While Omega-6 fatty acid is essential for health, excessive amounts in your diet can have negative consequences; they promote inflammation, allergic conditions, and blood clotting, as well as other conditions. They may also lower HDL (good) cholesterol and can interfere with the pro-inflammatory actions of Omega-3.

The amount of Omega-6 fats that you need is fairly small, about ½ to 1 tablespoon (7-14 grams) a day using corn oil or safflower oil. But, most of us get more than that. You can avoid consuming too much Omega-6 by paying attention to the source of these inflammatory fatty acids in your diet (animal fats raised on grain, vegetable oils, processed foods, cookies, and fast foods). This will help improve arthritis and other inflammatory diseases. Better yet, you should eat foods that are high in anti-inflammatory Omega-3 fatty acids, such as fatty fish, flaxseeds, flaxseed oil, dark green leafy vegetables, and nuts like walnuts.

## Gamma-Linolenic Acid (GLA) Is a Different Type of Omega-6 Fatty Acid

As a general rule, Omega-6 fatty acids are pro-inflammatory and you have been advised to pay attention to their sources and limit their intake, especially if you have chronic health problems. However, gamma-linolenic (GLA) acid is a different type of Omega-6 fatty acid that behaves more like an Omega-3 fatty acid – suppressing inflammation and also helping the body burn fat to create heat and energy, instead of depositing excess calories for storage as fat.

GLA supplements have been found to be beneficial in the treatment of diabetes, asthma, cystic fibrosis, allergies, hyperactivity in children, and loss of hair and nails. Other conditions that have also been shown to benefit from these supplements are listed below.

Weight control: GLA may help by stimulating fat tissue to burn calories
Arthritis: in some cases, some sufferers have discontinued use of non-steroidal anti-inflammatory drugs
Cholesterol: reduction in cholesterol
Blood pressure: reduction in blood pressure
Eczema and other skin disorders: may improve
Premenstrual syndrome (PMS): GLA may help reduce bloating and tenderness as well as depression and irritability
Multiple Sclerosis: GLA may help to relieve some of the distressing symptoms of the disease and may even reduce the severity and frequency of relapses
Alcoholism: GLA may help with withdrawal symptoms and reduce post-drinking depression

GLA is found especially in borage oil and evening primrose oil. Some borage oil contains 24% GLA or 240 mg per 1,000mg capsule whereas evening primrose may contain 10% GLA or 100 mg per 1,000 mg capsule. The recommended amount of evening primrose oil or borage oil by experts is about 500 to 1,000 mg taken two to three times daily. You will need higher doses of four to six times daily for conditions, such as asthma, eczema, or arthritis.

## Sources of Omega-6 and Omega-3 Fatty Acids in Our Diet

Heart disease and diabetes are two deadly diseases that may reflect the high consumption of Omega-6 fatty acids compared to Omega-3 fatty acids. To help you recognize the dietary sources of these two competing fatty acids, check the listing below:

| Omega-3 Sources | Omega-6 Sources |
|---|---|
| Fish oil (mackerel, salmon, regular tuna, herring, sardines, lake trout, halibut, anchovy, dogfish, sablefish, lake whitefish, bluefish) | Corn oil |
| Dark green vegetables (kale, collard greens, broccoli, cauliflower, chard, parsley, spinach) | Cotton seed oil |
| Flaxseed oil and seeds | Grape seed oil |
| Walnuts and walnut oil | Meat |
| Soybean oil | Peanut oil |
| Canola oil | Poultry fat |
| Hemp oil | Safflower oil |
| Wheat germ | Sesame seed oil |
| Hard red winter wheat | Soybean oil |
| Pumpkin seeds | Sunflower seed oil |
| Some brands of eggs- Eggland's Best | Borage oil |
| Seaweed, Spirulina, dried | Primrose oil |
| Purslane | Sesame oil |
| Butternuts | Egg yolk, chicken |
| Chia seeds, dried | Corn, germ |
| Beechnuts, dried | Rice, bran |
| Cowpeas, dry | Margarine |
| Cod liver oil | Salad dressings |
| Menhaden oil | Shortening |
| Oats germ | Chickpeas, dry |
| Oyster, Pacific | Soybeans, dry |
| Oyster, European | Processed foods |
| Organic eggs | Fast foods |
| | Almonds |
| | Cashews |
| | Macadamia |
| | Pine nuts |
| | Filberts |
| | Pistachio |
| | Walnut oil |

Some seafood and fish are good sources of lean protein; however, they may be low in fat, particularly the Omega-3 fatty acids. These include light canned tuna fish, fresh water bass, pacific halibut, flounder, Atlantic cod, Pacific cod, grouper, shrimp, snapper, whiting, catfish, sole, croaker, haddock, perch, pike, swordfish, lobster, clam, mussels, octopus, Eastern oyster, scallop, tilapia, and crab. In most cases, you will have to consume 2-3 serving sizes (6-9 ounces) to meet the required Omega-3 fatty acids (500-1000 mg daily). This has the possibility of increasing calories beyond your need.

**Why so Much Omega-6 and so Little Omega-3 in Our Diets?**

Animals, like chickens, cows, pigs, and sheep, that are raised as free-grazing on green vegetation grass, wild plants, algae, seaweed and insects, instead of fattened with commercial grains, like corn, have a higher concentration of Omega-3 fatty acids in their flesh. Their eggs are also healthier to eat. Animals fattened with grains (such as corn and feed) that are high in Omega-6 fatty acids produce meat and eggs rich in Omega-6, but low in Omega-3 fatty acids. As a result, today's diet of beef, chicken, and eggs are high in Omega-6 fatty acids (inflammatory and tumor promoting) and low in Omega-3 fatty acids (anti-inflammatory and anti-tumor).

Studies of tissues and flesh of Americans show a similar ratio that has shifted in favor of Omega-6 fatty acids. Many Americans consume 4 to 5 times the recommended portion size of steak (12-16 oz.), eggs, Omega-6 dominant vegetable oils, and products made from them, causing body fat and tissues to become high in Omega-6 fatty acids. To make matters worse, most of us do not eat enough dark green leafy vegetables, low-glycemic fruits, legumes, seeds, fish, or seafood.

The probable reason for the high Omega-6 fatty acids and low Omega-3 fatty acids in our diet is that Omega-6 foods and products are relatively cheap and readily available. For example, margarine, cookies and crackers, snack cakes, frozen entrees, fried fast foods, and baking products are found in every supermarket. Inexpensive vegetable oils high in Omega-6 fatty acids are widely used in restaurants and homes.

On the other hand, sources of Omega-3 fatty acids are somehow scarce and expensive. These healthy fatty acids as you already know are found in fish, seafood, and the flesh of free-ranging animals whose diets are high in healthy fats. They are also found in plants and seeds, like flaxseeds, walnuts, pumpkin, and hemp. Others sources include canola oil, walnuts, algae, seaweed, and the leaves of dark green leafy vegetables.

**Too Much Omega-6 and Too Little Omega-3 Is Not Healthy**

As already stated, the biological action of Omega-6 and Omega-3 are in opposition to one another. These essential fatty acids are involved in reproduction, brain function, mood regulation, sleep, heart and lung function, and immune functions. These delicate activities and functions are carried out with the cooperation of both essential fatty acids. They seem to work smoothly when their ratio in the body is 1:1 or 2:1 The prostaglandins and other inflammatory substances produced by Omega-6 fatty acids are blocked or dampened by prostaglandins and anti-inflammatory compounds produced by Omega-3 fatty acids and vice versa. In this way, there is a natural check and balance system that coordinates all the body functions and makes things work smoothly.

Omega-6 fatty acids produce powerful compounds that are inflammatory and promote cell growth (including cancer cells and blood clots), as well as increase the risk of heart attack and stroke when the system runs out of control due to a deficiency of Omega-3. That is why consuming large amounts of Omega-6-dominant vegetable oils and animal fats at the expense of Omega-3 foods have serious health risks. Besides promoting tumor growth, vegetable oils (like corn and safflower), have other major health risks. These oils readily combine with oxygen and become rancid when exposed to air, light, or heat. Oxygen-free radicals are formed from the oxidation of vegetable oils that can cause damage throughout the body. Arterial walls, DNA, enzymes, and cell membranes could all be affected. In the absence of adequate antioxidants and phytonutrients, this damage can lead to inflammation, the root cause of most degenerative diseases.

In contrast, Omega-3 fatty acids keep our blood relatively thin and circulating well, as well as lubricate our blood vessels and help to reduce the risk of arterial plaque, heart disease, and stroke. They help to control high blood pressure, depression, mood swings, fatigue, aggressive impulsive behavior, and arthritis and may also lower the risk of cancer. The Omega-3 fatty acids help to control craving, appetite and stimulate fat burning. Other benefits include a youthful-looking, more resilient skin. But, on the downside, too much Omega-3 and very little Omega-6 can also increase health risk: the body is unable to mount an effective defense against invading bacteria, virus, fungi, parasites and foreign objects. The body is also unable to control bleeding – a small cut can quickly become life-threatening and menstruating women can easily bleed to death. But, none of these terrible things are allowed to happen when the two essential fatty acids are in their right proportions to one another.

Unfortunately, the American diet is generally too high in Omega-6 fatty acids and too low in Omega-3 fatty acids compared to the Asian, Mediterranean, and Inuit diets, where the incidence of heart attack and stroke is very low. People throughout the world who consistently eat a diet that is rich in wild plants, dark green leafy vegetables, fish, and products from either wild or domesticated free-grazing animals, have low incidence of heart disease, stroke and diabetes, probably because of the protective anti-inflammatory effect of Omega-3 fatty acids and antioxidants.

## SEAFOOD, THE RICHEST SOURCE OF OMEGA-3 FATS

### Fish and Seafood Are the Richest Sources of Good Fats (Omega-3)

If you are not eating fatty fish at least 3-4 times a week, you are missing out on one of the richest sources of Omega-3 fatty acids. Fatty fish, like regular tuna and mackerel, are high in Omega-3 fatty acids and should be eaten frequently to help burn fat and reduce inflammation. Leaner fish, like flounder, light canned tuna, and snapper, contain low amounts of Omega-3 fatty acids. You will have to eat large portions of these to get the required amount of essential fats; nevertheless, they are good protein sources that will help you burn fat and calories.

As you already know, the two major sources of Omega-3 fatty acids are fatty fish and plant flaxseed oil. Omega-3 fatty acids family of compounds is the EPA and DHA. Fish oils are the direct source of EPA (eicosapentaenoic acid) and DHA (decoshexaenoic acid), which are used as starting materials to build more powerful biological compounds that regulate thousands of metabolic functions through out the body. Omega-3 from plants (alpha-linolenic acid or LNA) is not active until it's further converted by the liver to the much more powerful EPA and DHA, in order for the body to use it. Some people lacked the enzyme to complete this conversion; thus, the importance of eating fish or products high in fish oil.

About 500-1,000 mg per day of Omega-3 fatty acids (EPA and DHA combined) from seafood is sufficient for most healthy people. You can easily meet this requirement by eating 3 to 4 ounce portions of a fatty variety of fish three or four times a week. However, you may need more if you have high cholesterol, heart disease, diabetes, high blood pressure, arthritis, or depression, including postpartum depression (such as 2- 4 grams of combined EPA/DHA or 6-8 ounce of fatty fish like salmon three to four times a week).

If you are interested in getting the maximum health benefit from fish, the best selections are those with high fat content per serving instead of the low-fat varieties whose Omega-3 fatty acids is low. When shopping for fish or canned seafood compare each product for total fat and polyunsaturated fat per serving. The higher the polyunsaturated fat, the higher the Omega-3 fatty acid content.

A three ounce serving of salmon has 1.4 grams of Omega-3 fatty acids (DHA and EPA) while a three ounce serving of canned white albacore tuna has an average of 1.3 grams of the same. By comparison, a three to four ounce serving of light tuna or flounder has about 0.2 gram of Omega-3 fatty acids, which is far below the daily requirement for an adult. To get an adequate amount of Omega-3 per meal, you might have to eat about nine ounces of light tuna or flounder. The disadvantage of increasing portion size is that calories are simultaneously increased and this could affect weight loss. For instance, a three ounce flounder contains about 100 calories, whereas, a nine ounce portion contains about 300 calories. You can find more information in the shopping list in Chapter 3 or in The Omega Diet by Artemis P. Simopoulous, MD (Harper Collins, 1999).

## Low Incidence of Heart Attack With Diets High in Fish or Olive Oil

In North America, the Eskimos and the older generations of Okinawa natives in Japan have a very low incidence of heart attack and stroke. These people eat very little meat and processed foods that are high in sodium and artery-clogging fats. Their main diet consists of fish and seafood (which are rich in Omega-3 fatty acids) and includes foods that are rich in protective antioxidants (dark green leafy vegetables, seaweeds, mushrooms, legumes, and soy).

In the well-documented Lyon (France) heart study, a diet that was high in vegetables, fruits, whole grains and healthy fats was found to be far superior in preventing heart attack and stroke than other well-established diets. The lesson learned is that we can reduce the risk of heart attack and stroke by increasing the dietary intake of healthy fats while, at the same time, keeping the amount of unhealthy fats in our meal very low.

## Insulin Resistance (Syndrome X) Improves With Fish Oil

Recently, Louisiana State University researchers studied the effects of Omega-3 fatty acids in people with insulin resistance, a condition in which the body fails to respond normally to insulin and often increases the risk for type 2 diabetes (see Chapter 5). Participants were given a daily supplement containing about 2 grams of DHA (Omega-3 fatty acid). After twelve weeks, people taking the fish oil supplements showed significant improvement in their bodies' ability to respond to insulin. These preliminary findings support previous observations regarding populations that eat more fish high in Omega-3 fatty acids, such as salmon, mackerel, and tuna. It is conceivable from these studies that even people who eat less fish or none at all can benefit from daily supplements of fish oils or flaxseed oil.

## Fish and Mercury Controversy

Fish are heart-healthy, but they may sometimes contain mercury, which, in excess amounts, can destroy brain cells, especially those of young children and developing fetuses. Industrial mercury pollution washes into waterways and ends up in fish that we eat. Over time, the mercury level may rise to dangerous levels in the flesh of those people who eat contaminated fish.

Mercury pollution is just one of the many environmental toxins that enter into our food chain. This is a major reason why you should eat more healthy foods, such as dark green leafy vegetables, fruits, mushrooms, seaweed, and legumes that are high in antioxidants – they can help neutralize the free radicals that trigger inflammation and cell destruction. The UDP template is designed to provide this protection.

## Not All Fish Have High Levels of Mercury

The good news for fish lovers is that not all fish contain high levels of mercury. Refer to the list below to help you make better choices:

**Low Mercury and High Omega-3 Levels**

| | |
|---|---|
| Freshwater trout | Sardines |
| Oysters | Sea bass |
| Salmon | Whitefish |

*(3-4 ounce portions provide the required amount of Omega-3)*

**Low Mercury But Low Omega-3 Levels**

| | |
|---|---|
| Canned light tuna | Flounder |
| Catfish | Pollock |
| Clams | Perch |
| Crawfish | Scallops |
| King crab | Shrimp |
| Croaker | Sole |
| | Tilapia |

*(If this group is your main source of Omego-3 fatty acids, you will have to eat bigger portions (6-9 oz.) from this group in order to get the optimum amount of Omega-3)*

**Medium Mercury Levels**

| | |
|---|---|
| Bluefish | Haddock |
| Canned white or albacore tuna | Lobster |
| Crabs | Orange roughly |
| Fresh tuna steaks | Salt-water trout |
| Grouper | Snapper |

**High Mercury Levels**

| | |
|---|---|
| King mackerel | Tilefish |
| Shark | |

*(The FDA advises pregnant women, lactating women, women of child bearing age and children to avoid this group because of the high concentration of mercury)*

If you are concerned about mercury contamination, you can reduce your risk by eating farm-raised fish. However, farmed-raised fish that did not eat algae and phytoplankton may have lower nutrients and Omega-3 fatty acids (it's cheaper to raise fish on a diet of grains, such as corn). The way around the problem is to eat a variety of fish instead of one type of fish all the time. This may help to increase nutrient quality, as well as reduce exposure to toxins. Secondly, try to limit fried and breaded fish (like fish sticks). The unhealthy saturated fat and trans fat could displace the available supply of healthy Omega-3 fatty acids.

# PLANT SOURCES OF OMEGA-3 FATTY ACIDS

## Flaxseed and Flaxseed Oil: The Richest Sources of Plant Omega-3

Flaxseed and flaxseed oil are two of the richest sources of plant Omega-3 fatty acids (alpha linolenic acid or LNA). *Barlean's* Forti-flax or flaxseeds, for instance, delivers about 3 grams of LNA per 2 tablespoons. If this is your main source of Omega-3 fatty acids, you will need about 2-4 tablespoons daily to meet your requirement for LNA, EPA and DHA. In addition, 2 tablespoons of flaxseed delivers 3 grams of dietary fiber and 1 gram of soluble fiber, including phytonutrients, such as lignans. There are also trace minerals, tocopherols (vitamin E), and B-vitamins.

*Barlean's* Forti-flax is made from cold-milled 100% organic flaxseeds and free of pesticide and herbicide. It tastes great and mixes easily in juice or water. Also excellent when used as a topping for yogurt, breakfast cereals, salads, and blended smoothies. It can also be added when baking breads, muffins, pancakes, and cakes. In baking, use 1 to 2 tablespoons of ground flaxseed per cup of flour. For cereal or vegetable salads, use 1 to 2 tablespoons per serving. Use ground flaxseed, since the whole flaxseed may not provide the same health benefits.

Dr. Simopoulos suggested that you should not consume more than 3-4 tablespoons of flax meal a day. Flaxseed contains thiocyanate (SCN), a chemical compound that, in high amounts, can block the function of the thyroid gland, causing an increased risk for goiter. However, SCN is inactivated during cooking for about 10-15 minutes. On the other hand, flaxseed oil does not contain thiocyanate.

Flaxseed oil is the world's most abundant source of plant Omega-3 fatty acids (LNA), delivering about 7 grams of LNA per tablespoon. Among the best is *Barlean's* organic Omega-3 and lignan-rich flaxseed oil – the richest and best-absorbed source of Omega-3 fatty acids. In addition to Omega-3 fatty acids, it's a rich source of lignans, plants chemicals that act like hormones in the body.

Plant LNA is only partially converted to EPA and DHA when you take flaxseed oil or other plant-based foods like flaxseeds and spinach and canola oil. As a result, you should eat a larger quantity of plant foods if you don't eat fish or take fish oil supplements – otherwise, you won't have the requirement your body needs for optimal health. To give you a rough idea, approximately 3-6% of LNA is converted to EPA and 2-4% to DHA. This is approximately the equivalent of 230-460 mg of EPA and 150-300 mg of DHA per tablespoon of flaxseed oil consumed. The recommended daily intake of combined EPA/DHA is around 500-1,000 mg. Taking 1-2 tablespoons of flaxseed oil daily can fulfill this requirement if this is your sole source of Omega-3.

Flaxseed oil can be added to vegetables, salad dressing, sauces, soups, rice, breakfast cereals, yogurt, and cottage cheese. If you can't tolerate the strong, fishy taste of the oil, you can take capsules instead (Omega-3 1,000 mg capsules, take 2-3 capsules 3 times daily). Other sources of plant Omega-3 are walnuts, walnut oil, butternuts, wheat germ, and pumpkin seeds. Flaxseed oil should be stored in the refrigerator and used within three months. It spoils easily because of its high content of unsaturated Omega-3 fatty acids.

**Flaxseed Oil – The Oil of Beauty**

Omega-3 fatty acids are not only protective to the internal organs, but also to the external organs, such as the skin – the largest organ in the human body (which is also usually the first tissue to feel the effects of aging and deficiency of nutrients and antioxidants). So many people are focused on body image and spend fortunes on topical cosmetic agents (such as lotions, creams, and anti-aging solutions) to keep their skin soft, supple, and lustrous.

Though these topical products can be helpful, for the most part, they only affect the superficial skin. The beauty and health of the skin really arises from within.

Topical moisturizing products and cosmetic agents may only mask underlying health problems and could delay appropriate medical interventions. Skin diseases, including dry and scaly skin, can only be healed from the interior. This means that skin tissues must be nourished and moisturized with proper cell nutrients that include clean water, essential fatty acids and the right amounts of vitamins and minerals (Beta-carotene, C, and E, as well as the minerals zinc, magnesium, and potassium). You probably recognized some of them as antioxidants that help the body to neutralize free-radicals that cause premature aging and wrinkling.

The key to healthy skin involves the same principles and practices that help to promote and ensure greater health and longevity. The skin requires optimal hydration within cells and adequate essential fatty acids on the cell membranes to keep it fluid and allow the passage of nutrients into the cells and waste materials out. Skin tissue also has sebaceous glands that secrete sebum onto the skin and hair strands. Sebum is made of fatty acids, triglycerides, wax, and other biological compounds that help to hold water and moisture within the skin. In addition, the essential fatty acids provide the building materials for the double layers of the healthy cell membrane and moisturizing sebum. This multiple layer of essential fatty acids provides protection and barrier against dryness.

Unfortunately, many people in the US over-consume the wrong fats – those found in animal products and processed foods (saturated fats, trans fat and Omega-6). These fats can lower the fluidity of cell membranes and prevent the smooth passage of nutrients into the cells and removal of toxic waste products into the external environment. These fats also raise levels of free-radicals and trigger inflammation that causes premature aging, wrinkling, and dry scaly skin.

Dry skin and hair, including premature wrinkling, are indicators of deficiency of essential fatty acids. A strong indication of deficiency is apparent around the heels, where the skin becomes cracked and dry. The irony is that even though so many of us are eating a high-fat diet, the fats are the wrong fats, which are not desirable for healthy skin.

On the other hand, having adequate amounts of essential fatty acids in the diet keeps the skin moist, soft, and well-hydrated. The Omega-3 fatty acids from fish or plant LNA from flaxseed oil work from the interior, deep inside the tissue, to heal and repair tissues and skin. This is the fundamental difference between topical skin products and getting the right fats and nutrients as part of a healthy meal. Again, the key are the Omega-3 fatty acids. You need these to keep the cell membranes and skin moist and fluid and to help fight inflammation and free radicals – thus slowing the aging process and keeping the skin young and resilient.

The good news is that it's never too late to reverse the process of dry skin, wrinkling, and premature aging. In order to correct the problem, you need to reduce the consumption of animal and whole dairy products, including deep-fried foods in vegetable oils that quickly become rancid and convert to trans fat and other unstable compounds that trigger inflammation. However, products and flesh from animals raised on organic, unpolluted green vegetation, or grazing in the wild have a desirable ratio of Omega-3 to Omega-6 and therefore are good for our health and longevity.

Once you start taking the Omega-3 fatty acids in the form of foods (fatty fish, fish oils, flaxseed oil, flaxseeds, and leafy vegetables), it may take a few months for the tissues and skin to respond to the new nutritional support. But, once the skin and tissues become rejuvenated and enriched in Omega-3 fatty acids, clean water, and antioxidants, the results can be dramatic – soft, supple, and lustrous skin. The overall result is a youthful-looking and desirable body image.

How much fish, fish oil, or flaxseed oil should you take? For fatty fish like mackerel, tuna or salmon; about 4 ounce per meal 3-4 times per week. For fish oil, like cod liver oil, about 1 tbsp daily. For flaxseed oil, about 1-2 tbsp per day. A good rule of thumb for children and adults is to consume 1 tbsp daily of flaxseed oil for every 100 pounds of body weight.

**Flaxseed Lignans: Key to Breast and Prostate Health?**

Lignans are insoluble plant phytonutrients that are concentrated in flaxseeds and act like hormones in the body. They have been shown to bind to hormones like estrogen in the body, lowering the hormone levels to the optimal balance needed for good health. Because of this property, lignans have been studied for their possible anti-carcinogenic properties. The lignan metabolites have a structural similarity to human estrogens and thus can bind to estrogen receptors and block the growth of estrogen-induced breast cancer.

Lignans have also been researched for their role in prostate cancer in which estrogen has been implicated. It appears that lignans block the enzyme necessary for converting testosterone to estrogen. When the enzyme is blocked, testosterone is not converted to estrogen and this favors higher levels of testosterone and a lower risk of prostate cancer and benign prostate hypertrophy (enlargement of the prostate gland).

Plant lignans are comparable to other well-known estrogen blockers that are clinically used to suppress the growth and proliferation of certain types of breast cancers. Some of the well-established estrogen blockers are tamoxifen and raloxifene. The isoflavones from soy are also well-studied and may have similar potential. Excessive estrogen has been implicated in the growth of breast, prostate, and colon cancers and, hence, understanding this process is a major research goal. This fact alone should be strong motivation for both women and men to consider including lignans in a regimen of healthy eating. But, before you do that, you should first consider consulting with your primary physician, especially if you are at risk for breast cancer. Some researchers believe that lignans and isoflavones can stimulate breast receptors and possibly increase the risk of breast cancer – but this is very unlikely. For instance, Chinese and Asian women eat a high amount of soy containing isoflavones throughout their lives and the incidence of breast cancer is relatively low. This is also true for the risk of prostate cancer in men.

## Summary of Omega-3 Fatty Acids

Before leaving this section, it's important to understand that the delicate balance between Omega-3 and Omega-6 is critically important in the control of inflammation, immune response, allergic reactivity, hormone regulation, myelin sheath development in the brain and nervous tissue, cardiovascular support, blood pressure health, and behavior. Westernized diets that provide abundant Omega-6 fats relative to Omega-3 fats promote inflammatory compounds in the body. On the other hand, diets that are high in Omega-3 fats promote anti-inflammatory compounds. As a result of these opposing roles, Omega-3 has been coined to be "good" and Omega-6 to be "bad". But the fact is that both are essential for our health and it's the delicate balance of the two in our bodies that is important.

Westernized diets are shifted towards more Omega-6 and lesser Omega-3 and this has created a situation of chronic inflammation that precedes multiple degenerative diseases (heart disease, stroke, diabetes, arthritis, auto-immunity, cancer and even obesity). These changes have only been seen within the last 50-75 years as a result of rapid industrialization.

Chances are we would increase our consumption of Omega-3 fatty acids and quickly restore a healthy balance. The numerous health benefits are outlined below:

- Omega-3 is a natural blood thinner that reduces threat of blood clots.
- Omega-3 is anti-inflammatory – reduces inflammation in the arteries and joints causing aches and pain, including arthritis.
- Omega-3 reduces arterial plaques and improves blood circulation.
- Omega-3 increases energy, concentration, and restful sleep.
- Omega-3 lowers LDL (bad) cholesterol and increases HDL (good) cholesterol.
- Omega-3 helps lower high blood pressure.
- Omega-3 increases insulin sensitivity and helps to control blood sugar levels.
- Omega-3 may help alleviate dry skin, eczema, and psoriasis.
- Omega-3 increases metabolism and help the body burn stored fat, such as belly fat.
- Omega-3 protects against cancers (such as breast and prostate).
- Omega-3 forms the primary building block of the brain and aids in the development of the delicate myelin sheath that is involved in the transmission of nerve impulses.
- Omega-3 is brain food and a key player in the development of the brain before and after birth. It increases our ability to learn and retain information.
- Omega-3 helps with Attention Deficit Disorder (ADD).
- Omega-3 helps fight depression, hyperactivity, impulsiveness, and aggression.
- Omega-3 help fights postpartum depression.
- Omega-3 helps in decreasing painful cramps before and during menstruation.
- Omega-3 helps control craving and compulsive eating.

# Other Healthy Fats That We Can Have

## Canola Oil is Rich in All the Good Fats

Cold-pressed canola oil is one of the healthiest oils available today. Canola oil and canola-based products like canola mayonnaise have some plant Omega-3 fatty acids (LNA). One tablespoon contains 120 calories, 14 grams total fat, 8 grams monounsaturated fat, 4 grams polyunsaturated fat, 1 gram saturated fat, and no cholesterol. It is rich in heart-friendly, monounsaturated fatty acids and has more Omega-3 fatty acids (LNA) than even olive oil. It also has the best ratio of Omega-6 to Omega-3 (2:1 or about 24% Omega-6 to 10% Omega-3).

You should use cold-pressed canola oil and extra virgin olive oil as your primary cooking oils. Unlike olive oil, it has a neutral taste and can be heated to high temperatures. Mixing the two oils – one part canola oil with one part of extra virgin olive oil – can give you the best quality oil possible. This mixture is also good with vegetable salads and greens.

## Olive Oil is Anti-Inflammatory

Olive oil is rich in monounsaturated fatty acids (MUFA) and squalene, an anti-inflammatory compound. Like aspirin and ibuprofen, olive oil has anti-inflammatory properties that are known to block the formation of blood clots and relieve pain. One serious advantage is that olive oil does not cause stomach ulcers and bleeding, which can be life-threatening – while aspirin does increase that risk.

Olive oil is believed to inhibit the formation of colon cancer and possibly breast cancer as a result of its inflammatory properties. Both olive and canola oils can help lower blood cholesterol and reduce the risk of high blood pressure and breast cancer. In some studies, people were able to lower the dosage of hypertension medication when they increased their consumption of olive oil.

The saturated fats in meat, whole dairy and butter spur inflammation – but when olive oil is a regular part of your diet, it may help to reduce inflammation. A combination of extra virgin olive oil with flaxseed oil, which is high in Omega-3, can result in very fine, healthy oil that can be used for vegetables, salads, and dressing. For cooking or baking, use olive oil or a combination of olive and canola.

Unsaturated oils (like olive or canola oil) are better fuel than saturated oils and they can help your body burn stored fat more efficiently. Saturated animal fats (grease, butter, lard, and Crisco) are notorious for being converted into body fat and depressing the body's ability to burn fat.

Other sources of MUFA include olives, avocados, almonds, macadamia nuts, soy nuts, cashews, pecans, pistachios, peanuts, and peanut butter. Almonds, cashews, soy nuts, pistachios, and peanuts, however, are high in Omega-6 fatty acids, so you should not eat too many of these if your HDL (good) cholesterol is low.

### High Heat Destroys Oil

Heating vegetable oils or other unsaturated oil (olive oil, canola oil, and flax oil) to high temperatures in deep-frying or reheating is not a healthy practice. However, heating oils at a lower temperature is safe. The unsaturated oils are very sensitive to oxidative damage that can lead to the formation of dangerous free radicals that may cause cancer. You can tell when an oil has gone bad if it is rancid and, for that reason, not good for consumption. To prevent oils from getting rancid, store them away from light or heat, preferably in the refrigerator. Never fry with the same oil more than once and don't keep oil more than three months.

To counteract and neutralize the destructive effect of free radicals, always eat abundant amount of foods that contain antioxidants, such as dark green leafy vegetables and supplements like vitamin E, C, beta-carotene, and selenium.

## TOO MANY NUTS CAN MAKE YOU FAT

### Nuts Are Good for You, but Eating Too Many Can Make You Fat

Nuts are a good source of healthy fats, proteins, fiber, vitamin E, and trace minerals like potassium, phosphorus, magnesium, zinc, calcium, and several important phytonutrients, including plant Omega-3 fatty acids. The amounts of plant Omega-3 found in nuts are arranged in descending order: butternuts or white nuts, English walnuts, and black walnuts. On the other hand, some of the other nuts are high in Omega-6 fats and extremely low or devoid of Omega-3 fats.

Nuts are generally high in fats and calorie dense, so don't eat too many at one time; otherwise, you could gain weight. A good rule of thumb is not to go by the recommended serving size listed on food label because the fat content may be too much for a snack. They are delicious and convenient snack foods and good on vegetables, salads, or cereals, but you have to take into consideration that they are loaded with fat. To make matters worse, the nuts containing the good Omega-3 are scarce and most people eat nuts that are predominantly heavy in Omega-6 fatty acids, such as almonds, pecans, soy nuts and peanuts. The brief discussion below of some common nuts will help you make healthier choices, as well as the appropriate portions that you should have for snack.

### Almonds

These nuts are relatively low in Omega-3 fatty acids and high in Omega-6 fatty acids, but they are a rich source of monounsaturated fats (the same fat found in olives and canola oils) and nutrients that may help reduce cholesterol levels. In some studies, eating a one-ounce snack (about 6 whole almonds, 167 calories, and 14.6 grams fat) has been shown to lower LDL (bad) cholesterol, thereby reducing the risk of heart disease. But, as a snack, this amount contains too much fat if you are trying to lose weight.

Therefore, as a snack, I suggest that you should have a smaller amount (about 1-2 tbsp whole, chopped, or sliced or 3 whole) or ½ ounce, which would reduce the fat from 14 grams to 6 to 8 grams. I have no doubt that even this reduced amount will help lower cholesterol and body fat if incorporated into a healthy meal plan. This same commonsense approach will apply to the other nuts, as well. Almond oil is used for flavoring, skin care and for buttery spread.

**Walnuts**

Walnuts are a concentrated source of protein, monounsaturated fats, vitamins B and E, calcium, phosphorus, folic acid, and fiber. In addition, they contain some amounts of plant Omega-3; however, the Omega-6 fraction is 3½ times the Omega-3 fraction. They are also rich in nutrients that may help reduce LDL cholesterol as well as fight cancer. An ounce of walnuts (5-6 whole or ¼ cup chopped), the standard serving size, delivers about 185-210 calories and 19-20 grams of fat. Instead, you should have a lesser amount for a snack. Four halves, ½ ounce or 1-2 tablespoon of chopped nuts, deliver about 50-100 calories and only 4 to 8 grams of fat.

**Peanuts**

This popular nut is also high in protein and fat and, although it contains heart-healthy monounsaturated fat like those found in olive oil, canola oil, and avocado, they could hinder your weight loss if you overindulge. Peanuts also have high levels of the pro-inflammatory Omega-6 fatty acids. Peanut oil is used in cooking, as salad oil, in margarines and the residue is fed to animals. Whole peanuts can be eaten raw, roasted, or made into peanut butter. A serving of 10-20 roasted, plain, whole peanuts delivers about 60-120 calories and 5-10 grams of fat and 12-25 roasted peanuts in their shell deliver about 55-110 calories and 5-10 grams of fat. Peanuts are actually legumes that are high in protein and contain 40-50% oil.

**Peanut Butter**

Two tablespoons of smooth peanut butter contains about 190 calories, 17 grams total fat, 4 grams of polyunsaturated fats, 3 grams of saturated fats, 6 grams of protein, 3 grams of sugar, and 2 grams of fiber. The Omega-6 fraction is high relative to Omega-3 and that's one reason why eating too much peanut butter may not be healthy for you. It can lower the protective HDL (good) cholesterol and may even raise inflammatory levels, especially if the diet is deficient in Omega-3 fatty acids. It may also have unspecified amounts of hydrogenated vegetable oil (look for brands which do not contain hydrogenated oils, which are highly saturated trans fats). By comparison, a slice of cheese (American, Swiss, Provolone, etc) has about 8-9 grams of fat and 5 grams of saturated fat – increasing cholesterol and health risk – whereas peanut butter is not only low in saturated fat, but also has a fairly moderate amount of monounsaturated fat acids (MUFA) that can help lower cholesterol levels. It's quite reasonable to assume that the beneficial effects of MUFA far outweigh that contributed by Omega-6 if you consume only a small amount at a time.

For a snack, try 1 tbsp peanut butter (about 95 calories and 8 grams fat and 1.5 grams saturated fat) with an apple or on a slice of toasted multigrain bread with a tablespoon of sugar-free jam or preserve. Also, select peanut butter that is low in sugar and free of trans fat, such as *Smart Balance* Omega Natural peanut butter.

**Cashews**

One ounce of this delicious nut contains 160 calories, 13 grams of total fat, 7.2 grams of monounsaturated fat, 2.4 grams of polyunsaturated fat, 2.4 grams of saturated fat, 0 grams of cholesterol, 4 grams of protein, and 1 gram of fiber. They also contain potassium, phosphorus, magnesium, and iron. For a snack, try 1-2 tbsp (50-100 calories, 4-8 grams of fat) or a half-ounce (80 calories and 6.5 grams of fat). They are generally high in protein and carbohydrate.

**Pecans**

They are high in phosphorus and potassium, which are good for lowering high blood pressure. They are also high in vitamin A and fat. One ounce (2 whole) contains 196 calories, 20 grams total fat, 11.6 grams of monounsaturated fats, 6.1 grams of polyunsaturated fat, 2 grams of saturated fat, and no cholesterol. For a snack, try ½ ounce or 1-2 tbsp chopped or sliced pecans (100 calories, 10 grams fat).

**Macadamia Nuts**

One ounce contains 204 calories, 21 grams of fat, 2 grams of protein, 2 grams of fiber, and 104 mg of potassium. These have the highest concentration of monounsaturated fats among nuts. They are good for lowering cholesterol, but their fat content is extremely high. They are low in carbohydrate and are expensive. For a snack, eat about 1-2 tbsp of dry roasted nuts (60-120 calories and 6 grams of fat) or 1-2 tbsp of chopped nuts (49-100 calories and 5-10 grams of fat) or ½ ounce (100 calories, 10.5 grams fat).

**Coconuts**

The coconut palm is common in the tropical regions of the world. The nut is covered in a fibrous outer coating. The unripe nuts contain coconut milk that is high in sugar. The nutmeat can be eaten fresh or dried (desiccated or flaked coconut). The oil is extracted from the nutmeat and used for cooking (it is high in saturated fat), margarines, soaps and detergents. The dried nutmeat is about 50% higher in fat than the fresh nutmeat. You should limit consumption of coconut meat and oil, because of the high saturated fat and Omega-6 fatty acids (increase risk of inflammation and heart disease).

## Palm Kernel and Red Palm oil

Red palm oil is an edible vegetable oil obtained from the fruit of the palm tree that grows in the tropical areas of the world (Africa, South East Asia, especially Malaysia-the world leader in exports of palm oil). Although, scarcely used in the United States as a dietary source, it's the second most common vegetable oil consumed in the world after soybean oil. In the United States, palm oil has been traditionally used for industrial frying, margarine and shortening; ice cream, chocolate, confectionery, non-dairy creamers, soap and detergent, and cosmetics, but that is changing as more people become educated about this versatile oil.

In its natural state, palm oil is red in color due to a rich source of phytonutrients (such as beta-carotene, alpha-carotene, vitamin E tocopherols and vitamin E tocotrienols and derivatives, lycopene and other carotenoids). The high concentration of carotenes is responsible for the striking red color of the oil (carrot color is also due to carotenes).

## Advantages of Red Palm Oil

Red palm oil is one of the healthiest oils in the world. Most oils and fats because of their molecular structure are susceptible to attack by atmospheric oxygen, resulting in rancidity or oxidation. Also important nutrients in vegetable oil and fats are broken down when food is cooked in high heat. Research has shown that red palm oil can be heated during cooking without destroying its rich phytonutrients and nutrients. It's also resistant to rancidity and oxidation.

## Difference Between Red Palm Oil and Palm Kernel Oil

Red palm oil (from the palm fruit) is physically and chemically different from the highly saturated palm kernel oil. For example, palm kernel oil (from the palm kernel or nut) is extremely high in saturated fat (1 tbsp of palm kernel oil contains 14 grams total fat and about 12 grams saturated fat). Therefore, foods made with palm kernel oil should be avoided because they can raise cholesterol levels and increase health risk just like animal fat.

Most of us have been sold the idea that palm oil is just as potentially harmful as animal fat because of the high saturated fat content. However, this is misinformation. There is a vital difference between palm kernel oil and red palm oil. Red palm oil is produced from the flesh of the palm fruit, and it is very healthy. Organically certified red palm oil is minimally processed using only steam, high temperature and a mechanical press; no chemical solvents or bleaches, so that it contains most of its phytonutrients in a natural and wholesome nutrient complex (these includes vitamin E derivatives, mixed carotenes, phytosterols, CoQ10 and squalene). It's distinguishable from the palm kernel oil by its distinct red color due to high content of carotenes. Red palm oil is low in saturated fat, Omega-6 fatty acids and is free of cholesterol and trans fat (1 tbsp red palm oil contains 14 grams total fat and only 3.5 grams saturated). By comparison, 1 tbsp of extra virgin olive oil has 14 grams total fat and 2 grams saturated fat.

Red palm oil contains a balance of polyunsaturated, monounsaturated and saturated fatty acids and including essential substances, such as linoleic acid, tocopherols and tocotrienols, which are powerful natural antioxidants against damaging free radicals. This is the reason why red palm oil has exceptional resistance to rancidity and oxidation. Red palm oil is particularly rich in tocotrienols, which are super-antioxidants. It's the only vegetable oil that has abundant amount of tocotrienols in nature. The vitamin E tocotrienols and carotene contents of red palm oil are superior to those of vitamin E tocopherol contents of other vegetable oils (such as corn oil, olive oil, sunflower oil and safflower oil). For example, the antioxidant activities of vitamin E tocotrienols are 40-60 times potent than that of vitamin E tocopherols that are widely used in vitamin supplements.

The health benefits of red palm oil are summarized below:

- Carotenoids and vitamin A (antioxidants)—1 tbsp of red palm oil contains about 8,480 IU of vitamin A and 9 mg mixed carotenes.
- Red palm oil is the largest natural source of tocotrienols, part of the vitamin E family, with a more potent antioxidant activity than conventional vitamin E supplements on the market. A tablespoon of the oil contains about 1.3 mg of vitamin E and 6 mg of tocotrienols (reduce cholesterol levels; reduce or reverse the blockage of the carotid artery, thereby reducing the risk of stroke; reduce blood clotting; inhibition of the growth of breast cancer cells, and enhancement of the efficiency of breast cancer drugs, such as Tamoxifen).
- Red palm oil is rich in plant phytosterols (12.8 mg per 1 tbsp of oil) that is used in spreads to lower cholesterol and reduce cardiovascular risk (about 0.5 - 1 tsp per day is more than adequate to get the health benefit). To get the full health benefits, you can use red palm oil in cooking, salad oil and meal preparations (mixing red palm oil with olive or canola oil or flaxseed oil gives a healthy blend of oil that is also flavorful). You can also take 1 tbsp per day to improve your overall health.

**Sunflower Seeds**

Sunflower seeds come from an annual plant belonging to the daisy family. They are a good source of potassium and phosphorous. The whole seeds can be eaten raw or cooked, and the oil can be extracted from the seeds and used in margarine, varnishes and soaps. They can be added to breads and cakes or sprinkled over salad or breakfast cereals.

The seeds are moderately high in fat, especially the Omega-6 fatty acids. One ounce contains 182 calories, 15 grams fat, 7 grams protein and 2 grams fiber. For snack, a reasonable amount will be ½ ounce serving (91 calories, 7.5 grams fat) or 1 tbsp (60 calories, 5 grams fat, 2 grams protein and 0.7 grams fiber).

**Pumpkin Seeds**

The pumpkin seeds can be eaten raw or cooked in both sweet and savoury dishes. They are delicious and the toasted seeds can be sprinkled, while hot, with Soya sauce and served on salads. They are rich in protein, iron, phosphorous and zinc. One ounce contains 126 calories, 6 grams fat, 17 grams carbohydrate, 5 grams protein and 1-gram fiber. Even though, the fat is low in comparison to other seeds, the Omega-6 fatty acids is dominant.

For snack, an ounce of toasted seeds will suffice since it's well balanced in fat, protein and carbohydrate (a perfect snack food).

**Sesame Seeds**

Sesame seeds originated from Africa, but are now common in tropical and sub-tropical Asia. The whole seeds can be eaten and are most often used as a decoration on cakes, confectionery etc. The oil is extracted from the seeds and used for cooking, salad oil and margarines. It is used as toasted sesame oil for Oriental cooking.

Sesame seed paste, Tahini, is used in many dishes (hummus). Halva, a sweet made from sesame seeds is often found in health food shops. Sesame seed is a good source of protein and calcium. As most of the other seeds, it is high in Omega-6 fatty acids. One ounce contains 161 calories, 14 grams fat, 5 grams protein and 5 grams fiber. For snack, a serving of ½ ounce (81 calories, 7 grams fat) or 1-2 tbsp (60-120 calories, 5-10 grams fat) will suffice.

**Soynuts**

Soynuts make good and healthy snacks that you can eat at the office or home, traveling or at your favorite activity. The roasted and lightly salted Soynuts are delicious, crunchy and great for snacks and as a salad topping. They are a good source of protein and fiber. They contain both Omega-6 and Omega-3 fatty acids, but the Omega-6 is by far more. They also contain isoflavones (genistein and daidzein) that have several health benefits. A typical serving is 1 oz or 1/3 cup and contains about 76 mg of total isoflavones.

*Good Sense* Roasted and Salted Soynuts (one ounce contains 140 calories, 7 grams fat, 10 grams protein, 10 grams carbohydrate, 0 gram sugar, 5 grams fiber and 90 mg sodium). They provide a complete snack that you can enjoy. The amount of fat in a typical serving should pose no problem, even with the Omega-6 fatty acids.

**Olives**

Olives are included in this section with the seeds, because they are common household items that are used in salads, sandwiches, hors d'oeuvres, snacks and drinks. Some people prefer Greek olives over the regular black olives for their sandwich because they give more of a salty, briny, slightly bitter taste, particularly if sour pickles are added.

Olives are a source of fat even though it is the healthy monounsaturated fat that olive oil is known for. Ten olives (3 oz) or 5 large Greek olives may contain as much as 110 calories, 12 grams fat, and 690-750 mg sodium, especially if they are canned. Therefore, use them consciously because they can add to the total fat and sodium intake, especially if a high fat and salty salad dressing is also used.

## Calories Count, Even Those That Come From Good Fats

Though I encourage you to add more good fats to your daily meals, it is equally important to be moderate in your fat intake. As with carbohydrates, keep fats in line with your level of physical activity and, of course, your medical health. Fats are much denser in calories than proteins or carbohydrates. One gram of fat contains nine calories, which is twice the amount found in a gram of carbohydrate or protein. One gram of fat releases 9 calories and one gram of alcohol releases 7 calories; whereas, one gram of carbohydrate or protein releases 4 calories.

It is very easy to eat too many fats because they enhance the flavor and aroma of food – but you should not overindulge; otherwise, you could sabotage your weight loss effort. A small amount of fat in a tiny serving can provide lots of calories. For example, a teaspoon of olive oil, 1 tablespoon chopped almonds, 1 tablespoon (4 walnut halves), or 1½ teaspoons of peanut butter all contain about 45-50 calories. Increasing the serving size of olive oil to 1 tablespoon, almonds to 1 ounce (6 whole), walnuts to 12 halves (1 ounce), or peanut butter to 1.5 tablespoons triples the calories.

In the UDP meal plan, you will eat primarily monounsaturated and polyunsaturated fats mainly from olive and canola oils, fish, nuts, flaxseed, flax oil, and non-starchy dark green leafy vegetables. These fats are nutrient-dense, readily converted into energy, and can help counteract the effects of saturated fats and trans fat in the body. They also help maintain the fluidity and integrity of cell membranes, allowing the passage of nutrients, toxic waste products, and chemical signals into and out of the cells.

You will eat about 20-35% of calories as fat, 80% of which is monounsaturated fat and 20% of which is polyunsaturated fat (Omega-6 to Omega-3 in a ratio of 1:1 or 2:1). Naturally, you would get saturated fats from various sources, but their impact should be less if you choose lean cut of meat and low fat dairy products. All fats and oil contain some saturated fat. Canola oil, for example, has a high percentage of monounsaturated fats but also contains small amounts of Omega-6, Omega-3 and saturated fats – but you won't have to worry about the bad fats if you eat appropriate portions.

Before leaving this Chapter, I would like to restate the health benefits of the essential fatty acids (Omega-3 and Omega-6). In the meal plans that you will see later in Chapter 16, they are incorporated into your daily food intake so that you will obtain their full health benefits.

## Summary of the Functions of Omega-6 and Omega-3

- They are the main structural components of the body's cell membranes.
- They help prevent oxidative stress to the body's cell membranes.

- They are precursors of eicosanoides, hormone-like compounds that regulate the nervous system as well as essential body functions, such as blood pressure, heart rate, blood clotting, and reproduction.
- They play an active role in the body's inflammatory process (Omega-3 is anti-inflammatory, whereas, Omega-6 is pro-inflammatory).
- Omega-3 lubricates blood vessels and prevents blood clots, whereas Omega-6 decreases bleeding by promoting the formation of blood clot. They work in opposition to each other in order to regulate the various body functions. They are both essential for the body's homeostasis. On the other hand, they can cause the body to dysfunction if your diet is too high in one and low in the other (as is the case with the westernized diet).
- They form structural components of the top layer (epidermis) of the skin; therefore, they play a vital role in slowing down wrinkling and aging.
- They provide a source of energy for the body. Unlike saturated fats, which are readily stored, essential fatty acids are readily burned for energy.
- Not having adequate amounts of these essential fatty acids in our daily meals can increase our risk of major health problems (such as depression, weight gain, diabetes, heart disease, high blood pressure, arthritis, premature aging, and wrinkling). Some other well-known problems are loss of hair, loss of skin elasticity, brittle nails, craving, and fatigue. Having too much of one in the diet can also shift the balance towards needless inflammatory response that can damage tissues and organs of the body or weaken the body's response to acute injury or microbial invasion. The key is balance and we can work to correct the imbalance in our bodies by making sure we get adequate amounts of both essential fatty acids in our diet or supplement as needed.

# Chapter 13

# Fast Food and Restaurant Meals

## Serving Calories, Fats, and Salt

The food industry, fast food, and other restaurants serve super-sized portions that are high in calories, fats, refined carbohydrates, and salts and no doubt have contributed significantly to the obesity crisis in America and around the world. Furthermore, these foods are lacking in fiber and healthy fats like Omega-3 fatty acids and monounsaturated fats found in extra virgin olive oil and cold-pressed canola oil.

For example, a 32-ounce bottle of soda, a large French-fries, and a double Quarter Pounder with cheese delivers about 1,560 calories in a single meal (65 grams fat, 24 grams saturated fat, 9 grams trans fat, 201 grams carbohydrate, 95 grams sugar, 2,680 mg sodium, 166 mg cholesterol, and 10 grams fiber – 70% of the fiber comes from the French fries). This is the amount of calories for the entire day for the average sedentary individual. Particularly disturbing is the high amount of fat, carbohydrate, sugar, and sodium – all of which can increase the risk of insulin resistance, fat storage, and sub-clinical inflammation.

Americans seem to be getting fatter in direct relationship with the increasing consumption of restaurant meals and fast foods within the last 20-30 years. About 1 out of 3 American adults are obese, compared to 1 in 6 in the early 1960's. Among children, 1 in 3 are overweight or obese, a rate that doubled in the last twenty years.

## A Deadly Combination

Eating too many calories (high in fats, salt, and refined carbohydrates) and minimum physical activity is a deadly combination that accounts for 400,000 US deaths in the year 2000, according to the Center For Disease Control (CDC). It is not surprising that obesity-related causes now represent the second-leading cause of preventable death (after tobacco, with 435,000). It seems like we are eating ourselves to death and fast foods and restaurant meals are fueling the metabolic meltdown in many ways.

Eating too much unhealthy fast foods that are high in calories, fats, and refined carbohydrates and not being active causes weight gain and obesity which, in turn, increases the risk of Syndrome X, heart disease, diabetes, and cancer (just to name a few). Besides health problems, there is the enormous psychological impact it has on people, young and old.

Young children are particularly vulnerable and could develop low self-esteem very early on. They are the subjects of ridicule by their fellow schoolmates. They often try to cope by withdrawing from social events, including sports that have definite positive benefits. This anti-social behavior often leads to poor school performance and poor social skills in adulthood. It is therefore mandatory to help these kids break this vicious cycle from a very early age (see the story of Natasha in Chapter 18).

Americans spend more than $33 billion a year on weight loss products and services and the United States government spends about four times that amount. Yet, the solution to the obesity crisis is far from being resolved.

**Global Expansion of Fast Foods and Obesity**

Globally, about 1.2 billion people are estimated by the World Health Organization (WHO) to be overweight. The irony is that most of these people live in developing, impoverished nations where malnutrition still exists. Most experts believe that the exportation of fast foods globally is the catalyst for this trend as seen in the United States. This is not so difficult to understand if we look at the facts closely: In countries where fast food consumption increases, so does the obesity epidemic. Unfortunately, most of these countries (particularly the developing ones) are replacing traditional whole foods for fast and convenient foods that are grossly deficient in nutrients (see the Okinawa experience in Chapter 7). Worst of all is the misconception that modernization means abandoning their basic ethnic foundation to acquiring something else that is foreign to their natural environment, but nevertheless, viewed as an upward movement in society and class. Perhaps early intervention at the local, grass-roots level in some of these countries could help to halt the trend.

**Type 2 Diabetes – A Global Disease**

Type 2 diabetes, which previously affected mostly adults 40 years of age or older, has reached an epidemic proportion worldwide (and young children are not exempt). This is a phenomenon only seen in the last twenty years and coincides with the growth and expansion of fast foods, as well as inactivity (brought about by computers, video games, and passive school policies).

**Super-Sizing (Big Portion Sizes)**

A typical fast-food restaurant portion is big, as pointed out in Chapter 8. Big portions give customers the satisfaction of getting more for their money. But, as the portion size increases, so is the temptation to eat more, causing Americans who eat fast-food meals on a regular basis to gain weight.

A *McDonald's* double Quarter Pounder with cheese delivers about 730 calories, 40 grams of fat, and 19 grams of saturated fat. This is about 50% of the total calories in an average 1,500 calorie diet. The fat is too high even for a 2,000 calorie diet (to give you an idea, the total fat in a double Quarter Pounder is 62% of the recommended daily fat intake and saturated fat is 93%). Mind you, this is just a single meal.

A *Burger King* double Whopper value meal delivers over 2,000 calories – more than the total daily caloric intake for an average, moderately-active individual. It is much too easy to eat more than an entire day's worth of calories and fat in a single meal.

### Over-Fed and Under-Active Kids

Kids are easy victims of super-sizing. Fast food restaurants serve kids' menus that are loaded with calories, saturated fats, trans fats, and salts. Big meals, coupled with gross inactivity, fuel the surge of childhood obesity that is not only growing into a public health crisis, but also a very costly one. A quick glance at what kids are being served in some of these fast food places will give you a realistic reason why this is a crisis that needs serious intervention at all levels. For example, the Applebee's grilled cheese delivers a whopping 520 calories, 26 grams total fat and 1,350mg sodium. Adding French-fries increases calories to 900 and 44 grams of fat and 2,050 mg sodium – nearly a day's worth. Some of the other culprits are listed below:

| Meal | Calories | Total Fat (G) | Sodium (MG) |
|---|---|---|---|
| Outback Steakhouse Spotted Dog Sundae | 730 | 42 | 180 |
| Outback Steakhouse Boomerang-Cheeseburger<br>W/French-fries | 470<br>840 | 32<br>56 | 940<br>1,450 |
| Denny's Cheeseburgerlicious<br>W/French fries | 350<br>760 | 17<br>39 | 490<br>610 |
| Denny's The Big Cheese<br>W/French fries | 310<br>720 | 16<br>37 | 790<br>910 |
| Red Lobster Popcorn Shrimp & Fries | 430 | 23 | 1,310 |
| Olive Garden Spaghetti and Tomato Sauce | 310 | 2 | 570 |

Source: Center for Science in the Public Interest

Inflaming the crisis is the fact that more kids are eating their meals away from home than ever before and it's getting very difficult to find outside locations where kids can eat healthy – school cafeterias are no exceptions. Fast food machines are readily available in some well-populated schools, making it hard to resist what they offer. Traditional school recreations are now reserved for the few who can measure up. It used to be that all the kids were required to be out in the field, playing like kids should.

## Smaller, Not Necessarily Better

Some of the major fast foods and restaurant chains are now making changes. For instance, *McDonald's* is phasing out super-sized fries (7 oz) and drinks (42 oz). *Burger King's* bun-less Whopper has 3 grams of carbohydrates compared to 52 grams for a regular whopper – but this does not necessarily make it better. In the case of the bun-less burger, the fiber is reduced from 4 grams to less than 1 gram. There is also a reduction of vital nutrients: protein from 30 grams to 22 grams, including vitamins A, C, calcium, and iron. Interestingly, the difference in total fat and saturated fat between the two burgers is very small.

Vital nutrients including fiber, minerals, and vitamins are lost when the carbohydrate fraction of a meal is lowered too much. This can have negative health consequences. Bear in mind that the average American diet is already low in fiber (about 10-12 grams a day instead of the recommended 20-35 grams). Lowering the fiber further only makes the situation worse (as appetite and craving is increased and satiety is decreased). The simple, practical solution is to introduce more foods with fiber that can be conveniently served.

*McDonald's* took the challenge with the new *Fruit and Walnut Salad,* but it too needs a major makeover: The fat is high (13 grams), carbohydrate is high (44 grams), and the sugar is 32 grams (about 8 tsp). Sugar, both natural and synthetic, has the potential to raise blood sugar and insulin level, leading to increased inflammation. Most diabetics are well aware that even fruits can raise blood sugar quickly when the amount eaten surpasses the body's capacity to use. Again, it goes to the core of the problem that we should eat foods (regardless of their health benefits) based on our level of physical activity – and this should apply to all foods, particularly those that deliver energy (such as fruits, starchy vegetables, whole grains, and fats).

## Fast Food and Restaurant Salads Are Not Synonymous With Healthy Eating

Most fast food and restaurants are now offering salads in response to growing criticism of dishing out unhealthy foods. But most of these ready-made salads do not measure up to sound nutrition. Among the 34 surveyed from a variety of chains recently (including *McDonald's, Wendy's and Subway*), only a few salads met healthy standards. The study conducted by the Physicians Committee for Responsible Medicine (PCRM) found only two to be healthy salads – "Veggie Delite Salad" from *Subway* and the "Garden Salad" from *Au Bon Pain. McDonald's* crispy chicken bacon ranch salad with dressing scored the least with about 600 calories, 49 grams fat, and 1,530 mg sodium. Not surprising, the salad dressing adds extra fat – as it is a major source of fat in the American diet. However, it appears *McDonald's* has replaced it with the Bacon Ranch Salad with Crispy Chicken (340 calories, 16 grams fat, and 1,140 mg sodium).

Simply omitting the salad dressing in fast food restaurants will cut out significant amounts of bad fats and calories. The amount of sodium in fast foods is also a serious concern and poses serious health risk for those who have heart disease, stroke, and high blood pressure.

The fact is that healthy choices of salads are hard to find in fast foods and restaurants. The *Subway* Veggie Delite salad is discussed in detail later. The *Wendy's* Homestyle Chicken Strips salad delivers 440 total calories, 22 grams fat, 8 grams saturated fat and 1,180 mg sodium even without the salad dressing. Although this salad is made of fresh Romaine instead of nutrient deficient iceberg lettuce, some questions still remain. The ingredient list includes products with suspected health risks, such as high fructose corn syrup (dextrose, modified corn starch, fructose, and maltodextrin) and partially hydrogenated oils.

## Fast-Food Can Drain Energy and Depress Mood

You might have wondered why sometimes when you eat fast-food meals, you feel good initially with an instant boost of energy but, two to three hours later, you may feel exactly the opposite: tired, depressed, headache, and feeling hungry and empty again. Well, this has to do with the rapid spike in blood sugar and insulin level as a result of the soda, fries, or the buns – most of this has been covered previously. Some people may even experience abdominal bloating, severe pain, discomfort, and constipation due to lack of adequate fiber from non-starchy leafy vegetables, fruits, whole grains, beans, and lentils.

### Fast-Foods Are Highly Processed Foods

Fast-food meals are designed for convenience and consistency, flavor and texture, as a result, they are typically frozen, dehydrated, and highly processed. Typically, the foods you eat in fast food restaurants are mostly reheated frozen foods that have lost essential nutrients. To compensate for these artificial flavors, preservatives with unknown health risks are usually added (for more detail read the *Fast Food Nation*: *The Dark Side of the All-American Meal* by Eric Schlosser).

### Fast Foods and Processed Foods Are Heavy in Sodium (Salt)

Sodium makes food taste good and helps to regulate water balance and equalize the blood pH along with potassium. Both minerals are also involved in muscle activity. The average person eats more than 4,000 mg a day, most of it from restaurants and fast-food meals, including processed foods like frozen dinners, spaghetti, potato chips, and French-fries. The current federal recommendation is about 2,300 mg per day, the equivalent of a teaspoon. Some experts are even suggesting reducing the salt requirement to 1,500 mg a day for health reasons. A similar change in the blood pressure reading is also suggested. A blood pressure between 120-139/80-89 is considered pre-hypertension and likely to progress to full-blown hypertension without a healthy weight, exercise, and reduction of salt intake.

### Sodium (Salt) Raises Blood Pressure

There is a strong link between salt and blood pressure. Eating less salt lowers blood pressure and decreases a major risk for heart disease and stroke. Also, too much salt may cause fluid retention and swelling of the face and legs and increases the risk of developing high blood pressure, especially in people with a family history of high blood pressure. Too much salt in your diet can increase your risk or aggravate existing high blood pressure.

### Sodium (Salt) Is Found in Virtually All Foods

For those of us who are at risk, the challenge is to decrease our intake of salt. But this is not so easy considering the fact that sodium is found in virtually all foods (including seafood, milk, poultry, meat, and soft water). But the most troublesome sources of sodium most of us don't suspect are found in fast-foods and processed foods, including others about which we have not the slightest clue (soy sauce, MSG, baking soda, baking powder, sodium nitrate, nitrite, alginate, sulfite, citrate, and propionate).

Too much salt in your diet may lead to loss of potassium in the urine, causing potassium deficiency, which can increase the risk of heart attack, especially if you have heart disease and are on medication that depletes potassium (such as the water pills used to treat high blood pressure). Too much salt can also contribute to liver and kidney damage.

The simplest way to reduce salt intake is to measure out a small amount of table salt used in cooking, cut back on fast foods and processed foods, and cook with herbs and natural spices that are salt-free. Mrs. Dash claims to have no salt or MSG and has recently introduced a line of marinades. You should read food labels carefully for sodium content and stay within the recommended range of 2,300 mg or less and, if you have high blood pressure, about 1,500 mg or less.

## Taking Personal Responsibility

There are no easy solutions. But one thing is clear for sure and that is that we all have to assume personal responsibility for our own health. The first step is to become an educated consumer. You need to learn how to evaluate nutritional information in order to determine whether it is appropriate for you. You should be able to roughly estimate or at least be aware of the number of calories, fat, and salt that you consume in each meal. In this way, you can budget your caloric and nutritional intake much better. This will allow you to make appropriate adjustments.

As consumers, we need to demand healthier foods that are reasonably priced from fast food manufacturers and the government. We need to hold food manufacturers and chain restaurants to the higher standards that we do other institutions such as the medical community. They should label food more clearly so that it is easy to figure out the amount of calories in a serving as well the total amount of fat and carbohydrate in the product.

For example, *Coca Cola Classic* (medium) contains 210 calories and 58 grams of sugar in a 21 ounce serving size. This is misleading and gives the wrong impression. It's actuality the content of two serving sizes. In other words, if you drink the entire content, you are consuming twice the recommended amount of soda and sugar. A twenty-one ounce of coke contains about 15 teaspoons of sugar, which far exceeds the daily allowance, even for a 2,000-calorie diet. On the other hand, a twelve-ounce coke provides about 29 grams of sugar or around 7 teaspoons. Consuming 29 grams (7 tsp) of sugar (of pure energy) is bad enough for a single serving. However, a small amount of sugar in the diet is not a problem, but too much sugar is bad for your health. Sugar and refined carbohydrates raise inflammation levels and also contribute to obesity as discussed in previous chapters.

### New Rules

The government now requests that fast food and restaurants list detailed nutritional information, such as total calorie, fats, salt, and fiber counts for standard menu items in order to give customers important tools with which to make better choices about the food they consume. Some restaurants already provide nutritional information sheets at their retail locations and websites – but this is not enough. It is best if the calorie count and nutritional information is provided on menu boards. This will let consumers see at a glance how much calories and fat they are eating. Most health conscious consumers will be more likely to make healthier choices if they know the extent to which they are eating badly. Making the right information readily available will encourage health-conscious consumers to make healthier choices as well as cut back on extra calories and bad fats. It will also encourage restaurants to compete on the basis of nutrition and not just on their hefty portion sizes.

### The Heart of the Problem

Fast food and restaurants are not interested in the health and well-being of their customers. Their primary concern is profit and there is really no compelling reasons for them to replace a winning formula. Unless consumers demand more healthy foods (such as the use of healthier fats in cooking and food preparation), the fast food and restaurants really have no legal obligation to offer them. Morally they do! Taking personal responsibility means educating yourself about the foods that you are eating and their consequences on your mood, focus, energy, memory, and health. Now I will move on to discuss some common fast food meals.

## Common Fast Food Meals

### Criteria for Choosing Healthy Fast Food Meals

Eating out on a regular basis is a real challenge, but it doesn't have to be if you follow simple guidelines – provided that the nutritional information is available (or if you know what you want ahead of time). If you are a woman who is sedentary to slightly active (burning about 150- 250 calories a day in exercise or physical activity, such as walking casually daily) aim for 1,300-1,500 calories and for men 1,600-1,800 calories:

## Carbohydrates

Women should aim for about 1-2 servings (15-35 grams) of carbohydrate per meal, mostly whole grain, and no more than 10 grams of sugar per meal. For men, about 1-3 servings (15-45 grams) per meal should suffice. Sugar less than 15 grams per meal or serving. For your reference, a slice of bread contains about 15 grams carbohydrates and ½ cup cooked rice, pasta, mashed potatoes, corn and breakfast cereal contains about 22 grams carbohydrates.

## Fats

Fats are a major source of calories in the American diet. Therefore, pay close attention to the amount of fat in your diet. Women will do well if they cut fat intake to less than 19 grams per meal or a total of not more than 56 grams per day and men less than 23 grams per meal or a total of not more than 70 grams per day. Reference: 1 tbsp of any oil contains about 14 grams fat and 120 calories; 3 oz lean meat contains about 7 grams fat; 3 oz fatty fish like salmon contains about 9 grams fat, whereas, low fat fish like cod contains 0.5 grams fat. For comparison, a slice of full fat cheese (American, Swiss, etc.) contains 8-9 grams fat.

## Protein

Women, keep protein intake to 24-38 grams per meal or 65-114 grams per day (the equivalent of about 3-5 servings or about 8-14 ounces per day). Men will need about 24-48 grams of protein per meal or 80-140 grams per day (the equivalent of 3-6 servings or about 10-17 ounces per day). The key is to have good quality protein and enough in each meal to help boost metabolism and control craving. Reference: 3-ounce meat or fish contains about 24 grams protein.

## Cholesterol

Both women and men should keep dietary cholesterol levels around 100 mg per meal or 300 mg per day, the equivalent of a single medium whole egg.

## Fiber

You are eating healthy if you are getting about 20-35 grams of fiber per day and making sure that you are also getting soluble fiber and not just roughage. You can achieve this by making sure that you get about 7-10 grams of fiber per meal. Just remember that it doesn't matter how good and tasty a meal is – if it doesn't have enough fiber, it is like driving a car without brakes. Fiber supplements like Benefiber and Clearly Fiber can be useful in places where you suspect the fiber is low.

**Sodium**

Fast foods are notoriously high in salts and I have already discussed some of the health risks. Keep salt below 800 mg per meal or 2,300 mg or less per day and even lower if you have high blood pressure or at risk. Meals that contain over 800 mg of sodium should not be a regular part of your menu – though, occasional usage is not going to cause serious problems.

Staying within these rough guidelines will help you to choose low calorie, low-fat, and low-salt options and not risk eating more than an entire day's worth of calories, fat and salt in a single meal. Now that you know what to look for, let's begin the analysis of some of your favorite fast foods to see if they still meet your expectations:

## Salad Choices

***Wendy's* Mandarin Chicken Salad**

| S. Size | Cal | Fat (g) | Chol (mg) | Sodium (mg) | Carb/Sugar (g) | Protein (g) | Fiber (g) |
|---|---|---|---|---|---|---|---|
| 1 each | 170 | 2 | 60 | 480 | 17/11 | 23 | 4 |

*Wendy's* Mandarin Chicken salad is a good pick without the high fat and salt dressing. It also has adequate protein. The *Wendy's* Spring Mix salad – with 11 grams total fat, 12 grams carbohydrate, 5 grams fiber, and 230 mg sodium – appears to be a healthy choice too. It has 11 grams protein, which can be further improved by adding one boiled egg, egg whites, textured vegetable protein or light mozzarella string cheese stick. You can also reduce the total fat and saturated fat by omitting the cheese. The Chicken BLT Salad and the Taco Supreme Salad are also reasonable choices, provided you omit the cheese. In the case of the Chicken BLT salad, this will significantly reduce the fat (18 grams) and the sodium (840 mg). Choosing a low-fat, low-sodium salad dressing is critically important as well (see *Wendy's* dressing below).

*Wendy's* Homestyle Chicken Strips Salad has 22 grams fat and 1,180 mg sodium and, therefore, is not a healthy choice. The *Wendy's* Fresh Fruit Bowl Salad seems to be healthy, but has 28 grams sugar (about 7 tsp) per serving and, even though it has romaine lettuce, the pineapple, cantaloupe, honeydew, and grapes are contributing to the sugar – three of the four fruits are high-glycemic.

You recall that these tropical fruits can raise blood sugar and insulin levels rapidly if the concentration of carbohydrate or sugar is high. This is exactly the case here and I have pointed out before that it really doesn't matter where the sugar comes from – it may still raise inflammation levels, especially if you are not eating adequate non-starchy dark green leafy vegetables like kale, collard greens, and broccoli with your meals. This is not easily feasible in a fast food restaurant, but you can still overcome this problem if you are seriously concerned about your health.

On the other hand, the *Wendy's* Fresh Fruit Cup Salad and the Mandarin Orange Cup Salad have 17 grams sugar (4 tsp) and eating half the serving is not a bad idea at all (reducing sugar to 8.5 grams or about 2 tsp).

Other *Wendy's* Side Salads (Caesar Side Salad and the Side Salad) are also recommended without the fatty and salty dressings and croutons. For example, the Caesar Side Salad has 4.5 grams fat, adding a pack of Caesar Dressing raises total fat to 20.5 grams, and adding a pack of croutons brings the fat to 23.5 grams. The total sodium count contributed by the salad, dressing and croutons is 515 mg, compared to the salad alone (150 mg).

***Subway* Salads With 6 Grams of Fat or Less: Veggie Delite**

| Serving Size | Cal | Fat (G) | Chol (MG) | Sodium (MG) | Carb (G) | Protein (G) | Fiber |
|---|---|---|---|---|---|---|---|
| 11.5 oz | 60 | 1 | 0 | 85 | 12 | 3 | 4 |

The *Subway* Veggie Delite is among the best choices of *Subway*'s "under-6 salads," but it is not filling. Nevertheless, it's a good side salad. The major problem is that the protein is very low, but you can improve it by adding an extra protein source, such as 2 egg whites, a slice of lean low sodium meat (ham, turkey, chicken), ½ cup low-fat cottage cheese, low-fat mozzarella string cheese, or 3 ounces of canned tuna if you are ordering out.

Other favorite *Subway* picks are salads with 6 grams of fat or less:

- Grilled Chicken Breast and Baby Spinach
- Grilled Chicken Breast Strips
- Roast Beef
- Savory Turkey Breast
- Turkey Breast and Ham
- Ham (salt 850 mg)
- Subway Club (salt 880 mg)

Most of these salads are low in calories, fat and salt. However, the protein is low in some of them and adding an extra protein source will enhance nutritional quality (roast beef, ham, and turkey breast).

Another area that needs improvement is the fiber fraction, which is bare minimum. You can overcome this drawback by adding to your salad extra fiber sources (such as ¼ cup of textured vegetable protein, 1-2 tbsp ground flaxseeds, wheat germ, oat bran, fruit, or a side dish of broccoli, etc). These also add nutrients that help to enhance the quality of the meal (such as Omega-3, vitamin E, folic acid and lignans).

The rest of the *Subway* salads are not recommended because they are very high in fat and salt. For example, the BMT Salad delivers 290 calories, 19 grams fat, and 1,360 grams salt without dressing or croutons. The Cold Cut Combo also has 1,140 grams salt. The Seafood Sensation Salad, which used to be in this group, appears to be discontinued. It delivered 480 calories, 36 grams fat, and 1,160 grams salt. This clearly shows that *Subway* is indeed seriously concerned about the health and weight of its customers.

***McDonald's* Salads: Caesar Salad With Grilled Chicken**

| Serving Size | Cal | Fat (g) | Chol (mg) | Sodium (mg) | Carb/sugar (g) | Protein (g) | Fiber (g) |
|---|---|---|---|---|---|---|---|
| 9.8 oz | 220 | 6 | 75 | 880 | 12/5 | 30 | 3 |

The *McDonald's* Grilled Chicken Caesar Salad is a favorite pick, although the sodium is slightly high. The trick is to use a salad dressing that would not add extra fat and salt. Unfortunately, there is no such dressing in the *McDonald's* franchise; so, you would have to bring your own (such as lemon and herb dressing). The Newman's Own Cobb dressing is the best *McDonald's* has – a pack of the dressing contains 440 mg sodium and 9 grams fat. Using the entire salad dressing on the grilled chicken Caesar salad will raise the sodium to 1,270 mg, which is undesirable. The proper strategy will be to use only half of the dressing, as this will reduce the sodium content (1,050 mg) and will make the salad slightly better than the first presentation.

You will also get a healthier nutritional profile if you omit the cheese and the croutons (the cheese contributes most of the fat: A slice of Swiss, American, or Provolone contains 8-9 grams fat). The *McDonald's* Caesar Salad without Chicken is a very light salad with a salt content of 170 mg. It has only 90 calories per serving, therefore you can double the serving size or use as a side dish. The Bacon Ranch Salad without chicken is also a good side salad (290 mg salt), whereas the California Cobb Salad without chicken is not – because of the salt (410 mg per serving).

*McDonald's* new arrival, the Fruit and Walnut Salad, delivers 310 calories, 44 grams carbohydrate and 32 grams sugar in a single meal – this is problematic (as already pointed out for *Wendy's* own Fresh Fruit Bowl).

Below are the *McDonald's* salads that I do not recommend because they are either high in fat, salt, or both. However, it doesn't mean that you can't have them occasionally as long as you avoid adding other ingredients that will increase health risk significantly, such as soft drinks and French fries. These are the ones that can potentially raise serious health risks or worsen already existing medical conditions, such as heart disease, diabetes, arthritis, and high blood pressure. For example, the California Cob Salad with Crispy Chicken has 360 calories, 18 grams fat, and 1,250 mg salt. Here are others that fall under this category:

- The Bacon Ranch Salad with Grilled Chicken (1,000 mg sodium)
- Bacon Ranch Salad with Crispy Chicken (16g fat, 1,140 mg sodium)
- Caesar Salad with Crispy Chicken (1,020 mg sodium)
- California Cobb Salad with Grilled Chicken (1,110 mg sodium)

***Burger King* Salads: Fire-Grilled Chicken Caesar Salad**

| S. Size | Cal | Fat (g) | Chol (mg) | Sodium (mg) | Carb/sugar (g) | Protein (g) | Fiber (g) |
|---|---|---|---|---|---|---|---|
| 10.3 oz | 190 | 7 | 50 | 900 | 9/1 | 25 | 1 |

This *Burger King* Fire-Grilled Chicken Caesar Salad is definitely a favorite pick, even though the sodium content is slightly over the cutoff point. Again, avoid the dressings that are high in fat and sodium (see *Burger King* dressing below). I also recommend that you cut your salt intake in subsequent meals, in order to be within the recommended amount per day.

The *Burger King* Side Garden Salad is a good choice for a side salad (20 calories, 0 fat, and 15 mg sodium). The Fire-Grilled Shrimp Caesar Salad is also a good pick (180 calories, 10 grams fat, and 20 grams protein); however, the fiber is low (2 grams) and the cholesterol (120 mg) is high due to the shrimp – but this is no real concern (you will have to eat a lot of shrimp for your blood cholesterol to be adversely affected).

Similarly, the *Burger King* Fire-Grilled Shrimp Garden Salad is a reasonable option (200 calories, 10 grams fat, and 21 grams protein) even though the sodium is slightly high (900 mg) and so is the cholesterol (120 mg). Another choice that is worth considering is the Fire-Grilled Chicken Garden Salad (210 calories, 7 grams fat, 26 grams protein, and 910 mg sodium). Across the board, the salads are all low in fiber and it would help if you have your own extra source of fiber as a security policy.

Below are the *Burger King* salads that I would not recommend – they are either high in fat, salt, or both.

- TENDERCRISP Chicken Caesar Salad (390 calories, 22g fat, 1,160 mg sodium)
- TENDERCRISP Chicken Garden Salad (410 calories, 22g fat, 1,170 mg sodium)

## Salad Dressings

Salad dressings are a major source of extra fats, salts, and sugar and, therefore, it is important to read the labels carefully so you can make healthier choices. Sometimes, it is best that you omit the dressing if you can't get a healthy choice. You can save on calories, salt, and fat by reading the small salad dressing packets you are given. In this section, I will help you to pick salad dressings that are healthy if you are eating in a restaurant or a fast food place. If the nutritional information is not available, I will suggest that you skip the dressing for just vinegar or lemon juice and black ground pepper for flavor.

When choosing salad dressings, pay attention to the fat, sodium, and sugar, which could add many more unhealthy ingredients to your salad. For example, croutons add calories, fat and salt: ½ ounce delivers 70 calories, 3 grams fat and 200 mg sodium. Mayonnaise adds fat, sodium, and extra calories and so forth. It is important to know that fast food places serve a combination of healthy and unhealthy meals because they are in the business of making a profit. They have always defended their position by arguing that it is the customer's responsibility to make the choices that are right for them. To some extent, they are right. The fast food franchises are not responsible for the bad choices you make, provided that they also have healthy food choices that you can pick from.

On the other extreme, there are those who hold the view that everything that comes from a fast food place is bad for your weight and health. Frankly, you can find some healthy selections of meals if you know what to look for and, more importantly, what to avoid. The salad dressing area is the obvious pitfall for most people and one reason for this is that the small packages usually look so nice and non-threatening. Some are given names of celebrities we love and admire – making them seem less threatening. As we go through the different salad dressings that are offered by the major fast foods places, you should be well-equipped to make better choices.

***Subway* Salad Dressings**

| S. Size | Cal | Fat (g) | Chol (mg) | Sodium (mg) | Carb/sugar (g) | Protein (g) | Fiber (g) |
|---|---|---|---|---|---|---|---|
| **Ranch** 2 oz | 200 | 22 | 10 | 550 | 1/0 | 1 | 1 |
| **Fat Free Italian** 2 oz | 35 | 0 | 0 | 720 | 7/4 | 1 | 0 |
| **Atkins Honey Mustard** 2 oz | 200 | 22 | 0 | 510 | 1/0 | 0 | 0 |

Clearly, you can see that these three popular *Subway* salad dressings have major problems: either the fat is very high or the salt is too high. If the small salad dressing gives you so much fat and salt, it's obvious that additional fat and salt from your main meal will throw you off the curve. Now this is what you do:

The Fat Free Italian dressing has the least calories, but the salt is a concern. However, if you use only half of the content, you can decrease the salt by 50% (360 mg), which makes it slightly better. The Ranch and the *Atkins* Honey Mustard are poor choices. They are high in calories and fat. Even half the package will still give enough fat for a major meal and, yet, this is only the dressing.

***McDonald's* Salad Dressings**

| S. Size | Cal | Fat (G) | Chol (MG) | Sodium (MG) | Carb (G) | Sugar (G) | Fiber |
|---|---|---|---|---|---|---|---|
| **Newman's Own Low-fat Balsamic Vinaigrette** 1 pack | 40 | 3 | 0 | 730 | 4 | 3 | 0 |
| **Newman's Own Cobb Dressing** 1 pack | 120 | 9 | 10 | 440 | 9 | 5 | 0 |

Newman's Own Low-fat Balsamic vinaigrette dressing is low in fat and calories, but the salt is problematic. One way around the salt is to use only half the pack and make sure that you choose a meal that is low in salt. The Newman's Own Cobb Dressing has the lowest salt (440 mg), but it has 9 grams fat. I suggest that you use half a pack, as this will reduce both the fat and salt – a remarkable improvement.

Newman's Own Low-fat Family Recipe Italian Dressing is low in fat (2.5 grams), but high in salt (680 mg). It could be a reasonable pick, provided you limit usage to a half pack and only with low-salt meals. Newman's Own Creamy Caesar dressing is high in fat (18 grams) and calories (190 calories) and should not be a choice.

***Wendy's* Salad Dressings**:

The favorite picks in the *Wendy's* salad dressings are listed below. However, I suggest that you use half the serving in order to reduce fat, sugar, and salt.:

- Fat Free French Style (1pkt, 80 cal, 0 fat, 210 mg sodium, 16g sugar)
- Low-fat Honey Mustard (1pkt, 110 cal, 3g fat, 340 mg sodium, 16g sugar)
- Reduced Fat Creamy Ranch (1pkt, 100 cal, 8g fat, 550 mg sodium, 3g sugar)
- Salsa (1 each, 30 cal, 0 fat, 440 mg sodium)

I do not endorse the following *Wendy's* salad dressings because they are loaded with fat, sugar, and salt:

- Creamy Ranch Dressing (1pkt, 230 cal, 23g fat, 580 mg sodium)
- Oriental Sesame Dressing (1pkt, 250 cal, 19g fat, 560 mg sodium, 18g sugar)
- House Vinaigrette Dressing (1pkt, 190 cal, 18g fat, 750 mg sodium)

***Burger King's* Salad Dressings**:

- Honey Mustard, Fat-Free Dressing (1pkt, 70 cal, 0 fat, 230 mg sodium)
- Garden Ranch Dressing (1 pkt, 120 cal, 10g fat, 610 mg sodium)
- Tomato Balsamic Vinaigrette (1 pkt, 110 cal, 9g fat, 760 mg sodium)
- Sweet Onion Vinaigrette (1 pkt, 100 cal, 8g fat, 960 mg sodium)

The Honey Mustard, Fat-Free Dressing appears to be the best choice, but the sugar (15g or 4 tsp) could be a problem for some people with diabetes, insulin resistance syndrome, or obesity. Using only half the dressing is suggested if it's your favorite pick. You can do the same for both the Garden Ranch Dressing and the Tomato Balsamic Vinaigrette. As for the Sweet Onion Vinaigrette Dressing, the sodium would still be a problem even for half the serving. It should not be your choice if you have high blood pressure or history of it.

## Sandwich Choices

***Subway* Sandwiches (Low Sodium) With 6 Grams of Fat or Less: 6" Veggie Delite**

| S. Size | Cal | Fat (G) | Chol (MG) | Sodium (MG) | Carb (G) | Protein (G) | Fiber |
|---|---|---|---|---|---|---|---|
| 5.9 oz | 230 | 3 | 0 | 520 | 44 | 9 | 4 |

The *Subway* 6" veggie Delite is a good pick, however, the carbohydrate fraction may be too high for individuals with Syndrome X or sedentary. The carbohydrate is high glycemic – eating only half of the bread reduces the carbohydrate by 50% and this may be suitable for someone who is sedentary (to give you a reference point, 1 slice of bread contains about 15 grams carbohydrates, 2 slices contain 30 grams, and 3 slices 45 grams carbohydrates. Most people don't normally eat three slices of bread in one setting, so why should you eat the carbohydrate equivalent of 3 slices or more?). You recall that a high carbohydrate load meal is mostly suitable for a physically active individual who can burn the calories. On the other hand, sedentary individuals risk storing body fat and gaining weight, as well as raising inflammation levels, especially if it's high glycemic.

The fiber is low, but can be enhanced by the addition of a fiber source (such as alfalfa sprouts, flaxseeds, raw carrots, cucumber, berries, other small fruits, or Benefiber or Clearly Fiber). The high ratio of carbohydrate to protein is not nutritionally balanced. Adding diced egg white, tofu, or soy protein can help to increase the protein fraction. Increasing the protein content could help to stabilize blood sugar levels.

The 6" Roast Beef Sandwich is a reasonable choice and has the second lowest sodium content of its group (920 mg). However, like the other sandwiches in this group, the carbohydrates range from 44-59 grams. For this reason, you should choose a sandwich made from a low glycemic grain, such as sourdough bread, multigrain, or oat bran bread (you can take your own). Highly refined breads, such as white Italian bread, deli roll, or wrap (made with bleached enriched wheat flour) can trigger craving and compulsive eating, especially when the carbohydrate load is high.

The rest of the 6" low-fat sandwiches are far from being heart-friendly meals if you have chronic health problems. The sodium ranges from 1,020-1,310 mg and even some favorites like the Turkey Breast Sandwich and the Oven Roasted Chicken Breast Sandwich are no exceptions (see the chart below). A simple solution is to eat only half the serving size, as this will reduce the salt and carbohydrate load, but this will also reduce the protein and fiber. You could compensate by adding some extra protein and fiber sources.

***Subway* Sandwiches (High Sodium) With 6 Grams of Fat or Less**

| S. Size | Cal | Fat (g) | Chol (mg) | Sodium (mg) | Carb (g) | Protein (g) | Fiber (g) |
|---|---|---|---|---|---|---|---|
| **6" Turkey Breast** 7.9 oz | 280 | 4.5 | 20 | 1020 | 46 | 18 | 4 |
| **6" Subway Club** 9.1 oz | 320 | 6 | 35 | 1310 | 47 | 24 | 4 |

Other *Subway* 6" low-fat sandwiches that are not recommended are:

- Ham (47g carb, 1,230 mg sodium)
- Oven Roasted Chicken Breast (47g carb, 1,020 mg sodium)
- Turkey Breast (46g carb, 1,020 mg sodium)
- Turkey Breast and Ham (47g carb, 1,230 mg sodium)
- Sweet Onion Chicken Terriyaki (59g carb, 1,310 mg sodium)

### *Subway* Deli Sandwiches

Unlike the Cold Sandwiches, the *Subway* Deli Sandwiches are relatively low in calories, fat, and sodium. The carbohydrate portions are appropriate for individuals who are physically active or eat only half of the sandwich if you are sedentary. However, there are two concerns: the protein and fiber are low and need to be boosted.

- Ham Deli
- Roast Beef Deli
- Turkey Breast Deli
- Tuna Deli

### *Subway* Cold Sandwiches

They are all high in fat, salt or both and not good choices. For example, the Cold Cut Combo is 8.9 oz and contains 410 calories, 17 grams fat, and 1,550 mg sodium. The 6" Tuna Sandwich has 31grams fat, which is extremely high – the mayonnaise adds to the fat and salt (1,030 mg). The fiber is almost consistently low. This is usually true of fast food meals.

### The *Subway* Hot Sandwiches

The sandwiches in this group are not recommended because they are uniformly high in calories, fat, or sodium. The Cheese Steak (360 cal, 10 grams fat, 1,100 mg sodium) would make the cut if you omit the cheese. To give you a better understanding why you should avoid this group, consider the stats of the Meatball Marinara (561 calories, 24g fat, 63g carb, 1,610 mg sodium) and the Italian BMT (560 calories, 21g fat, 47g carb, 1,790 mg sodium). The others are just as bad.

- Chicken Bacon Ranch (25g fat, 1,400 mg sodium)
- Chipotle Southwest Cheese Steak (25g fat, 1,200 mg sodium)
- Spicy Italian (25g fat, 1,670 mg sodium)
- *Subway* Melt (12g fat, 1,600 mg sodium)

***Burger King* Original Whopper Jr.**

| S. Size | Cal | Fat (G) | Chol (MG) | Sodium (MG) | Carb (G) | Protein (G) | Fiber |
|---|---|---|---|---|---|---|---|
| 5.6 oz | 390 | 22 | 45 | 550 | 31 | 17 | 2 |
| 5.3 oz w/o mayo | 310 | 13 | 40 | 490 | 31 | 17 | 2 |
| 2.7 oz low carb | 140 | 10 | 40 | 140 | 1 | 11 | 0 |

The *Burger King* Original Whopper Jr. is high in fat. However, if you omit the mayonnaise, it is possible to reduce the fat by almost half. Omission of the cheese also reduces calories, fat, and salt. Even though this burger is intended for a child's meal, it is quite adequate for an adult if you use a low sodium lite mayonnaise. The fiber fraction is low, but can be improved by adding extra fiber. The low-carb version of the Whopper Jr. is the lowest in fat, sodium, and carbohydrates, but it lacks fiber. It may not be a good choice.

The Chicken Whopper Sandwich is high in calories, fat, and sodium (570 cal, 25 grams fat, and 1,410 mg sodium). Omission of the mayonnaise decreases calories and fat substantially, but not sodium (1,280 mg). This sandwich should not be on your list.

***Burger King* BK Veggie Burger**

| S. Size | Cal | Fat (G) | Chol (MG) | Sodium (MG) | Carb (G) | Protein (G) | Fiber |
|---|---|---|---|---|---|---|---|
| 6.6 oz | 380 | 16 | 5 | 930 | 46 | 14 | 4 |
| 6.3 oz w/o mayo | 300 | 7 | 0 | 870 | 46 | 14 | 4 |

This meatless sandwich is preferred without the mayonnaise dressing, which adds extra calories, fat, and sodium. It is best that you eat only half of the bun if you are inactive in order to prevent sugar overload. If you are active, then it is proper to eat the whole burger in one meal. For dressing, use reduced fat dressings, such as low sodium light mayonnaise, ketchup, and mustard.

***McDonald's* Sandwich**

| S. Size | Cal | Fat (g) | Chol (mg) | Sodium (mg) | Carb/ Sugar (g) | Protein (g) | Fiber (g) |
|---|---|---|---|---|---|---|---|
| **Hamburger sandwich (plain)** 3.7 oz | 260 | 9 | 30 | 530 | 33/7 | 7 | 1 |
| **Double Quarter Pounder w/cheese** 9.9 oz | 730 | 40 | 160 | 1330 | 46 | 9 | 3 |

The plain hamburger is the best choice among the *McDonald's* sandwiches – it is low in fat, cholesterol, and sodium and the carbohydrate portion is modest. However, the fiber is very low and the protein is average to poor. At any rate, you can still have it, preferably with a dressing that is low in fat and sodium (such as low sodium lite mayonnaise or mustard) and omit the whole fat cheese. Follow the methods described earlier to increase protein and fiber, including using fiber supplements (Benefiber or Clearly Fiber) and even ground flaxseeds or textured vegetable protein.

Other *McDonald's* sandwiches that are modest in fat and sodium and therefore meet healthy standards are listed below (* these are high in fat):

- Cheeseburger (310 calories, 12g fat, 740 mg sodium)
- Quarter Pounder (420 calories, 18g fat, 730 mg sodium)
- Filet-O-Fish (400 calories, 18g fat, 640 mg sodium)
- Big N' Tasty (470 calories, 23g fat, 790 mg sodium)*
- McChicken (370 calories, 16g fat, 810 mg sodium)
- Hot'n Spicy McChicken (440 calories, 24g fat, 920 mg sodium)*

The *McDonald's* Double Quarter Pounder with cheese is a health hazard with a fat and salt content of over 50% of an entire day's needs. The total fat is 40 grams, saturated fat is 19 grams, and, to make matters worse, the fiber is only 3 grams in a meal that delivers 730 calories. The rest of these *McDonald's* sandwiches fall under the cautionary category, if not the 'completely avoid' category:

- Quarter Pounder w/Cheese (510 cal, 25g fat, 1,150 mg sodium)
- Double Cheeseburger (480 cal, 23g fat, 1,140 mg sodium)
- Big N' Tasty w/Cheese (520 cal, 26g fat, 1,010 mg sodium)
- Big Mac (560 cal, 30g fat, 1,010 mg sodium, 46g carb, 3g fiber)
- Premium Crispy Chicken Club (660 cal, 29g fat, 1,800 mg sodium, *63g carb*)
- Premium Crispy Chicken Classic (490 cal, 29g fat, 1,800 mg sodium, *62g carb*)
- Premium Grilled Chicken Ranch (480 cal, 13g fat, 1,590 mg sodium 53g *carb*)
- Premium Grilled Chicken Club (580 cal, 21g fat, 1,660 mg sodium)
- Premium Crispy Chicken Ranch (570 cal, 20g fat, 1,730 mg sodium, *64g carb)*
- Premium Grilled Chicken Classic (410 cal, 9g fat, 1,210 mg sodium)
- Chicken McGrill (400 cal, 16g fat, 1,010 mg sodium, *52g carb*)
- Crispy Chicken (500 cal, 23g fat, 1,090 mg sodium, *50g carb*)

Note the differences between a double Cheeseburger and a single Cheeseburger: The single Cheeseburger is a much smaller portion and thus contains less calories, fat, and sodium (4.2 oz, 310 cal, 12g fat, 740 mg sodium). As a rule, you tend to eat healthier when the portion size is reduced.

***McDonald's* Fruit 'n Yogurt Parfait**

| S. Size | Cal | Fat (g) | Chol (mg) | Sodium (mg) | Carb/Sugar (g) | Fiber (g) |
|---|---|---|---|---|---|---|
| 5.3 oz | 160 | 2 | 5 | 85 | 31/21 | < 1 |
| 5.0 oz w/o granola | 130 | 2 | 5 | 55 | 25/19 | 0 |

Both items are high in sugar and I suggest that, for a treat, you have only half the serving. This will reduce sugar intake to about 5-10 grams per meal, the equivalent of 1-2 teaspoons.

## Eating Out Without Sabotaging Your Weight Loss Goal

### Plan Ahead

Choose a restaurant location that offers a variety of healthy options. This will increase the chance that you will eat healthy, especially if you plan ahead and know what you want. Snack or eat something nutritious, but light before going out to eat, such as a fruit, vegetable salad or vegetable soup. This may help you avoid the temptation to overeat. This step is particularly important if you are going to a party. It is difficult to think rationally when you are hungry and your emotions are out of control. Do not wait until you are hungry before going out to a fast food place or restaurant since you may be tempted to make some bad choices. This is one moment when will-power will let you down.

### Snacking

When snacking, read the label carefully in order to determine the actual serving size of the product as it may contain more than one serving size – and eating the entire package may deliver two or three times the calories and fat you need. To avoid the temptation to overeat, measure out your snacks into small serving portions that you put aside. Another trick is to buy snacks in small individual packages that contain small portions so that you limit the amount you eat.

## Reducing Fat and Calories

### Avoid Value Meals

Proportion your calories so as to avoid eating an entire day's worth of calories and fat in a single meal. This is very easy to do since fast food and restaurant meals are high in fats and calories and are served in large portions. One way to avoid this problem is to order regular size meals instead of jumbo sizes. For example, order a plain hamburger and small French-fries with water or a small diet soda instead of a *McDonald's* Quarter Pounder with large fries and large soda.

Avoid value meals and economy-size meals and drinks unless you are willing to share with someone else or take home some of the meal for the next day. Choose an appetizer, such as a non-starchy green vegetable salad, fresh fruits or fruit cocktail, steamed seafood, or shrimp cocktail. For dressing, use lemon juice, vinegar, or another reduced fat dressing instead of a high sodium cocktail sauce, salsa, or full fat dressing.

Begin your meal with a vegetable salad or vegetable soup (without white pasta, potatoes, corn, too many beans, or high-sodium broth). This will help to fill you up so that you reduce your portion of the main course. Ideally, you should avoid soups made of cream and high cholesterol egg yolks (including creamy chowder because of its high fat and starch content). Choose low sodium broth or canned tomato-based soups with low sodium. Also, limit butter sauce, cheese, meat, and whole eggs in your salad and other entrees, except when you are in control of the preparation itself.

**Salads**

Choose romaine, arugula, red leaf lettuce, spinach, or other leafy vegetables with high nutrients for salad without the croutons, cheese, whole eggs, or bacon. Iceberg lettuce is very low in nutrients in comparison to romaine or arugula. Choose a dressing with low fat, low sugar, and low sodium. Use lemon juice or vinegar if you can't find a suitable dressing with fresh black pepper. Don't fall into the trap of using more than you need of mayonnaise or other dressings made with olive oil or canola oil that are healthy – they too can add extra calories and cause weight gain. Limit the traditional chef salads, Caesar, Greek, and taco salad, since they usually contain large amounts of meat, cheese and eggs and can be high in calories, fat and cholesterol. However, you can also specify the ingredients you want in your salad.

**Entrée**

Better choices are items that are baked, grilled, poached, roasted, steamed, or broiled without added butter, gravy or cheese sauce. Lean meats and non-starchy green vegetables (not including potatoes and corn) are usually low in fat if sautéed or stir-fried in a small amount of oil, water, or low-sodium chicken or meat broth. These include fish or un-breaded chicken breast (broiled or grilled).

A veggie sandwich or garden salad with low-fat or fat-free dressing without the eggs and cheese are also good choices. Avoid fried dishes and others that are creamed, fricasseed, sautéed, or stir-fried in heavy oil, especially vegetable oil or butter. Even foods fried in healthier oils (olive and canola oil) can also add extra calories. Also avoid dishes that are stuffed, broasted, buttered, breaded, or basted. Ask for the sauce to be served on the side.

**Side Dish**

Steamed, non-starchy green vegetables, fresh vegetables, or a small amount of rice (½-1 cup *Uncle Ben's* or brown rice if they have it), a small 2-3 oz baked sweet potato or boiled new potato (2-4 small round potatoes – eat with the skin), or ½ cup or a few tablespoons of beans or lentils are all good choices. Avoid French-fries, fried onion rings, potato chips, potato salads, and macaroni salads (heavy in mayonnaise and high-glycemic). You can also request that your dish be prepared without butter, margarine, salt, or high-sodium seasonings like soy sauce.

### Desserts

Desserts are a source of fats and empty calories that you should limit. But, if you must have desert, make sure you budget the calories, fat, carbohydrate, and sugar that it contributes into your overall meal. Always keep portion size small and make healthy choices, such as fresh low-glycemic fruits (apples, fruit cocktail, baked or grilled fruits, plain cake with fruit puree, and sorbet). Flavored, decaffeinated coffee with skim milk or green or herbal tea is good too. Avoid milkshakes, sugary cakes, pies, and sundaes with syrups, except for occasional treats.

### Condiments

Limit olives, salty pickles, and sauerkraut, which can be high in sodium, especially if you have high blood pressure. Other high sodium sources that you can reduce are ketchup, mustard, mayonnaise, commercial salsa, and other sauces. For flavor, use spices, herbs, dried peppers, ginger, black pepper, paprika, or lemon juice. Avoid adding extra table salt. Mrs. Dash has seasonings without salt and MSG.

Paying attention to the condiments that you add to your sandwiches can also help to reduce fat, salt, and calories. Below are some healthy choices that you can pick from:

- Vinegar (1 tsp) and olive oil blend (1 tsp): 5 grams of healthy fats, 0 sugar and 0 sodium
- Light mayonnaise (1 tbsp): 5 calories, 0 sugar and 100 mg sodium
- Mustard yellow or deli brown (2 tsp): 0 fat, 0 sugar and 115 mg sodium
- Fat free red wine vinaigrette (2 tbsp): 0 fat, 3 g sugar and 340 mg sodium

## Controlling Your Appetite

### Bread

In a sit-down restaurant, do not be tempted to start your meal with bread and butter. Most of the bread served in fast food restaurants is made with refined white flour and can cause a surge in insulin levels that increase your appetite and make you eat more food. It's best to have the bread after your vegetable salad or greens – this will give you better control.

It is also better if you have a multigrain, 100% whole-wheat bread or sourdough bread instead of white refined bread (such as rolls, garlic bread, French bread, Italian bread, biscuits, croissants, muffins, bagels, or bread sticks). These are usually high in fat and calories and mostly served in large portion sizes. Also limit crackers – they can be high in both trans fats and sodium and it is easy to eat more than you need.

Ideally, bread and carbohydrates are best eaten with the main course as a side dish and not as a starter. This gives you a better control of your energy source, especially if your bread is refined white flour bread.

### Buffet

Avoid going to buffets since you may be tempted to eat enormous portions of high-calorie foods that you didn't intend to, especially if you are hungry. Buffets are cheap, but the price you may have to pay afterwards is many times more. There is also the risk of contacting infectious diseases, such as the flu causing virus and the fecal bacteria that causes serious upset stomach and weakness (E. coli). Contaminations of food by direct contact or airborne is more common in buffet environment than we would like to believe.

## Beverage

### Limit Sodas

They are loaded with sugars and empty calories. So are juices that are sweetened with sugar. Remember that an 8 oz serving of grape juice may contain 40 grams or 10 teaspoons of sugar and an orange juice, 22 grams or 6 teaspoons of sugar – they have no fiber or nutrients. You are better off if you choose water or water with lemon or flavored sparkling water (non caloric), juice spritzer (half fruit juice and half sparkling water), iced tea, low sodium tomato juice, or diet soda with splenda. However, there is nothing harmful in occasionally having unsweetened juices, such as apple and orange juice but, nutritionally, the whole fruit is always the best.

### Coffee

It's a huge problem and can easily add extra calories and fats because of the serving size and the added ingredients – whole milk, cream, and sugar. For example, coffee mocha with low-fat milk has 302 calories and 16 grams of fat; whipped cream and coffee mocha with whole milk has 340 calories and 20 grams of fat. The whipped cream and one tablespoon of half and half have about 50 calories and 5 grams of fat.

If you must have coffee, ask for the regular 8 oz size and use fat-free milk instead of whole milk and a small amount of sugar or substitutes such as Splenda or Stevia (1 pack). Also order coffee without whipped cream, flavored syrup, chocolate, or candy pieces.

Caffeinated or decaffeinated green tea with high levels of antioxidants is a good choice – it can help fight diseases. It also has compounds that help burn body fat.

**Alcohol**

Occasional drinking is not harmful as long as you control the amount that you drink – but that can be challenging sometimes. A glass of wine is rich in antioxidants and has health benefits – however, alcohol is empty calories and could also affect your mood so that you are more inclined to eat out of control. Even beer can add more calories than you think. A can of beer (light or regular) has 100-150 calories; an 8 fl oz serving of wine has about 170 calories, and 4 fl ounces of whiskey, rum, or vodka contain about 257 calories. If you must drink, have it only after you've eaten and keep it to only a few drinks on weekends (keep in mind that 2 servings of wine deliver about 400 calories---empty calories that the body converts to fat unless you burn them off by exercising).

Food slows the absorption of alcohol and helps to dampen its effect on your metabolism. Most people who drink alcohol repeatedly find it very hard to lose weight despite their best efforts. Furthermore, they are usually very moody and depressed and this is due largely to the depletion of the B-vitamins (see Chapter 7). Alcohol can drain your energy and worsen high blood pressure. In some circumstances, alcohol can trigger deep and buried, unresolved emotions and anxiety that can invoke craving, impulsive behavior, and even aggression.

## Eating in Ethnic Restaurants

Ethnic restaurants are not immune to high fat, sugar, and sodium cuisines, especially if they are prepared to suit the American taste. So, approach them in the same cautionary manner you would fast food places and restaurants. It's always appropriate to ask questions and also request that food be prepared in methods that you prefer (such as grilled instead of fried). Below are a few tips that will help you make healthier choices that are low in calories, fats, salts, and sugars.

**Oriental**

Ideally, their cuisines tend to be very rich in vegetables, seafood, noodles and white rice. Steamed or mixed vegetable soups that are low in fat and calories are the norm. However, salt can be a problem. The steamed cuisines with lots of vegetables, poached fish, and steamed rice are good choices. Stir-fried entrees with little or no oil with mixed vegetables, seafood, or chicken are usually delicious and low in fats and calories.

Wanton soup and shrimp cocktails with non-fatty sauce or dips are good appetizers. Spring rolls wrapped in lettuce are a good choice. On the other hand, avoid fried dishes that are soaked in fats, such as fried rice, egg, or spring rolls. Spring rolls that are not fried are acceptable. Ideally, you should ask for items that are low in salt instead of those high in salt, such as soy sauce or monosodium glutamate (MSG) and other salty sauces.

## Japanese

Japanese dishes are known to be low in fat and calories and contain lots of vegetables, fish, and a small portion of white rice as a side dish. The nutrient density is quite high, but you have to be careful with the excessive amounts of salts due to seasoning with soy and other salty sauces. But this may not be a problem if you talk to the chef ahead of time.

Some of their favorable dishes are tofu, steamed white rice, sushi, chicken teriyaki, vermicelli noodles, stir-fried noodles, steamed dumplings, and steamed vegetables and rice. Sushi is also a good choice, but bacterial contamination is a concern – make sure the place is clean and proper hygiene is followed by the cooks and attendants. Avoid vegetable tempura or shrimp, fried pork, fried tofu, chicken katsu, and shrimp agemono.

## Italian

Italian dishes are centered on pasta, usually white flour that is highly refined. In addition, the pastas are often served in huge portions with fatty and salty sauces. However, you can always ask for smaller portions of pasta with low-fat and low-salt tomato sauce. Better choices of sauce are red or clam sauces and fresh tomato-based sauces like marinara that are high in vegetables and nutrients. In general, you should limit the amount of pasta you eat whether at home or in a restaurant because of the high starch, regardless of its glycemic index.

Other favorable Italian dishes are seafood or chicken dishes, such as shrimp marinara, chicken in wine sauce, or grilled fish. Pizza is highly refined white flour and you should avoid ordering it with sausage and cheese. A better choice is a thin crust (1-2 slices) without the extra cheese and meat and containing lots of vegetables (veggie pizza). You could order a side salad to accompany it, but without the fat-laden dressing.

Avoid dishes with cream or butter sauces, such as pasta stuffed with cheese, fatty meat, or fettuccine alfredo. Also avoid Italian bacon, sausage, and ham. These are all high in fat and usually served in large portions.

## Mediterranean Dishes

The traditional Mediterranean (Crete) diet is among the world's healthiest dishes, but the American version may be high in calories and fats. However, good choices are seafood broiled with lemon, herbs and spices, or pan-roasted meats and dishes coated with herbs and spices. The Greek salad is a favorite selection, granted that the right amount of olives, olive oil, and cheese are used. Meals are often prepared with fresh vegetables and include okra and dark green leafy vegetables (some of our favorite and healthy recipes have come from *Andreas* restaurant in Rhode Island). Avoid dishes prepared with butter, cream, cheese, and fatty meats because they are high in fats, calories, and salt.

## Hispanic Cuisines

The common link with all these somewhat diverse dishes is that they are traditionally high in fats due to the addition of full fat cheeses, sour cream, and guacamole. The foods are usually fried with lots of Omega-6 dominated vegetable oils, including fish, beef and chicken, making them saturated with fat. Good choices are fajitas with lots of grilled vegetables and less sour cream, cheese and guacamole (guacamole is high in heart-healthy monounsaturated fats, but you don't want to eat too much of it because it is high in calories and fat).

Beans and white rice are staple carbohydrate sources and are better choices than refried beans and rice, which can be high in fat and salt. Fried plantains with fried fish and meat are delicious and quite tempting, but they are loaded with fats and high glycemic carbohydrates.

Avoid fried chips and white flour tortillas. The plain tortillas or corn tortillas are better choices, but keep the portion small because they are highly refined white flour carbohydrates. By far the best choices are the oat bran/whole-wheat tortillas and pita pockets (*Joseph's*) that are high in fiber. Also avoid meals loaded with full fat cheeses.

## African Dishes

Typical African dishes tend to be hot, spicy and based primarily on white rice, cassava, potatoes, yam, plantain, and various green leaves that are often over-cooked (potato greens, cassava leaf, spinach, or other leafy green vegetables). There is a liberal use of fats, particularly palm oil, vegetable oils, and high fat meats like pig foot, cow skin, and internal organs. Peanut butter is also widely used in cooking. In fact, there are similarities between the African and Hispanic dishes and ingredients, including preparation methods (the two cultures have a common ethnic background).

Most foods are stewed, boiled, or fried instead of baked, broiled, or grilled. Tomato paste is used in almost every dish for flavor and coloring. Bread, white rice, fufu (highly refined flour made from cassava or potatoes), plantain, and cassava root are the main sources of starch and often dominate the meal. White rice is often served in big portions—3 or more cups per meal.

African cuisines are loaded with flavor and taste, but you have to watch out for sodium due to the liberal use of salty seasoning, such as bouillon cubes and broths. The dishes are also hot and spicy (cayenne pepper, paprika, habanera, ginger, jalapeno, and chili peppers), but you can ask for milder dishes.

Healthy choices include fish soups, okra soup, spinach, and greens with fish, chicken, or meat. Most of the restaurants serve a variation of African cuisines that are designed to suit the American taste and you should try these first before going for the ethnic dishes.

Ask for limited use of oil in cooking green vegetables (such as spinach) and keep portions of rice and fufu small (side dish). Plantain is starch-dense and the fried plantain adds both carbohydrates and fats. Avoid other fried foods, such as fried pork, beef, and chicken because they are high in fat and calories.

# Chapter 14

# The Food and Exercise Connection

## Physical Activity Is Imperative

When you decide to lose weight or stay healthy, you have to consider eating healthy as the first line of defense and being physically active, the second. In a recent study, people who lost weight and kept it off for five years exercised religiously. They burned around 400 calories a day – the equivalent of walking briskly 4 miles per hour daily. Research does show that it can help to significantly reduce intra-abdominal (belly) fat, which is linked to Syndrome X, heart disease, stroke, high blood pressure, type 2 diabetes, and certain forms of cancer, including breast, colon, and uterine.

You may not see a dramatic weight loss on the scale when burning off belly fat with regular exercise – but don't be discouraged. This type of fat may not register immediately on the scale, but you are improving your health and adding years to your life. Furthermore, research shows that regular exercise improves insulin resistance, blood glucose, and lipids (cholesterol and triglycerides), including cardiovascular disease, osteoporosis, and bone fractures.

Exercise must be regular in order to be effective and improve blood sugar levels and insulin response. As you might recall, insulin spikes promote fat storage and food craving. Exercise does not only improve blood sugar after the last meal, but it can also improve insulin sensitivity and glucose metabolism for an extended period of time.

Exercise is more effective at improving insulin response if it is done daily or at least every other day. Skipping exercise for more than two days loses its benefits. As a matter of fact, the insulin response associated with physical activity is lost in a short time once you stop regular exercise. This is one reason why you should keep up your exercise routine on a regular basis, even if it is not at the same intensity and duration.

## Sedentary Lifestyle Is Unhealthy

In a large study recently presented to the American Association for Cancer Research, it was shown that moderate physical activity prevents breast cancer recurrence. Dr. Michelle Holmes and her colleagues from Harvard University followed the health of almost 122,000 female nurses since 1976. The researchers analyzed the physical activity of 2,167 women who were diagnosed with breast cancer after the study began.

During a period of 14 years of follow-up, it was clearly evident that those women who engaged in regular, modest physical activity were more likely to survive their cancer. Most of the women walked for exercise. Those who walked 1-3 hours a week at a leisure pace of 3 miles/hour, reduced their risk of dying from breast cancer by 25%, compared to women who were sedentary. Women who walked between 3-8 hours/week reduced their risk by 50%. This latter result is comparable to the benefits of treatment with tamoxifen in women with breast cancers that are estrogen receptor positive. It's very important to emphasize that, in the study, those women who lived a sedentary lifestyle did not survive their cancer well.

Exercise probably helps to protect women against breast cancer because it can affect the amount of estrogen hormone produced in the body. Estrogen promotes the growth of breast cancers that are estrogen receptor positive and, therefore, less estrogen means a lower risk of breast cancer. Women who are overweight or obese have increased risk of breast cancer or recurrence of cancer even after treatment. And this is due to the fact that the extra fat tissue makes extra estrogen that stimulates susceptible breast tissue to grow into cancer. Regular exercise helps to reduce body fat as well as cellular inflammation. This is the reason why women who exercise or keep physically active after being treated for breast cancer have a better chance of staying alive compared to women with a sedentary lifestyle.

Regular physical activity, even modest exercise, can have major health benefits in preventing as well as decreasing the risk and complications of chronic diseases. It is associated with both lower insulin levels, as well as increased insulin response in muscle and fat tissue and this can be an effective tool in reversing the insulin resistance associated with the development of chronic diseases, such as heart disease, stroke, diabetes, some cancers, and even obesity.

Regular exercise may also help to reduce the levels of low-grade chronic inflammation that precedes heart disease and other degenerative diseases. In a study at the Fred Hutchinson Cancer Research Center in Seattle, obese menopausal women who exercised regularly saw their inflammatory marker, C-reactive protein fall about twenty percent after a year, even if they did not lose a significant amount of weight.

If your intention is to lose weight so you can also decrease the risk of major health problems, besides eating proper meals, regular exercise activity that breaks a sweat should be a high priority as well as stress reduction. Losing weight by eating healthy alone without exercise can cause your body fat percentage to go up because of loss of muscle tissue. Muscle is a high water tissue composed of 70% water, 7% fat and 23% protein and, unless stimulated by exercise, it breaks down quicker than fat tissue, which is composed of 22% water, 72% fat, and 6% protein.

Even if you are overweight and exercising, regardless whether you lose weight or not, you may be healthier than a person of normal weight who is sedentary. In fact, it is proper to keep physically active whether you are overweight or lean. Young women should be more than encouraged to engage in physical activity at a very early age – as they can reduce their risk of developing breast cancer by 50% in their menopausal years.

The good thing is that your exercise routine does not need to be high-intensity. For example, a simple 60 minute period of brisk walking each day can help to burn body fat or maintain desired weight, provided that you cut down your caloric intake. Furthermore, it is the cumulative effect of your physical activity throughout the day, rather than a single exercise routine, that seems to truly matter – taking the stairs instead of the elevator or parking farther from your destination, for example. Every activity that breaks a sweat counts and could make a difference between developing common health problems, such as heart disease, diabetes, high blood pressure, cancer, and osteoporosis. It could also help you live longer as well as healthier.

Moderate intensive exercise routines that will help you burn body fat, especially belly fat are: swimming, brisk walking (4 miles in 1 hour), cycling, running, jogging, biking, jumping rope, ballroom dancing, Hoola Hoops, skiing, table tennis, mowing the lawn with a push mower, stair climbing, or brisk walking uphill with or without a load.

As you burn body fat, it is equally important to strengthen or build muscle tissue – the more or better tuned your muscles are, the more calories you burn, and the better chance you have of losing weight and keeping it off. Strength or resistant exercise can be easily performed in the convenience of your own home or work place, such as weight lifting, push-ups, sit ups, or using free weights or weight machines (available at the gym). Some people prefer to walk during their lunch break, including parking a good walking distance from work, and taking breaks to stretch.

You will see better results if you do a combination of aerobic and resistance exercises. At the start of your weight loss program, do more aerobic (70-80%) to burn fat and some resistance training (20-30%) to build and maintain muscle. This order can be reversed in the maintenance phase. Don't forget to stretch your body (flexibility exercise) to loosen ligaments and joints and prevent injury before and after a major exercise routine, including walking. You should also get approval from your health provider, of course, before starting any exercise routine, especially if you have a medical problem.

Begin your exercise routine at a pace that is comfortable for you and always choose a routine that you enjoy. The first few minutes are the hardest – muscle, bones, and ligaments tend to ache and it is easy for you to get tired and discouraged. But you should not give up. Stay the course and you will feel better gradually and in the long run you will be happy that you did not give up. It gets better with time and in fact "sedating" and "addictive".

*When Patricia started the UDP program, she had all the right excuses not to exercise: she was 100 pounds overweight, ached all over, her legs were swollen, she didn't have the energy and the motivation, and she was quickly out of breath. So, she concentrated on eating proper meals, but that was not enough. However, with repeated encouragement she began to exercise gradually, walking for about 10-15 minutes 2-3 days a week. A couple of months later she added light swimming. Eventually, she joined the gym, began enjoying it, and would not miss a day. "I don't feel good when I don't exercise and it has become therapeutic for me," she said (she was presented previously in Chapter 8).*

## A Brief Note on Maximizing Your Exercise Routine

### When Is the Best Time to Exercise?

Experts advise that it is best to exercise first thing in the morning to boost, energize and jumpstart your metabolism for the day and in the evening shortly after dinner to help reduce overnight fat storage when your body metabolism has slowed down.

Timing your exercise routine to coincide with the release of certain hormones in the morning can help you burn more body fat. If your goal is to burn body fat, it is best that you exercise first thing in the morning before you eat. Your body is already in a starvation mode since your last meal was about 12 hours ago and probably all or most of your stored carbohydrate reserve in muscle and liver has been used up.

As a result, your body will be forced to turn to its stored fat for energy. When you exercise aerobically during this period, your body will release a significant amount of growth hormones in order to speed up the burning of stored fat to meet the new energy demand.

The burning of body fat requires a great deal of oxygen, which is used up in the process. During the first 20-30 minutes of aerobic exercise, your body uses mostly the sugars stored in liver and muscle (glycogen), which is only a small amount. Amino acids from protein and fatty acids from fat already in the bloodstream also contribute to the energy source. But the entire process, which does not require oxygen, only releases a small amount of energy. This process is called anaerobic respiration or metabolism. It releases a burst of energy for only a short period of time and is favored by fast, short distance runners (such as the 100-yard dash) and weight lifters.

The small amount of carbohydrate stored in the body as glycogen and fatty acids in the blood stream has to be used up before the body can tap into its huge fat reserve. There is a catch. Fat reserves are not released for energy without the availability of oxygen. In other words, burning body fat is powered by oxygen fuel.

There must be an abundant supply of oxygen fuel for the body fat to begin burning and releasing energy that muscles and body cells can use. To get the level of oxygen required to do the work, we must breathe faster – this implies working our lungs and heart faster – breathing rapidly to circulate more oxygen and nutrients to our muscles and cells and fat storage sites. This is exactly what we are doing during aerobic exercise (we are increasing oxygen uptake).

During aerobic exercise (breathing fast), our muscles and cells burn the fat that is released at a faster rate and, therefore, we can burn a considerable amount of body fat as long as the supply of oxygen continues. This is the reason you lose body fat and weight faster when you do aerobic exercise on a regular basis first thing in the morning. As a rule of thumb, aerobic exercise must be done for at least 30 minutes in order to burn body fat efficiently. Short aerobic exercises would be ineffective in burning body fat. On the other hand, the longer you exercise aerobically, the more body fat you burn.

Once the switch to fat burning is made (about 20-30 minutes into your exercise), your body will begin to burn stored fat, especially belly fat, if you continue breathing rapidly and getting an adequate amount of oxygen to fuel the process. You will burn more body fat if you do 60 minutes of aerobic exercise as opposed to 30 minutes. Perhaps, you might have already experienced that it takes significant amount of work (energy and time) to burn body fat, whereas accumulating body fat is quite easy. This is because the storage of fat requires less energy compared to the burning of fat.

As you burn or melt body fat, you will immediately see more muscle definition and will look physically fit. Aerobic exercise also helps to increase your body metabolism so that you continue to burn body fat as much as 48 hours after the exercise. It also helps you to improve the performance of your heart, lungs, and blood vessels (cardiovascular systems). Other benefits include lowering of blood glucose and total cholesterol levels, increasing HDL (good) cholesterol and controlling high blood pressure, depression and arthritis.

During aerobic exercise, you should monitor your breathing and heart rate in order to determine if you are exercising effectively. You should be breathing rapidly but, at the same time, comfortably enough to speak a sentence. But the most accurate method is to measure your heart rate – your heart rate is influenced by your age, physical condition, and sex. You can calculate your target heart rate by using the formula below or heart rate chart:

***General formula:*** *220 minus your age and then multiply by 0.65 and 0.85. Your target heart rate during aerobic exercise is a range of 65% to 85%. For example, a 36-year-old female target heart rate will be 220-36=184; 184 x 0.65 and 184 x 0.85=120-156.*

You should strive to keep your heart rate within your target range when you do aerobic exercise. If you are below your minimum range, you probably won't burn fat because you may not be in an aerobic state. Likewise, if you are above the upper limit, you could be straining your heart and muscles and probably not burning fat either (you may be probably in an anaerobic respiration).

Sometimes exercising too vigorously and not getting enough oxygen can cause your body to switch from aerobic to anaerobic state. Therefore, your body stops burning fat. This can happen when you run out of breath and become extremely exhausted. To avoid this, you should refrain from strenuous exercises that take away your breath and render you unable to breathe enough oxygen. Before going any further, here are the important points you need to keep in mind:

*To be successful in burning body fat, you need to focus your exercise routine on aerobic exercise that is done first thing in the morning during the weight loss period until you reach your goal weight or your body fat percentage. Aerobic exercise is less intense than strength training but, to be effective, it must be done for longer periods – at least over 30 minutes 5 or more times a week. For maximum results, you should do aerobic exercise at least 1 hour daily (in the morning), along with strength training 10-20 minutes, 3-5 days a week (shortly after dinner in order to prevent fat storage).*

*If you are unable to exercise in the morning, then the next best thing is to exercise whenever you can. For instance, walking briskly during your lunch break is beneficial as long as you are consistent and not skipping days. If you can't exercise because of pain or injury, move your individual body parts (such as hands, legs, feet, etc) – just about anything that can cause you to sweat if repeated for an extended period of time. The worst thing you can ever do to your body is to do nothing!*

A much more practical way to look at the importance and value of aerobic exercise is to try to understand how the world famous cyclist, Lance Armstrong does it. First of all, he works very hard and could easily burn 6,500 calories or more per day when he is training (probably trains for about 6 hours daily).

We can assume that he takes in a lot of oxygen during training and his food intake is also increased quite a bit. But the mystery is that he doesn't gain weight despite increasing his food intake. The simple reason is due to the fact that he is burning off the calories during training. On the other hand, if Lance Armstrong eats the same amount of food when he is not training hard, he will definitely store fat and gain weight. This is exactly the scenario with a great number of professional athletes who were once in great shape and physique until they retired and continued to eat as if they were still very active. Unfortunately, most people think that way.

The truth is that you do not have to train like Armstrong or professional athletes to be in shape. All that is required is consistency and a daily exercise routine that is right for you. This will keep your body working well and burning off extra calories and fat.

In very simple terms, you learn how to tailor the amount of food and calories you eat daily to your exercise routine. In other words, any time you eat too much or cheat, you should exercise more vigorously and longer to burn it off. Again, it is aerobic exercise that will help you burn body fat more efficiently.

Most people with a personal trainer or training at a gym fail during the first few months because they concentrate too much on weight lifting and resistance exercises instead of aerobic exercises. I hope you don't make the same mistake. Once you understand this simple concept and put it into practice, you will have no further need to diet or starve. You will lose weight, body fat and, most importantly, keep it off for good by eating proper meals, and keeping a level of activity that is suitable for you.

| Aerobic exercise is sustained activity that makes your body deliver more oxygen to your muscles. |
|---|

Aerobic exercises include activities that increase your breathing and heart rate so that you can increase the metabolic activity within the fat reserves and muscles and also remove poisonous waste materials from the body. Fat burning aerobic activities include:

- Brisk walking (about 4 miles in 1 hour)
- Fast ballroom dancing
- Running/jogging
- Biking/Stationary bicycle
- Strong swimming
- Jumping rope
- Kickboxing
- Hoola Hoops
- Steps aerobics (10,000 steps/day)
- Skiing
- Treadmill
- Ball – it is believed to help reduce belly fat
- Elliptical machine
- Pilates – It is good for toning, shaping, strengthening, flexibility, and mobility. However, it may not be the best choice for burning body fat during the initial phase of weight loss. It is more effective after the initial weight loss or maintenance phase.

## Resistance or Strength Exercise (Anaerobic Exercise)

These are exercises to strengthen and build muscles as well as strengthen and increase bone density. Strength exercises do not directly burn body fat because oxygen is not involved. Strength exercises stimulate the growth of muscles and, the more muscle mass you have, the more calories your body burns to keep you fit and lean. But, at the same time, you will have to eat more calories to support the growth of your new muscles – and that is why it's not proper to concentrate on it during the early phase of weight loss.

Strength exercises do not require oxygen as long as sugars, amino acids, and fatty acids are available in the blood stream. But, since these energy sources are present in only small amounts in the bloodstream at any given time, strength exercises are usually done for only a short period of time; whereas aerobic exercises, which burn body fat, can go on for a longer period of time because the body fat reserve is huge.

Strength exercises are very important for maintenance of weight loss after you have reached your target weight or body fat percentage. During the weight loss period, you should focus on doing more aerobic exercises to burn body fat and a small amount of resistance exercise to strengthen and build muscles.

If you are trying to burn body fat and lose weight, you do not want to waste too much energy and time focusing on building muscles. Building muscle too early in your weight loss program can cause you to eat more calories to fuel your muscle growth (at the expense of burning body fat). This can sabotage your weight loss effort and prevent you from reaching your goal. Most people who go to a gym to work out fall into this trap.

> Anaerobic exercise or strength training is used to build and strengthen muscle. It does not directly burn body fat. It also does not require oxygen.

During the late phase of your weight loss program, it is perfectly fine to begin to focus on resistance exercise or weight training. At this time, you can either choose to do your resistance exercise in the morning, noon, or shortly after your dinner to prevent overnight fat storage as well as to help keep your body metabolism in high gear when you are sleeping. This is particularly important if you missed your regular dinner and ate a late one, like after 8 pm.

Typically, you should not eat a full meal after 8 pm or 3 hours before your bedtime. If you do, most of the calories you ate will be converted into body fat because your body is not burning calories efficiently at this time. This is a recipe for storing belly fat and gaining weight, including failure to reach your goal weight. Simply changing this type of eating pattern can greatly help you to be successful.

It is also very important to point out that most people lose weight and gain it back quickly because they stop doing resistance exercise. A simple 5 to 10 minutes five or more times a week can help prevent fat storage and weight gain. There are many sophisticated machines and trainers. But all you need are the basics:

- Push ups
- Sit ups
- Ball
- Weights/Weight lifting
- Kickboxing
- Yoga/Karachi – may help in building muscles. It is probably more effective in sculpting muscles, flexibility, toning, and strength. It may be also effective for relaxation and stress reduction. This could help to reduce toxic levels of cortisol that trigger the breakdown of muscle mass.

## How Active Are You?

### What Does It Really Mean to Be Sedentary or Active?

Perhaps the single most important question is, "How active are you?" In other words, how many calories do you burn per day as a result of being active or using your muscles and moving your body. For instance, if you are sitting or lying down most of the day, the amount of calories your body burns is very small compared to being active and moving your muscles frequently.

It's intriguing how some people overestimate their level of activity and most don't even have a clue as to whether they are active or not. Sometimes, even those that are sedentary most of the time think they are fairly active. That's why it is necessary to clarify the different levels of activities, so that you will know where you fit in with respect to your level of activities. I believe this will force you to make real changes and to eat what your body is capable of burning by way of muscle activity. This is one of the cornerstones of the UDP program. The question whether you are sedentary or active can be reached in so many ways but, for our purpose, we will keep it simple.

As you already know by now, the more you move your muscles and body, the more active you are and, hence, the more calories your body burns to keep you lean and fit. On the other hand, the less active you are, the less your body burns fat. This link between the amounts of food you eat and level of muscle activity (physical activity you engage in) is the key to controlling your weight and body fat irrespective of other factors, such as age, sex, and weight. This information can be used to roughly establish how much food or calories you should be consuming in order to maintain a healthy body fat percentage and weight at all times. This is the crucial difference between this program and other traditional weight loss programs.

> The amount of food you eat should depend entirely upon how active you are, instead of your weight.

## Committed to a Lifelong Endeavor

Even before you embark upon your quest to lose weight and improve the quality of your life, there are other important considerations to think about: Are you committed to a lifelong endeavor? To be absolutely committed, you need to have a clear purpose of why you are doing it. Hopefully, relatives or friends are not pressuring you. For no one can force you to do anything. It has to come from your own desire. You must have thought about it deeply and reached a decision on your own. Oprah Winfrey simply defined it as a 'decision' – a very personal decision whose ultimate purpose is to help transform your life into a healthier and happier one. If you haven't made such a compelling commitment to yourself, staying the course and reaching your goal can be very difficult, if not impossible. But it's more attainable if your decision is based on a commitment towards a lifelong process of self-discovery and happiness instead of a short term gain. The story of Kathleen is inspirational:

*Kathleen is a healthy 83-year-old woman whom for me became a model of optimum health and longevity. This quite spoken elderly woman is not only in the best of health, but her memory is sharper and intact for her age. It seems that she and husband had discovered the secret to aging gracefully---eating for as long as she could remember, an anti-inflammatory diet (salmon, tuna, walnuts, beans, fruits, whole grains and leafy vegetables), and not letting a day go by that she didn't exercise for the past forty years. She also understood the importance of de-stressing. In addition, she and her husband maintained a very active life.*

*When Kathleen came to see me in my office 3 years ago, I had no idea what she really wanted me to do for her. From the very moment that I met her I liked her instantly, and she did too. She was 5' tall and weighed about 95 pounds – she had maintained this weight for the past 40 years. Her diet was flawless and she was in excellent shape for her age. As our conversation progressed, she told me she had heard of me and wanted to learn the new things about health. She didn't want to lose or gain weight—she was quite content with her life. But she wanted more knowledge.*

*She seemed to be fine and in control, until she started talking about her twin sister who suffered from Alzheimer's and other chronic health problems. Kathleen did her best to help her, but it was too late. She often wondered whether her only sister could have been alive today had she followed the same path that she had – proper meals, exercise, and relaxation.*

*Kathleen projected her mind and thoughts into this future and beyond even before she embarked on this journey. She had a long-term view of health. Do you?*

Once your mind is made up, the next important thing to find out is whether the amount of calories or food you are eating daily is in line with your activity level. You can easily figure this out by adding the total calories you burn per day doing aerobic and resistance exercises and then multiply by 7 to estimate the total calories burned in a week. This is very important for you to know – it will give some idea of what you need to do in order to get where you want to be. Secondly, it will help to remove unrealistic expectations that may crush your ego.

*For example, you need to know and fully understand that in order to lose a mere pound of body fat, it requires a level of activity that burns about 3,500 calories per week. This is the equivalent of burning about 500 calories a day and doing it for at least six to seven days. But there are other things you can do to help maximize your efforts and that is to cut back on the amount of food and calories you eat on a meal-to-meal basis. This is the key to healthy weight loss and optimum health that can be sustained as a lifestyle endeavor.*

Most sedentary people are usually physically inactive and most of the food and calories they eat are stored as fat and very little body fat is burned. As a result, it is easy to gain weight and body fat, but much more difficult to lose weight or body fat. The solution to their problem is simply to cut back on food and calories and then gradually add aerobic activity, such as brisk walking for short distances with gradual increments. The cliché, "Tell me how active you are and I can tell you the state of your health and body fat," is one for you to think about. It's that simple. So, let's find out where you fit.

**You Are Sedentary**

Consider yourself sedentary if your days are spent primarily sitting at a desk job and simply don't make any real effort to engage in some form of exercise or strenuous activity. On the other hand, you might be involved in some form of light physical activities (e.g. daily chores, such as cooking, light cleaning, light yard work, slow walking, driving, and inconsistent light aerobic or weight training). You may even try to engage in some form of exercise for less than 2 hours in a week. But is this enough to work your muscles and raise your body metabolism? There is no question that, if you're not, the answer is, you are sedentary.

Most people who are sedentary barely burn enough calories and body fat and, at most, may burn about 1,000 calories or fewer per week – the equivalent of about ¼ pound of body fat. Because it's so small, even this positive change may go unnoticed. However, it's possible to register the change if your physical activity is in line with the amount of food you consume. One serious mistake people often make is that they continue to eat the same amount of food they ate before trying to lose weight. However, the results can be dramatic if you cut back the extra calories (about 500-1,000 per day and you will be losing an extra ¼ -1 pound per week in addition to burning fat from exercise).

There are obvious reasons why you don't want to belong to the sedentary group (unless you are disabled or incapacitated). Being in this group (sedentary), regardless of your weight, squarely places you at a higher risk for inflammation, Syndrome X, diabetes, heart disease, stroke, cancer, depression, premature wrinkling, aging, and early death. However, it may console you to know that chronic diseases like diabetes and heart disease may predate the onset of full-blown diseases by a decade or more. Therefore, the chance that you could prevent this from happening to you is pretty good in spite of your genetic predisposition. And, if you already have heart disease or any other chronic disease, your chance is still good that you can have a high quality of life and enjoy health and vitality no matter what your age. It's an opportunity for a life that you do not want to miss.

The good news is that it doesn't require heroic measures to change the course of inflammation and sub-clinical diseases to become full-blown diseases or to slow the progression of an existing disease. For example, small changes like eating anti-inflammatory meals that are high in nutrients and antioxidants and low in bad fats and refined carbohydrates will help to boost metabolism so that you burn body fat and reduce insulin resistance and inflammation. This will also help to control craving and binges, which is often the biggest obstacle to overcome. If, in addition to proper eating, you engage in some consistent level of exercise routine (such as brisk walking for 30-60 minutes daily), you will notice a dramatic increase in your energy as long as your food intake is in line with your activity level.

It may take a few months for your body to fully respond to the new nutritional support and physical activity that you are engaged in. As the body adapts, the results can be so dramatic that you would never have the need and desire to go back to bad foods and bad habits. Once you are committed, you should continue to consistently make these wiser choices and never have to concern yourself with the scale or dieting again. You should also reinforce your progress by setting up new goals and gradually increase activity daily or weekly and, soon, you will be in the next category.

**You Are Slightly Active**

You are here if you are engaged in light exercise that slightly increases the heart rate: volleyball, golfing, gardening, walking at a moderate pace, sailing, baseball, light strength or weight training, light manual labor, moderate housework, calisthenics, curling, etc. You are considered to be slightly active if you spend about 240 minutes (4 hours) doing light to moderate activities per week. The chance is that you may be burning around 250 calories per day (1,750 calories per week; the equivalent of about ½ pound of body fat). At this level of exercise, you may be able to reduce some health risk, improve cardiovascular, and bone health. But it may not be enough for significant weight reduction, unless it is accompanied by reduction of calories (500-1,000 daily) and incorporating healthy foods choices. Theoretically, you should see a weight reduction of about ½ -1 pound or more per week. In general, people in this group represent those who have made a substantial leap from a sedentary lifestyle to one that is more active and they can ensure greater health. But the greatest reward is yet to come and can be realized when you advance to the next level.

**You Are Moderately Active**

This is the category you should aim for regardless of age or sex (regular exercises or activities that break sweat). You can claim to be moderately active if you're engaged in moderate to intense activities that get you feeling warm, including increase in heart rate and breathing: brisk walking with or without weights (doing 4 miles per 1 hour), aerobics, skiing, ballroom dancing, treadmill, elliptical machine, skating, tennis, canoeing, rowing, roller-skating, cycling, moderate swimming, machine operating, shoveling, loading boxes, and other moderate physical labor.

A moderate intensity aerobic exercise of about 60 minutes for five to seven days per week will ensure the burning of about 3,500 calories; the equivalent of one pound of body fat per week. Again, reduction of calories in order to balance level of activity will ensure effective weight loss, reduction of body fat, and, most importantly, improvement of general health (such as substantial reduction of total blood cholesterol, blood sugar, and triglycerides and increase in the protective HDL cholesterol). In addition, you might be able to reduce or get off medications with serious side effects that you may be taking for health reasons. Most people in this category lose about 2-3 or more pounds of body fat per week.

Furthermore, your new whole foods and regular physical activity will help reduce the risk for some of the most deadly common health problems, such as diabetes, heart disease, and high blood pressure. If you are lucky enough to have not gotten the disease yet and you are genetically predisposed, you have a fairly good chance of beating it (and this is something to strive for).

Once you have developed and gotten used to the idea of eating healthy meals with regular exercise, it's very difficult to give that up for meals that are loaded with bad fats, refined carbohydrates, and coupled with a lifestyle of inactivity. Yet, it is easy, however, to reverse into your old ways if you are dieting and relying on chemical stimulants instead of eating healthy. That's why UDP does not encourage dieting or the use of chemicals that are unsafe (some of these may even increase free radicals).

You should have nothing to worry about as long as you stay the course and regard your progress as a lifelong ongoing process of learning and personal discovery instead of a quick fix. Also, remember that for aerobic exercises to be effective in burning body fat, you need to keep it up continuously for at least 30-60 minutes and make sure you are breathing within your target range. Otherwise, your effort could be wasted.

The key to optimal health and longevity at any age is simply to tailor your food intake to your level of activity. For example, as you grow older, you might not be able to perform physical activity at the same level of intensity that you did as a younger person. Nevertheless, cutting back on calories and energy food (replacing these with more antioxidants, nutrients and lean proteins), will allow you to ensure greater health and longevity at a lower activity level.

**You Are Very Active**

You are in this category if you are engaged in strenuous and vigorous activities that cause you to sweat, breathe heavily and get your heart beating rapidly: jogging, distance swimming, cycling, football, basketball, soccer, racquetball, squash, hockey, mountain climbing, heavy manual labor, soccer, tennis, and cross-country skiing. Athletes, military personnel and very active young people are generally in this category. Losing extra body fat or maintaining a lean and fit body is quite feasible at this level of activity.

However, it's very important that you continue to maintain a reasonable level of activity in case of a retirement from a professional sport or heavy-duty work; otherwise, you could be at an increased health risk, particularly if you continue to consume the same amounts of food that you had when you were quite active. Unfortunately, this is the path that most professional athletes often take – but it doesn't have to be this way.

### How Many Calories Do You Burn per Day?

Take a guess and, most likely, you don't know or are overestimating. To be in a healthy range, you should burn about 400-500 calories per day and this squarely places you in the company of people who are considered moderately active. That's the reason why you should aim to accumulate 60-90 minutes of moderate intensive physical activity daily and incorporate proper meals – under these circumstances, you will lose weight and keep it off for good, including maintaining a healthy body fat. Use the guide below to estimate the number of calories you burn per week. Some exercise machines have built-in calorie calculators. Make sure they are properly calibrated and working correctly.

| Activity | Total Calories Burned/HR |
|---|---|
| Swimming w/crawl stroke | 790 |
| Running, 10 min per mile | 720 |
| Bicycle, 15 mph | 720 |
| Martial Arts | 720 |
| Skiing, cross country | 575 |
| Hockey, ice or field | 575 |
| Tennis | 505 |
| Aerobics, high impact | 505 |
| In-line skating | 505 |
| Racquetball | 505 |
| Hiking | 430 |
| Water skiing | 430 |
| Dancing, nightclub | 395 |
| Kayaking | 360 |
| Walking, 4 miles in 1 hr | 325 |
| Lawn mowing | 325 |
| Golf, played w/cart | 250 |
| Volleyball | 215 |
| Weightlifting, non vigorous | 215 |
| Sitting | 80 |

Sources: Fitresource.com, Caloriesperhour.com

## What You Eat

### What Is Important in a Meal?

Once you decide to lose weight and improve your health, it is important to focus on making better food choices and eating proper meals most of the time. The good news is that it's never too late to make the transition, although at first it may seem strange or uncomfortable as you learn to acquire new tastes, flavors, and techniques of evaluating and preparing proper meals.

The UDP food plan is really not a diet (dieting or starvation is not healthy; it can cause muscle loss), but rather a conscious way of eating that you can adapt to your lifestyle (the key is to learn a new and better way of eating and physical activity habits that is tailored to your preference). It's a gradual process that is aimed at empowering you to make better food choices and to eat proper meals for the sole purpose of improving your health and maintaining a healthy body fat percentage and weight. To this end, UDP puts nutrients and antioxidants first over calorie- and nutrient-poor foods and encourages you to make every meal count. Other important aspects of the UDP program are food timing, food combination, and tailoring food intake to the level of physical activity on a meal-to-meal basis.

In this chapter, I will emphasize some of the important things I covered in preceding chapters in order to re-enforce the UDP program objectives. Most of these are probably well known to you, but there are those you may be hearing for the first time:

- Eat 3 balanced meals with snacks.
- Proportion your calories throughout the day.
- Eat a balanced breakfast of high fiber carbohydrates, lean proteins, fats, and fiber.
- Keep lunch modest, but balance in carbohydrate, protein, fat, and fiber.
- You must have a healthy snack between lunch and dinner.
- Eat a light, but high quality dinner not less than 3 hours before bed.
- Always balance carbohydrates with non-starchy vegetables, proteins, or fats.
- Eat more nutrient-dense foods, including high fiber rich food in each meal.
- Eat your meals in courses (4-5 course meals, particularly lunch and dinner).
- Eat appropriate portion sizes (this requires knowledge of serving size).
- Limit refined carbohydrates, sugars, and starchy vegetables.
- Eat each meal in line with your current level of physical activity.
- Tailor your food and carbohydrates to your level of physical activity.

**Eat 3 Meals With Snacks**

For most people, it is extremely important to eat 3 meals and at least a snack between lunch and dinner in order to provide a more consistent energy level so you do not have strong blood sugar lows that drain energy and stamina. The goal is to keep your blood sugar and insulin level even keel as much as possible throughout the day and night. This will stimulate your body to burn stored fat as well as give you better control over craving and compulsive eating.

It is also important to not skip meals. Many people make the mistake of skipping meals and then eating a large dinner later on. This stresses the body and can trigger emotional eating. If you go long hours (4-6 hours) without food, the body's blood sugar level will drop too low, causing a rise in cortisol. In order to prevent this, you should eat a good snack between meals, especially if your main meals are too far apart.

## Proportion Your Calories Throughout the Day

In order to keep your blood sugar and insulin under control, you should not eat the majority of your calories (especially carbohydrates) for the entire day in a single large meal, even if you are hungry. This can create a carbohydrate and fat overload, causing your body to store fat. When you eat a large meal containing carbohydrates, it will raise insulin levels, except when you burn it off immediately. If you are athletic or physically active, this may not be a problem. In fact, you may need more food and energy to fuel your active lifestyle. On the other hand, if you spend your time primarily being inactive or exercise sporadically, this can cause fat storage and weight gain. A single heavy meal that is loaded with carbohydrates and fat is a sure way to store belly fat and gain weight. It is best that you spread your calories throughout the day; ideally, eating more of your calories during breakfast and lunch and a very light dinner. This is something that most Americans don't understand.

## Eat a Balanced Breakfast

The typical American breakfast of cereal, bread, milk, fruit, and juice is carbohydrate-loaded and not balanced (refer back to Chapter 7). There are too many carbohydrates and not enough protein or good fats to prevent a spike in blood sugar and insulin levels and may predispose susceptible people (Syndrome X or insulin resistant, sedentary individuals) to accumulate body fat and gain weight. Likewise, a breakfast high in bad fats, such as saturated fats (sausage, bacon, cheese, whole fat milk, muffins, bagels, croissants, etc.) is also fattening and unhealthy.

It is beneficial to eat a high quality breakfast that consists of adequate amounts of carbohydrates (whole-grain and low-glycemic) and, most importantly, good proteins and good fats (olive oil, canola oil or flaxseed oil), including adequate fiber to slow down the carbohydrate and fat surge. By contrast, the combination of highly refined cereal, bread, fruit, milk, and juice for breakfast could cause rapid and strong blood sugar insulin response that drains energy and causes fatigue and craving. On the other hand, you could have the fruit for a snack instead – and this would probably not cause your blood sugar to spike.

Eating a balanced breakfast will also help to jumpstart your metabolism and build up your energy for the entire day, particularly if you exercise in the morning. You may not even need a snack before lunch if your breakfast is adequate and balanced in terms of carbohydrates, proteins, fats, and fiber (see Chapter 7). I will use Darlene to explain this point:

*Darlene thought she was eating a healthy breakfast consisting of a hefty bowl of cereal with milk, a glass of orange juice, and a banana. To her surprise and frustration, she found that, midway between her breakfasts and lunches, she was hungry again and feeling lousy.*

*Obviously, she was not aware that she was overloading on carbohydrates and having a major sugar spike that was draining her energy. Darlene is not alone – this is the typical*

*American breakfast and it's not at all healthy. There is not enough protein or fats to help slow down the heavy load of carbohydrates. But when Darlene began adding proteins, fats and extra fiber to her breakfast cereal, her energy was good throughout the morning, and she did not need to snack. You really don't need too much protein, fat, or fiber – just enough to counterbalance the carbohydrate load.*

You should never skip breakfast, especially if your last dinner was light. You must provide your body with enough nutrients to help burn its fat reserve. If you do not eat breakfast, your body will be extremely stressed since you would have been fasting too long (about 17 hours), which is bad for your health. Cortisol levels may be dramatically increased, leading to increased muscle breakdown. Ideally, you should never go without breakfast or other meals. Even if you are not hungry, you don't have to eat much, but you do have to eat something no matter how small and this will keep your blood sugar from plummeting.

Skipping meals also tend to make you bloated and gassy as a result of increased bacterial activity. It can also affect your breath (bad breath). Your body appears to go into metabolic shutdown when you go without breakfast on a consistent basis and, for the rest of the day, you are literally trying to play catch up. Even when you eat later, your body may not feel right. It may even take several days for your body to get back on track. And, if the trend continues on a regular basis and becomes chronic, it may be difficult to reverse.

**Keep Lunch Modest**

Keep your lunch modest but, again, have an adequate amount of carbohydrates, proteins, fat, and fiber to help maintain a steady blood sugar level and energy level. Avoid having too many carbohydrates with inadequate protein, fats, and fiber as this can make you feel sluggish and lethargic because a carbohydrate-loaded meal stimulates serotonin release.

If you are prone to insulin resistance, obese, or your lifestyle is sedentary, it is very important to have an adequate protein portion with lots of non-starchy dark green leafy vegetables. Keep your carbohydrate portion small to moderate, especially if you are eating a late lunch. Otherwise, you tend to get a sugar surge that could make you sleepy and tired.

Basically, the rule of thumb is to have more carbohydrates than protein for breakfast and, for lunch, an equal portion of protein to carbohydrates, or slightly higher carbohydrates to protein. You should also pay close attention to your sources of fat, as this may add extra, unwanted calories.

For lunch, start with a generous serving of 1-2 cups of non-creamy vegetable soup and non-starchy dark green leafy vegetables (about 1-2 cups cooked or 2-3 cups raw or more) for your template. Use olive oil/vinegar dressing (1-3 tsp extra virgin olive oil + 2 tbsp red wine vinegar or any other vinegar per serving. You can prepare a large batch with your favorite spices, herbs, and minced garlic) or a low-fat, low-sodium commercial dressing (such as Italian fat-free dry dressing by *Good Seasons* that you prepare yourself per specification). One of my favorites is fresh lemon juice with herbs, spice, black ground pepper, and minced garlic to taste. You can also use Mrs. Dash seasoning and *Goya* vegetable seasoning.

Your main course could be a sandwich, wrap, or cuisine that you brought from home or purchased from a restaurant or fast food place. Where you get your meals from is not all that important as long as the meals have adequate nutrients. Even fast food places and restaurants have some healthy, decent meals that you can pick from (refer to Chapter 13).

Always make sure that you have high quality carbohydrates (such as 100% whole-grain or high fiber multigrain bread, barley, oats, brown rice, long grain white rice, sweet potato, new potato, or whole-grain pasta). It is always safer to eat a smaller portion of carbohydrates for lunch if you are planning on eating a dinner that calls for more carbohydrates like pasta, potatoes, or rice. This also applies if you are eating out.

For protein, emphasize lean and low-fat high nutrient types, such as seafood (water or oil parked regular canned tuna, mackerel, sardines, and salmon); white chicken or turkey without skin; legumes, nuts, and low-fat dairy and lean meat of appropriate portion size (3-4 oz or 24-32 grams of protein). It is all right to have deli meat as long as they are low in fat and sodium and devoid of trans fat (such as 3-4 oz ham, turkey, roast beef, etc.).

### You Must Have a Mini-Meal Between Lunch and Dinner

Emotional stress can lead to eating when you are not hungry and you are most vulnerable midway between lunch and dinner (2:30-3:30 pm) when cortisol level is on a decline. This has been covered in Chapters 1, 7, and 8. Cortisol steadily increases in the morning, peaks at noon, and thereafter declines to low levels by dinnertime. Cortisol controls our energy level and its decline is usually followed by fatigue, low energy and lack of concentration, irritability, restlessness, and confusion. The worst thing for you to do is to eat highly refined and sugary carbohydrate foods like sodas, juices, sweets, and potato chips. These tend to cause a rapid rise in blood sugar and insulin levels followed by a sudden drop in blood sugar, which triggers craving and an increase in appetite.

You are more likely to be vulnerable if you skip meals or eat a refined carbohydrate dominant meal and not enough protein, fat, and fiber in your meals. You may be also susceptible if your blood sugar is low most of the time or you have diabetes, Syndrome X, are obese, or your lifestyle is sedentary.

You can prevent the drastic sugar swings that naturally occur at mid-afternoon by making sure you have a snack or "mini-meal" between your lunch and dinner in order to prevent a sudden drop in your energy level, which will trigger craving, emotional eating, and poor food choices. To be effective, your snack should consist of carbohydrates with proteins or fat (such as an apple with a tbsp peanut butter, a boiled egg, or low-fat mozzarella string cheese). Other choices that do not require too much effort to prepare are the snack size low-fat, low-sugar yogurts, or ½ cup 2% cottage cheese – adding 1-2 tbsp ground flaxseeds, wheat germ, or fruits, such as berries can greatly enhance nutritional value. Adding a small amount of fat (such as 1 tbsp flaxseed oil) helps to restore energy and provides another means to get the healthy fats that our bodies need. Eating the carbohydrate alone (such as oranges or bananas) without the stabilizing protein or fat can trigger craving and hunger pangs shortly thereafter. Secondly, a balanced lunch and late noon snack will give you a much better control over dinner, which is problematic for most people.

## Eat a Light But High-Quality Dinner

Eat a protein-rich but smaller dinner, emphasizing lean proteins and nutrient-dense high fiber foods, such as non-starchy dark green leafy vegetables and limit highly refined foods and fatty foods. Your dinner is proper if it reflects your body metabolism – meaning that your body burns fewer calories and fat at dinner. Therefore, you should eat a light meal consisting of an abundance of non-starchy vegetables and non-creamy vegetable soup, lean protein and minimal whole grain carbohydrates and healthy fats. This type of regimen will give your body a better chance to process and use the calories – so that most of it is burned and not converted to fat.

Some people voluntarily omit pure carbohydrates (rice, pasta, or potatoes) at dinner a few times a week (using alternative sources of carbohydrates, such as fruits, beans, lentils, edamame, whole-wheat crackers, carrots, beets, green peas, green snaps, etc.). This is only justified if you felt that you had adequate amounts of carbohydrates for breakfast and lunch. I would like to clarify that the UDP program is not a low-carbohydrate or a high-carbohydrate diet, nor do I endorse the elimination of carbohydrates in your major meals. But it's really up to the individual to decide the amount of carbohydrate that is suitable for them based on their level of activity. This is not a number that can be accurately calculated. The individual's experience is more reliable than any calculations – provided carbohydrates are consumed according to ones ability to burn them. Truthfully, the source of the carbohydrate doesn't matter as long as it meets energy needs and there is enough fiber in each meal.

It appears that some people tend to lose weight and reduce body fat with ease when the carbohydrate portion is kept to a minimum at dinner (for example, ½-1 cup brown rice or ½-1 cup whole-wheat pasta, instead of 2-3 cups) and, most importantly, it's whole grain (not starchy or refined). This makes good sense since at dinner our body metabolism is at a low point and it's easy to convert carbohydrates into fat. Another very important consideration that will help to facilitate weight loss and burning of body fat is to have adequate fiber in your meals at dinner. Strive for 8-10 grams of fiber, of which the soluble fiber is 3-5 grams (soluble fiber is high in okra, carrots, apples, oat bran, oats, broccoli, cactus, beans, lentils, soybeans, okra powder, etc). You will only need about ½ cup of these to reap the benefits. This is a very effective means to decrease your cholesterol and also control your blood sugar levels (particularly the fasting blood sugar). The more soluble fiber in your meals (especially at dinner), the better your metabolic profile.

Whenever you decide to reduce or omit carbohydrates, make sure you increase your protein portion (for instance, from 3 oz to 4-5 oz), otherwise, you could be hungry a few hours later. Overall, the dinner calories should be kept low most of the time – this is consistent with eating less when your body is resting.

The mantra for dinner is quality as opposed to quantity. The payoff is enormous: a peaceful sleep and rest, less snoring and improvement in sleep apnea. In fact, it's not unusual to see people less dependent or totally off oxygen therapy during sleep or daytime activities. The good news is that achieving these benefits requires very little effort on your part – simply follow the simple format of eating your meals in courses (this will be described in greater detail later).

Non-creamy vegetable soups with chunks of seafood, chicken, turkey, or lean meat are not only convenient and easy to prepare, but provide effective means to cut back calories and fat without compromising nutrients as well. You will find light vegetable soups very useful when you do not feel like having something heavy or it's close to bedtime. However, make sure to have a generous serving of non-starchy leafy green vegetables in your soups.

Sandwiches and wraps are also a great idea for dinner, especially when you are not in the mood to cook or eat a conventional meal. But, before you have your sandwich or wrap, make sure you have your template first (lots of non-starchy dark green leafy vegetables and soup). We all know that eating salad can be boring and far from inspiring. However, this shouldn't be a problem if you have variety and also prepare vegetables in different ways: steamed vegetables, baked vegetables, grilled vegetables, stir-fried vegetables, vegetables in soups, and fruit cocktails, etc. The possibilities are unlimited if you use your imagination and are not afraid to learn new things. I hope this illustration will help: After I directed one of my patients to the local Asian market, she reluctantly went. Not very long, her apprehension turned to curiosity and excitement finding so many different varieties of fresh and exotic leafy vegetables that she has never seen before in Westernized supermarkets.

She decided to pick a wide variety of leafy green vegetables (baby bok choy, Chinese broccoli, watercress, bamboo shoots and many more). After she paid at the counter, she realized that she didn't know how to prepare the vegetables she had bought. So, she turned to the pleasant Oriental lady who was working the counter and politely asked, "How do you cook your vegetables?" The Oriental lady politely answered back, "I turn my vegetables into soup" Since that day, my patient has never gotten bored eating vegetables. She has literally replaced the boring salads with delicious and tasty vegetable soups that are simple and quite refreshing. She no longer complains about eating vegetables, instead she eagerly looks forward to have them as the centerpiece of every meal. Following the advice of the store clerk, unless she stir-fries, she uses all her vegetables in soups that are cooked for only about 3-5 minutes to preserve the nutrients. You too will like eating vegetables once you learn new and better ways of preparing them (see recipes in Chaper 17).

At dinner, you should limit foods that are high in bad fats, such as those found in fatty red meat, full fat cheeses and milk products, deep fried foods, processed meats, cream sauces, butter, cookies, and ice cream – the tendency for your body to store fat at this time is extremely high because your metabolism is at a low point. This is one of the reasons why it is generally not a good idea to eat a heavy meal less than 3-4 hours before bed.

Timing is very important and can actually make the difference between gaining and losing weight. When circumstances arise that force you to eat a meal closer to your bedtime, have a very light, protein-rich dinner with abundant non-starchy vegetables or vegetable soups as pointed out above. Avoid eating large amounts of refined carbohydrates and high-fat foods, as these tend to cause quick fat storage. Ideally, have no food after 8:00 pm except water or non-calorie dense foods, such as pickles, cucumbers, celery, tomatoes, and very light non-creamy soups or vegetable soups.

*Most people gain weight over the years, making dinner their biggest meal. Your metabolism works best in the earlier part of the day (breakfast and lunch) and appears to be at its lowest point closer to your bedtime. That's why eating most of your calories at breakfast and lunch and a smaller meal at dinner can help you lose and maintain weight. On the other hand, the typical American pattern of eating (in which you eat a small breakfast, a modest lunch, and a large dinner) promotes fat storage and weight gain because the body is unable to burn the calories off.*

Dinner is also the worst time to eat a large amount of refined carbohydrates and refined white flour (such as pizza and pasta) and starchy carbohydrate (such as potatoes, white rice, plantain, fufu, and even sweet potatoes).

Some of the worst dinners are combinations of a large steak (8-12 oz), mashed or baked potatoes (12-16 oz) smothered with butter and sour cream accompanied by juice or soda and a sugary dessert (this is usually served in restaurants). To top it all off is the beer or alcohol – all delivering empty calories and depriving your body of vital nutrients and B-vitamins.

If your dinner looks this horrible, rather than watching television or going to bed, the least you can do is exercise vigorously in an effort to prevent overnight fat storage (for instance, you could do 50-100 pushups, walk briskly at least 30-60 minutes, or do 30-60 minutes on the treadmill or stationary bicycle). And you should make all efforts to eat healthy and exercise more the following day. The bottom line is that you should avoid having large meals at dinner, especially foods that are high in saturated fats and refined carbohydrates or even complex carbohydrates like potatoes that break down to sugar rapidly. These foods tend to raise blood sugar and insulin levels as well as cholesterol quickly and strongly. It doesn't mean that you can't have bad foods at all. If you do have them, you must keep their portion small and limit your exposure to earlier in the day when your metabolism is working at optimal level.

## Always Balance Carbohydrates With Lean Proteins or Good Fats

Carbohydrates (even whole grains or fruits) have the highest potential among all foods to raise insulin levels. That's why eating a balanced meal in which all three macronutrients are present is a proper way to eat. As you already know, proteins, fats, and fiber slow down the digestion and absorption of carbohydrates, thereby preventing blood sugar and insulin spikes that trigger fat storage. Protein, fat, and fiber also help to keep you full and satisfied for a longer period of time, which will keep you from getting hungry too soon. The good fats also help to control your appetite as well as help your body burn stored fat.

The proportion of carbohydrates, proteins, and fats in your meal doesn't have to be in the appropriate ratio for every meal you eat as long as you have a reasonable intake of these macronutrients throughout the day. However, it is important to vary the proportion (especially of carbohydrates) along the lines of your body's metabolism or level of physical activity. For example, eating most of your carbohydrates at breakfast and lunch, and the least amount at dinner can greatly help your metabolism to burn rather than store fats.

It is extremely important to eat protein or fats whenever you have your carbohydrates – even fruits and vegetables that are starchy either during your main meals or snacks. Protein is particularly important with the mid noon snack and dinner when your metabolism is at a low point. The problem with snacks is that it is sometimes not easy to find a good protein source. But the various types of proteins that you can use are easy to find and include hard boiled eggs or eggbeaters (if cholesterol is persistently high on medications), a slice of low-fat cheese, like mozzarella string cheese, ½ cup low-fat cottage cheese, and plain or low-fat yogurt with low sugar, slices of deli meats (lean turkey or ham), chunks of tuna and smoked salmon, soy protein, peanut butter, nuts (almonds, peanuts, and walnuts), seeds (sunflower, pumpkin, and sesame), hummus, vegetables, textured vegetable protein, beans, edamame, and lentils. Beans and lentils are excellent sources of lean protein, but they are also high in starch – but this is not a problem if you keep your portion small (such as ½ cup).

### Eat More Nutrient-Dense Foods

UDP emphasizes nutrient-dense foods because they are low in calories and bad fats and, most importantly, they are wholesome and not over-processed (as opposed to highly refined and processed foods). The UDP meal plan is based on eating more of these nutrient-rich foods with every meal – they help to fill you up that so you eat less. In addition to low calories, they are high in phytonutrients and antioxidants that help to reduce the risk of cardiovascular disease and cancer. They also help to keep blood sugar and insulin levels under control; they suppress appetite, speed up metabolism, and increase fat burning, as well as help in converting food into energy (refer to Chapter 7).

Focus on incorporating a number of nutrient-rich foods with every meal. Fresh is always better and choose organic whenever possible if the nutitional profile is better or you have major health concerns (multiple sclerosis, cancer). Some variety of frozen vegetables and fruits are also convenient and beneficial. The less refined and closer to nature they are, the more nutrients and health benefits they have.

When making protein choices, always remember that fish, beans, lentils, and lean meats are nutrient-dense and are better for your health and weight than fatty red meat, poultry with skin and full fat dairy.

### Include Fiber-Rich Food in Each Meal

Apart from eating high fiber foods, your meals should contain adequate soluble fiber in addition to insoluble fiber. You will get this information on food labels. Typically, the soluble fiber fraction is the one that is usually missing in the meals and you should make a conscious effort to have a sufficient amount (about 3-5 grams per meal).

One mistake people often make is to assume that they are getting enough fiber because they may be eating more vegetables than they did before. Let me clarify. The non-starchy vegetables are providers of antioxidants and nutrients, but their contribution to fiber is small except you eat huge amounts. On the other hand, you can get enough fiber from whole grains, multigrain products, oats, oat beans, fruits, beans, and lentils just by eating a small amount. Therefore, if you are not eating an adequate amount of these, your meals would be low in fiber – this can have some major health implications that I have already pointed to in previous chapters. The soluble fiber found in oats, oat bran, beans, broccoli, carrots, and apples can help to lower cholesterol and may help maintain healthy blood sugar and insulin levels, as well as boost body metabolism. On the other hand, the insoluble fiber found in wheat bran, whole-grains, oats, vegetables, and fruits help promote bowel regularity.

Eat enough fiber-rich foods (instead of meat and cheese) and you will not only lose weight, but also decrease your risk of colon cancer and other health problems as well. Aim for about 7-10 grams of fiber per meal and at least 3 grams soluble fiber (have a side dish of foods that are high in soluble fiber, such as ½ cup steamed broccoli, lentils, beans, carrots, or okra, etc.).

When eating out, carry fruit, vegetables, or fiber supplements if you are going to a place where the serving is likely to be low. You can also ask for extra vegetables if they have them. And also include vegetables or fruits in your snacks (such as apple with skin, strawberries, blackberries, blueberries, grapefruit, pear, raw carrots, broccoli, cauliflower, celery, cucumber, or cherry tomatoes).

Buns are sometimes seeded with sesame seeds to add fiber. However, sesame seeds and oils are high in Omega-6 fats and can trigger allergic reactions in sensitized individuals. On the other hand, flaxseeds, and oils are rich in Omega-3 fats that are anti-inflammatory. Therefore, sprinkling one or two tablespoons of ground flaxseeds to your salad or bun to increase your fiber intake is a good idea. Two tablespoons of ground flaxseed *(Barlean's)* delivers 3 grams of fiber in addition to Omega-3 fatty acids. The idea is to make sure that every meal that you eat has adequate fiber, particularly soluble fiber. Sometimes, you might even have to use soluble fiber supplements like Benefiber and Clearly Fiber.

## Eat Your Meals in Courses

As a rule, eat your meals in courses except when you are in a hurry (4-5 course meals whenever possible). Eating your major meals in courses is easy to do and can help you control your portion size and prevent overeating. This simple technique is unique to the UDP program: Start your major meals with a glass of water to which you add 1-2 tbsp lemon juice, apple cider vinegar or any other vinegar and drink half of that and the other half at the end of the meal. Next, have 1-2 cups of light non-starchy leafy vegetable soup and then your food template of nutrient-dense non-starchy vegetables greens or salad – only then do you eat the main course. I will explain how this works by illustration.

Upscale Japanese restaurants or five star hotel restaurants serve their meals in precise courses, like a well-organized symphony playing beautiful music that is pleasing to the senses. The first course: I was served a choice of water or green tea with lemon wedges. My second course was a bowl of light soup containing vegetables with small chunks of fish. Contrast this experience with that of a typical American restaurant, where they start you off with a basket of highly refined white bread and butter – which only serve to reinforce one of the obvious reasons we overeat.

Starting your meals with refined breads can trigger your appetite and force you to eat more than you intended to. From the very beginning, you are fighting a losing battle – you can see how difficult it is to control your appetite. From there onward, it will take a strong willpower to put you back in charge of your food intake. And this is one instance in which willpower fails to work in your favor most of the time.

The third course: My third course was a generous portion of fresh green leafy vegetable salad with vinegar and olive oil dressing. Doubtless, this part of the meal was the most important of all the courses that were served to me. Here was the powerhouse of nutrients and antioxidants that wage battle with free radicals, and help convert food into enengy, as well as curb craving. It was this portion that made me felt quite satisfied and content. It was as if they were reading my mind. As I sat and glanced at some of the faces that were going through the same ritual, I couldn't help wondering: Do they even grasp the power of serving food in this orderly manner, or is it just their culture? I wondered silently, trying to understand the reason the Japanese and Chinese people have a lower incidence of obesity and cardiovascular disease. The irony is that they lose the protection when they eat like Americans.

Finally, the main course arrived. It was a 4-6 ounce portion of steamed white fish garnished with steamed mixed vegetable greens. In a separate, small bowl was a small amount of white rice (probably about ½-1 cup at most). By all appearance, it was a side dish. It was clear that the majority of the food that I was eating was non-starchy vegetables and lean protein instead of white rice and fat. In other words, the meal was not dominated by carbohydrates (rice) and fat, which would not go well for dinner. The bottom line was that I did not finish my main meal and neither did the people sitting in front of me. I ate to fullness and satiety and was able to take some food home.

It was gratifying that I didn't have to wrestle with my appetite. Instead, I simply enjoyed the food and made every taste and aroma count.

Eating your meal in courses is a practice that you can do at home. Just pretend that you're being served and the meals are presented to you in courses. Eating in this format allows your brain to process your food intake and then determine with accuracy when you have had enough. Unlike the eyes, the brain depends on sensors in the stomach and specific hormone massagers to carry the signal of satiety back and forth. It takes about twenty minutes for the brain to get the signal that that you are full and that's why it is important to eat food slowly. If you rush through your meals, you would be finished eating by the time the brain sends signal of satiety.

Eating in this orderly fashion can be learned and it's not based on willpower, but rather on the body's biology, which is more predictable and reliable. The difficult part is learning to listen and interpret the signals correctly. For example, you stop eating when the first instance or sensation of feeling full strikes you, regardless of whether the food is finished or not. If you are hungry a few hours later, it could be an indication that your protein portion was inadequate and needed to be increased. Symptoms like headache and fatigue, especially during exercise could be an indication that your carbohydrate portion was inadequate and may need to be increased slightly, or may indicate that your choice of carbohydrates was poor.

One last thing to consider is that, had the entire meal been served all at once in one plate (as is often the case), there is no doubt that I would have cleaned my plate – this is exactly what happens time and time again with people who are giving their best effort to lose weight.

### Eat Appropriate Portion Sizes

There is no doubt that this is the most difficult thing to conquer. Nevertheless, eating appropriate portion sizes is simple if you get into the habit of reading serving sizes that are readily available on food labels. With time the serving sizes of your favorite foods will become a second nature to you. Familiarity with the serving sizes eliminates the need to count calories or diet. It also gives you a tool to gauge what you eat with a reasonable degree of certainty, particularly if you are listening to your body. But most importantly, you must learn to eat your meals in courses. This will help you to control portion sizes with minimal effort and certainty.

It's easy to lose weight or maintain your desired weight by keeping your food portion sizes in line with your level of activity. For example, eating 2 cups of pasta or rice instead of 1 cup when you are relatively inactive can increase the chance of storing belly fat and elevating cholesterol levels. On the other hand, 1 cup may be appropriate for your body to handle without triggering abnormal levels of blood sugar and insulin. This is the reason why eating the appropriate portions of meals (carbohydrates, fats, protein and fiber) is so critical in determining whether your body is going to burn body fat or store it. Likewise, you should be concerned about not starving or eating small portion sizes that are inappropriate for your level of activity. This could result in loss of muscle tissue and cause your metabolism to slow down.

Eating large portions of food at times when you are sedentary and physically inactive is bad for your weight and health. In contrast, you would do fine if your food portion was in line with your activity level on a meal-to-meal basis. You can apply this principle to any food that you eat (carbohydrates, protein, fruits, nuts, meat, fish, poultry, and fats). Eating a big portion that is suitable for an active person is a major reason most sedentary and inactive people gain weight over and over again. If, by error, you eat more than you should, you could take immediate action to burn it off by walking or exercising shortly thereafter. You could also reduce the portion and calories in your next meals, as this will probably give you a much more favorable overall profile for the entire day.

### Limit Bad Carbohydrates

Limit bad carbohydrates and starches that break down to sugar quickly, such as highly refined white bread, sodas, ice cream, sweetened or sugar-loaded cold breakfast cereals, highly processed baked goods, white flour pasta, French fries, and calorie-dense fast foods. This list also includes starchy vegetables, such as potatoes and fruits like overripe bananas and plantains. By contrast, carbohydrate foods that are high in fiber and not over-refined, such as multigrain bread, oat bran breads and cereals, brown rice, or whole-wheat flour pastas tend to produce a lower blood sugar response than their highly refined counterparts. They are more metabolically appropriate for people who are obese, sedentary, or those with diabetes, heart disease, or high blood pressure.

Some of the common household items that pose serious health risks are often held in high regards in our food chain. These include fruit juices, sweetened and unsweetened juices, fruit punch, and lemonade. They all cause very strong blood sugar and insulin response, just as strongly as sodas. That is the reason why orange juice and apple juice are among the standard treatments for people with diabetes who need to raise their blood sugar quickly when it falls too low.

The take-home message is that you risk raising your blood sugar to dangerous levels rapidly when you consume these highly refined carbohydrates, especially on an empty stomach. Perhaps, occasional usage would not be as damaging as regular usage in quantities that far exceed the body's capacity to process. This is also true if you accompany them with protein, healthy fats, or a full stomach.

Whole fruits are by far a better choice than fruit juice, which is devoid of fiber. For example, a medium apple has about 16 grams sugar and 5 grams fiber whereas 1 cup unsweetened apple juice has 28 grams sugar and 0 grams fiber. It's for this reason that you should choose the whole fruit over the juice, except when you are trying to furnish your body with instant energy. Whenever possible, eat your fruits with the skin, which has the fiber and most of the nutrients that will help to slow down the sugar response.

One of the justifications for the repeated use of juices is that they are fortified with minerals; but there are definitely better and safer means to get minerals in our diet. Indiscriminate use of low-nutrient juices and sodas is a major hindrance to weight loss in America and these items are cheap and readily available. Stop drinking them and you will soon notice the difference in your energy and concentration.

Consider the health and psychological benefits of not having sweetened juices and sodas as a major component in your diet: improvement in food craving, boost of energy, and concentration. In fact, you will be surprised to realize that once you start eating healthy, your tolerance to low-nutrient-density foods, such as sweetened juices and sodas, will become extremely low. In other words, your body rebels against the inferior foods once it gets use to high quality, nourishing foods. You can relate to this experience if you are a heavy soda and coffee drinker.

People with insulin resistance, polycystic ovarian syndrome, or are sedentary usually fair well if they limit intake of refined carbohydrates and eat more whole grains and whole foods. Again, their bodies adapt very quickly and they often display very low tolerance for highly refined foods once they have stopped eating them. This is a good thing since they have a higher risk for developing heart disease and diabetes.

Don't forget that even complex whole foods like potatoes, corn, plantain, garri, farina, and fufu behave just like highly refined carbohydrates and can cause very strong spikes of blood sugar and insulin levels. Therefore, you should not eat large portions of these foods at one time. Secondly, you should eat them infrequently and make sure they are accompanied with lots of non-starchy leafy vegetables, some good low-fat proteins, and healthy fats.

It is better that you eat potatoes (sweet or new potatoes) with the skin because the fiber will help to slow down blood sugar spikes and it also contains most of the nutrients. Sweet potatoes are better eaten without the brown sugar or marshmallows. Sweet potatoes and new potatoes break down to sugar relatively slowly, but you still have to eat small amounts at a time. For example, a 4-ounce sweet potato contains about 28 grams carbohydrate (the equivalent of about 1.5 serving) and would be appropriate to satisfy the energy requirement of a sedentary woman. By contrast, an 8 ounce sweet potato will contain about 56 grams carbohydrate (about 2.5 servings) and carries a greater potential to flood the body with extra blood sugar that will be immediately converted to fat.

Similarly, 2-3 new potatoes and ½ cup mashed potatoes (contains about 20 grams carbohydrate) will be well-tolerated by the body of a sedentary woman, but 3-6 new potatoes and 1 cup mashed potatoes will be very close to the tolerance threshold and anything above that will be far beyond the body's capacity to handle effectively. As a result, the body stores fat and cholesterol goes up.

Before leaving this section, another important point to be aware of is that the time of the day that you eat these starchy foods makes a big difference whether they get stored as fat or processed for energy. Heavy, starchy carbohydrate meals at breakfast or lunch are likely to be burned for energy, whereas, those consumed during dinner are likely to be converted to fat. The reasons for this should be quite clear to you by now. It also explains why those who are prone to insulin resistance, are obese, sedentary, or have diabetes (including high cholesterol and tryglycerides) should avoid eating large portions of starchy carbohydrates at dinner (in spite of the low glycemic index).

The same arguments for potatoes equally apply to rice and pasta, which are major sources of carbohydrates and starches in the American diet. It's no exaggeration that we normally eat too much of these foods in one sitting. As a result, they play a critical role in the development of obesity and its associated health problems in this country. The fundamental difference between societies that eat a whole lot of carbohydrates and Americans is the simple fact that most of these societies still depend solely on manual labor instead of machinery. In short, Americans' professional and personal lifestyle is sedentary in comparison to developing societies that are relying heavily on carbohydrate as the dominant energy source.

A friend of mine returned to West Africa to attend the funeral services of his father. He was only there for a week and lost 10 pounds, which he quickly regained when he came back to the United States. Traditional African funerals like those of African Americans in the United States are well known to be festivities of food and celebration of life, and so, my friend's weight loss was definitely not from the lack of food. The simple reason was the fact that he had to walk just about everywhere he went (like visiting relatives and friends). When he returned to United States, he practically drove even short distances, instead of walking.

But the fact is that you wouldn't have any metabolic problems if you were to simply tailor your carbohydrate intake to your level of physical activity. You will see how this is done shortly. For now, it will suffice to say that you will prevent a severe carbohydrate overload if you keep your portions of pasta and rice to about ½-1 cup cooked (22-44 grams or 1-2 servings) when you are physically inactive, instead of 2-3 cups (about 44-66 grams of pure starch or carbohydrates).

You will also fair well if you keep your selections to those that break down to sugar slowly. Among your better choices are whole grains that are minimally processed. Brown rice is the best and has the lowest rise in blood sugar. The second best is basmati rice and the long grain white rice (such as *Uncle Ben's* and parboiled rice) is the third best. The worst rice is jasmine rice. It can raise blood sugar more than twice the other rice. The short grain rice also breaks down to sugar quickly.

Traditionally, the white flour pastas have dominated people's choice, even though it shares the fate of other highly refined carbohydrates, such as white bread and breakfast cereals. However, that too is changing. Pastas made from nutritionally superior whole-wheat flour are now available in different shapes and sizes with textures and taste that are very similar to refined white flour pastas. In addition to whole-wheat pastas, there are the whole-grain pastas made with brown rice, buckwheat, spelt, quinoa, faro, and kamut.

When shopping for pastas, look for those that are made with whole-wheat or whole-grain and those enriched with protein (refer to the shopping list in Chapter 3). Chinese vermicelli pasta and noodles are also good. You can find them in many Oriental dishes and Asian food markets. Pizza is made from white flour pasta and it's highly refined and can quickly flood your body with sugar.

Again, keeping your portion size in line with your level of physical activity is the key – instead of omitting these highly tasty and nutritious foods. Unfortunately, most people tend to eat large portions at one time and are virtually unable to control their urge for pastas. As a result of this weakness for pastas, some people go to the extreme and omit pastas altogether – but this is not the solution.

Controlling your portion size of these staple foods is quite easy if you eat your food in courses and, most importantly, regard pasta as a side dish instead of a main dish. Following this format will help to prevent carbohydrate overload and dangerous sugar spikes that can lead to fat storage and weight gain. Even a fairly low glycemic index may not adequately protect you if you eat pastas like most people do (such as a plate full or about 4 cups – 176 grams carbohydrates). You have to be a professional athlete to absorb all that energy.

On the other hand, a portion size of ½-1 cup cooked pasta can be well-tolerated by your body, even when your exercise routine is not up to standard yet. You can eat a portion that is far less than what you previously ate only if you eat your food in courses, otherwise, you will succumb to the powerful pasta weakness. You will be amazed by how satisfied and content you will be after eating lesser amounts of these starchy foods (and you will be losing weight too). The good thing is that you can always increase your portion size as you become more active and your body demands more fuel (think of demand and supply).

Ethnic foods like fufu, garri, and farina (garri and fufu are highly refined cassava flour) are loaded with starch and can cause an intense blood sugar spike, especially given the fact that they are usually eaten in large portions. So is a ripe medium plantain, which could have as much as 60 grams carbohydrate (about 3 serving sizes). The green plantain tends to create a lesser sugar response than the ripe one. Boiling a green plantain or one that is not overripe instead of frying is a reasonable idea, provided you eat only a small amount at a time (such as ¼ - ½ medium plantain).

Limit or eat sparingly (only in small amounts) all convenient foods that are loaded with carbohydrates and fat, such as croissants, bagels, muffins, sugary desserts, ice cream, yogurt, and bean burritos. If you do indulge in these types of foods, be aware that they can create a vicious cycle of craving, and hunger. You are more prone to these attacks if you are obese, sedentary, or have Syndrome X, diabetes, and heart disease.

Tropical sweet fruits like mango, pineapple, orange, nectarine, dried dates, dried figs, and overripe banana can all cause strong blood sugar rise when a large portion is eaten at once. It's best to eat these fruits with lean protein, lemon juice, or vinegar. Very ripe bananas break down to sugar quickly, but not the green and just ripe ones.

Raisins are notorious for eliciting one of the strongest sugar responses, yet, they are widely used to sweetened breakfast cereals. The raisin brand of cereals is often the favorite cereal for young children because of the sweetness. Others, like cantaloupe, oranges, papaya, and watermelon, also give a rapid blood sugar rise, but their carbohydrate content is so small that the sugar response (glycemic load) is weak if you eat only small amounts (1 cup diced watermelon has about 10 grams carbohydrate). These foods are packed with nutrients, including vitamin C and potassium.

Limit your intake of carbohydrate foods that are also high in saturated fat, such as dairy products (full fat milk, cheese, and yogurt). Be careful in combining in a single meal full fat dairy products and other carbohydrate-loaded foods (such as fruits, lemonade, and sweetened juices) because this can create an intense blood sugar and insulin response, leading to belly fat storage even though milk has protein and fruit has fiber. Juices are the worst offenders since they lack fiber.

Reducing the fat content in the foods you eat will help you lose weight and decrease health risk, but make sure that you get adequate essential fats that the body cannot make on its own (Omega-3 and Omega-6 fatty acids). For instance, skim milk has a lower amount of fat than whole milk, but they both have the same amount of protein and sugar. Dairy products with reduced fat and sugar are better for your health and weight loss. They also contain calcium, which may help you shed the pounds. If you don't like cow milk, you can get calcium from soymilk, yogurt, cottage cheese, seaweeds, leafy green vegetables, and nuts, as well as a good quality multimineral supplement.

## Carbohydrates and the Weight Loss Connection

### Brain and Muscle Fuel

Our brain and muscle cells depend on carbohydrates for fuel. Without adequate amounts of carbohydrates, we lose muscle tissue and accumulate fat, which slows down our metabolism, spurs inflammation and weakens the body's immune system. Also, our ability to think and focus is impaired. Our body converts carbohydrates into blood sugar (glucose), which is used to fuel the body's energy need. Insulin aids the entry of glucose into muscles and body cells, thereby regulating the expenditure and storage of fat. Under normal conditions, there is a healthy balance between fat storage and fat burned. For instance, muscle tissue that is physically active is able to burn calories and carbohydrates more quickly and efficiently, so only a minimal amount of fat is stored. In contrast, physically inactive muscle tissue burns calories and carbohydrates slowly. As a result, large amounts of fat are stored.

Furthermore, the muscles and cells of people who are physically inactive resist insulin's signal to absorb glucose from the blood, causing high and dangerous levels of glucose in the circulatory system – a condition that can encourage the body to store fat, leading to a condition you're now familiar with: insulin resistance syndrome or Syndrome X. Syndrome X predisposes an individual to the development of diabetes, heart disease, obesity, and cancer, as you already know.

The capacity of our bodies to use calories and carbohydrates is regulated by our muscles and body cells, which, in turn, depend upon our level of physical activity. As you might expect, the more active we are, the more calories and carbohydrates we need and vise versa. A change in our activity level must be followed by appropriate adjustments in our calories and carbohydrate intake on a daily basis or, more precisely, on a meal-to-meal basis. This is very easy to do and it's explained later in this chapter.

### Low-Carb Diets Promote Short-Term Weight Loss

Studies show that most people on low-carbohydrate diets lose weight quickly during the first six months, but they also regain the weight quickly. This may be due to the fact that when they start eating carbohydrates again, they are not tailoring their intake to their level of activity. As a result, carbohydrate is readily converted into fat, which leads to weight gain. Studies comparing the low-carbohydrate diets and the traditional low-fat, high-carbohydrate diets also show that, in the long run, it is calories that matter. These findings are consistent with the UDP eating plan. But we go a step farther in promoting nutrients and antioxidants first and calories second.

### Too Restrictive

Low-carbohydrate and high-carbohydrate diets are too extreme and are based on the one-size-fits-all approach, which assumes that every individual is the same. They are severely restrictive and limit the amount of carbohydrates you eat regardless of your level of physical activity and special medical conditions (such as Syndrome X). This is the simple reason why most people fail.

Low-carbohydrate diets that are not in line with your level of activity may impose obstacles to high-energy performance and physical activity, both of which have many health benefits, including the development of healthy bones, muscles, and joints. Restricting carbohydrates from a person that requires it can cause intense cravings and fatigue as well as emotional and psychological problems. The feeling of deprivation can sabotage your best efforts to reach your goal weight. On the other hand, very high carbohydrate diets, especially the finely refined grains can increase health risks in people with metabolic syndrome and those living a sedentary lifestyle.

### Tailor Carbohydrates to Your Level of Physical Activity

The ultimate solution is to tailor your food, particularly carbohydrate intake, to your level of physical activity. You will solve the problem most people face on strict low-carbohydrate or high-carbohydrate diets. Understanding this connection between food and, particularly carbohydrates, the body's 'instant' and primary energy source, is the key to permanent weight loss and optimum health, including longevity. In simple terms, our survival and well-being is intimately connected to our muscle activity.

It was vital for the survival of our primitive ancestors from charging lions and a hostile untamed environment. But, in modern societies, there are no charging lions. Instead, there are hostile environments (such as highly refined grains, pesticides in foods, refined vegetable oils, stress, and so forth). Dealing with these problems on a daily basis requires boosting our muscle activities and bodily cells to absorb and neutralize these environmental toxins before they trigger inflammation and cause cellular destruction. So even though the conditions have changed, we must keep our muscles and brain active in order to survive. And eating more foods, especially carbohydrates, than our body can handle increases health risk substantially, as illustrated below:

*Sean, a 20 year old, was recruited by a college in New England to play football and was forced to eat about 5,000 calories or more a day to fatten him up as a defensive guard. "During the time that I was actively playing sports, I was in good shape, and fit," Sean said, "But when I couldn't play because of an injury. I gained weight rapidly and became ill."*

The irony is that Sean was dropped from the team as a result of his injury and returning to normal life was a huge struggle that he was far from winning – he was completely out of shape and gained too much weight.

The story of Sean is a good reason why it's important to eat food in line with your activity level. UDP does not require that you eat the same amount of food or carbohydrates at every meal, but that you adjust your intake on a meal-to-meal basis according to your level of physical activity. Making these appropriate adjustments on a consistent basis will allow you to eat the food and carbohydrates of your choice (such as bread, pasta, rice, potatoes, and fruits) and feel satisfied, instead of being deprived. This is what makes the UDP approach superior to the low-carbohydrate or high-carbohydrate diets that encourage you to eat a specific amount of calories and carbohydrates, regardless of your level of physical activity. As a result, most of us either eat too many carbohydrates or too few, and ultimately increase our health risk substantially.

## A Diet of Too Many Carbohydrates and Calories

It is not proper for a person to eat either a low carbohydrate diet or one that is high over an extended period of time with no regards to activity level. On the other hand, it is proper to base the amount of food and carbohydrates you eat on your activity level at all times. Unfortunately, most of us don't eat that way. The average American consumes about 200-330 grams of carbohydrate daily, regardless of whether he/she is sedentary or active. This is the equivalent of 13-22 servings of starches per day. And it doesn't matter whether the starches come from fruits, starchy vegetables, or whole grains. If too many carbohydrates are eaten at one time and they are not cleared from the bloodstream by the muscle in a short time, they could be converted to body fat for storage, the target being belly fat.

In previous chapters, I described the potential health risk of eating too many carbohydrates, especially if they are refined or starchy. On the other hand, there is Maryann who became sick eating a very small amount of carbohydrates, including the healthy whole grains. Hopefully, we can put an end to this trend and begin to eat carbohydrates based on our level of activity (really referring to muscle and body activity).

To fully grasp this concept, you may want to read this chapter over again. The theory is that carbohydrates from various types of food are the preferred energy source for our brain and muscles. Therefore, the more our brain cells and muscles are active, the more nutrients and carbohydrate and, to a lesser extent, the calories they require to carry out the vital functions of keeping us alive and well. The problem and confusion most people have with this idea is that they have been taught to plan their meals based on calories and this may cause some people to disregard what is really important – nutrients and antioxidants.

When we are active, our muscles and brain cells quickly use up most of the nutrients, calories and carbohydrates that we eat – this is the first line of defense. However, when we are inactive, the exact opposite happens – the brain cells and muscles are not working fast enough to use up the calories, nutrients and carbohydrates we consume in our meals. On the other hand, if we had only consumed just the right amount of calories and carbohydrates, our brain cells and muscles would likely absorb them, provided we have enough nutrients and antioxidants. As a result, only a minimal amount goes to storage and this helps to keep us lean and healthy.

It should be stressed again that the key driving force in the UDP model is not calories, but the nutrients and antioxidants that are found in the foods we eat. The second point is that while the total calories in a given meal are important, it's the individual components that hold the key. In this case, the carbohydrates are the body's primary energy source. Among the macronutrients (carbohydrates, fat and protein) that supply the nutrients and energy needs of our body, carbohydrates are the only ones that induce a strong insulin response – causing our body to store energy instead of releasing energy from fat depots. There is also another major difference that plays in favor of carbohydrates: They are readily transformed and stored as reserve energy in fat cells if they are not used up quickly by muscles and brain cells because there is not enough space, you might say, to safely store a huge quantity of carbohydrates as glucose (this is really what happens when we eat a huge portion of carbohydrates when we are inactive). Therefore, the rate at which the carbohydrates are cleared from the blood stream into the brain, muscle and body cells is directly linked to how active these organ systems are, particularly the muscles (since they are the powerhouse of the body). This explains why we can afford to eat more carbohydrates when we are active and using our muscles and fewer when our muscles are in a sedentary state.

## How Much Carbohydrate Is Adequate?

The question now is how do we know the amount of nutrients and carbohydrates that will be adequate for someone who is sedentary, slightly active and so forth. I solve that by giving a range of carbohydrate foods that a sedentary person can have instead of a fixed amount as is often done. Since most people are not fixed in their activity level, so is their intake of nutrients and carbohydrates. The activities of each individual changes from day to day. Therefore, food intake should reflect physical activity if we are concerned about overloading our muscles and brain cells. It is easy to tell whether a person is having adequate nutrients and carbohydrates by monitoring energy level, focus, concentration, hunger pangs and satiety. The examples below will give you an idea how this works.

| | **Sedentary** | **Slightly Active** |
|---|---|---|
| **Female** | 15-27 g/meal or 45-81 g/day | 27-38 g/meal or 81- 114g/day |
| **Male** | 20-33 g/meal or 60-100 g/da | 33-47 g/meal or 100-140 g/day |

The amount of carbohydrate you consume should be roughly proportional to your level of activity as shown above. It is very easy to use this system if you get into the habit of reading food labels because all the information you need is right there at your fingertips. My hope is that you will learn and strive to keep within your carbohydrate range when you are sedentary and gradually shift into a slightly higher carbohydrate range as your activity level increases. At the same time, your overall calories should shift back and forth in a similar fashion as your carbohydrate intake. The only difference is that your calorie intake changes much slower than the carbohydrate fraction.

For example, a sedentary female on 1,300-calorie diet will probably store fat and gain weight eating over 114 grams of carbohydrate per day (for reference: 1 slice of bread is 15 grams and ½ cup cooked pasta or rice is about 22 grams carbohydrate). But on days in which she is slightly active, she could consume up to 114 grams of carbohydrate (8 servings) while still on a 1,300-calorie diet. In due time, as her activity level picks up, she can afford to eat up to 140 grams of carbohydrate per day without inducing levels of blood sugar and insulin that will promote fat storage. Perhaps, this change would also require adjustments of calorie intake upwards, but this would solely depend upon the individual's energy level. Again, strictly speaking, the amount of calories is irrelevant as long as there is adequate supply of nutrients and antioxidants (in other words, you eat to fullness and not get bogged down with calories. After all, the Okinawa people don't count calories, yet they are lean and healthy and are one of the longest living people on the planet).

But in order to prevent braking down muscle tissue, it's important that your carbohydrate intake as well as calories parallel your activity level. For example, if you are moderately active, you could be starving your body eating less than 114 grams of carbohydrates a day. On the other hand, the probability of burning body fat and not muscle is greatest when you are eating carbohydrates within the range that is in line with your level of activity. This is the key and you can learn to master the process over time, making the necessary adjustments on a meal-to-meal basis.

*For example, if, on a given day, you decide to be inactive, your consumption of calories and carbohydrates should be reduced adequately enough to place you in the range that your body can still get enough nutrients without storing fat. In other words, you should never eat the same amount of food that you ate when you were active, when you are not. This is the major mistake most people make, especially on holidays and festive celebrations.*

*You can always return to the appropriate range of calories and carbohydrate when you start exercising again (slightly active) and are no longer sedentary. You will find out that on some days you will have to eat more and other days less, depending on your activity level. In some cases, you may only have to make the adjustment for a given meal, such as dinner.*

*I call this process "conscious eating" and it's like driving a car. When you drive a car that has a standard gear you will appreciate this more – you make adjustments according to the road conditions and if you simply drive on one gear throughout you will destroy the engine. Similarly, our bodies are biological engines just like vehicles and if we flood the engine with too much fuel (carbohydrates) when it is idle, it could destroy the engine.*

It is simple to roughly estimate the amount of carbohydrates you consume at a given meal without actually counting carbohydrates if you know the average serving sizes (see the average of calories and portion sizes for common foods in Chapter 15). For example, the serving size of cooked rice, pasta, and cooked cereals is a half cup and contains approximately 120 calories and an average of 22 grams of carbohydrate. Now you can see how such a basic knowledge can become a powerful tool that can help you to eat appropriate portion sizes just about any place (at home, restaurants, parties, etc).

It's easy to memorize the serving sizes of common foods that you like to eat and, if you forget them, you can always refer to the food label. In Chapter 15, you will find the simplified food serving sizes and averages of calories that will be very useful. In the near future, you may go to a restaurant and the nutritional breakdown will be right there in front of you.

Always keep in mind that your calorie and carbohydrate intake are not 'fixed' and are constantly changing to reflect your activity level and this fact should always be a consideration in planning your meals on a meal-to-meal basis. The chart below will help you to make your own adjustments as best fits your lifestyle and needs.

**Carbohydrate and Activity Connection**

| | **Sedentary (15%-25%)** | **Slightly Active (25%-35%)** | **Mod. Active (35%-45%)** | **Active (45%-65%)** |
|---|---|---|---|---|
| **Calories burnt/wk in activities** | **<250/day or 875/wk (¼ lb or less)** | **250/day or 1,750/wk (½ lb)** | **500/day or 3,500/wk (1 lb)** | **>500/day or over 3,500/wk** |
| **1,300 cal.** | **15-27 g/meal or 45-81 g/day** | **27-38 g/meal or 81-114 g/day** | **38-49 g/meal or 114-146 g/day** | **49-70 g/meal or 146-211 g/day** |
| **1,600 cal.** | **20-33 g/meal or 60-100 g/day** | **33-47 g/meal or 100-140 g/day** | **47-60 g/meal or 140-180 g/day** | **60-86 g/meal or 180-240 g/day or more** |

UDP does not require you to count calories as long as you eat to partial fullness and satiety and also eat your major meals in four-five courses. However, you are required to monitor your food template and carbohydrate intake, as this can directly influence your body's capacity to burn the calories from your meals or cause the conversion of calories into fat for storage. You keep track of your carbohydrate intake by using serving sizes. Later you will see how you can do the same for protein and fat.

As far as being active is concerned, it is the accumulative activity over the entire day and week that counts. That is why it is better to engage in regular physical activity rather than irregular physical activity. Most people assume that working out or going to the gym for a few hours once or twice a week is enough physical activity. This is wrong. Sporadic exercise doesn't work, but consistency does.

Hopefully, the guidelines above will help you plan your activity and carbohydrate intake for the purpose of effective weight loss and optimum health. And also help you to realize that being physically active throughout the day may be more beneficial than planned or scheduled physical activity that is done inconsistently, particularly if food intake is out of line.

**Your Calorie Needs**

As you learn to eat your calories or meals according to your level of physical activity, things will begin to make sense and you will be more likely to succeed. In other words, eat less food when you are physically inactive (burning less than 1,000 calories per week). And this is one of the ways to do it: If your lifestyle is sedentary, the first and foremost action you should take is to reduce your food intake by 25%-30% over a few weeks and, if that doesn't work, reduce by 40%-50% over the next few more weeks (reduce portion size of carbohydrates and fats and make sure that you are getting adequate lean protein and non-starchy leafy green vegetables that are abundant in nutrients and antioxidants). Keep in mind that you should only reduce or increase the energy foods (protein, particularly carbohydrates and fat) and not the non-starchy leafy vegetables. In fact, the more vegetables you have in each individual meal, the more you are likely to succeed. You are quicker to appreciate this idea if you regard the vegetables as " buffers". Continue this process until you feel full and satisfied, without being tired or sleepy after meals. You may be surprised to realize that you may feel more energy and satisfaction on lesser foods that are high in nutrients and antioxidants compared to inferior foods that are low in nutrients.

I arbitrarily recommend that sedentary adult females consume 1,300-1,500 calories per day and 1,600-1,800 calories for adult men. Children generally eat between 900-1,200 calories per day. You should begin your program at the lowest calories (1,300 calories for women and 1,600 for men) when activity level is low (burning less than 1,000 calories per week). As you shift from being sedentary to slightly active (burning about 1,750 calories a week in activities like walking briskly for 30 minutes daily or working on the treadmill), you can gradually increase portion size, carbohydrates, and calories. At the same time, be prepared to decrease portion size, calories, and carbohydrates anytime your exercise routine drops again. This practice should be carried out on a meal-to-meal basis.

## Adjusting Calories and Food to Your Level of Activity

First of all, you need to determine whether you are eating enough calories or to be exact, food for your level of activity. If you are not hungry between meals and your energy is high enough, it is likely that you are getting adequate calories. On the other hand, if you are tired and hungry between meals, you may be eating fewer calories than your body demands. Correct the situation and increase calories by increasing portion sizes slightly. The next thing to pay attention to after you have adjusted the quantity of the individual components in the meal (portion sizes of carbohydrates, fats, proteins, and fiber) is the quality of the meal. For example, are your carbohydrates choices mostly whole grains high fiber types or refined low fiber carbohydrates? Are you having adequate lean protein? Are you choosing the right types of fat? Are you getting enough leafy vegetables and fruits? Do you have adequate soluble and insoluble fiber in your meals? And are you drinking enough water? Perhaps, most importantly, are you increasing your level of physical activity?

I can't stress enough the need to increase your level of activity even a small notch upwards. It shouldn't regress or stay the same and it should go hand in hand with the amounts of food you are eating. Set your distant goal to burn about 500 calories daily doing mainly aerobic exercises in order to burn body fat. If you are doing about 30 minutes of moderately intense aerobic exercises daily you are half way there – burning about 250 calories per day. When you are at the lowest level of activity, make sure you are not eating more than you need to. The problem is that if you eat more food and calories than your body needs, you will have to exercise more (and longer) in order to burn it off. If you don't, you will store body fat and gain weight, instead of losing weight.

A good number of people have joined this program unable to engage in any form of exercise initially as a result of arthritis, muscular dystrophy, lack of energy, and excessive body weight. But even people in this situation lose body fat and weight if they make the efforts to eat enough nutrients and antioxidants and have enough soluble fiber in each meal.

Before leaving this very important chapter, I will summarize some of the major points that have been covered. Always aim to keep your portion of food in line with your level of physical activity. Eat less food or smaller portion sizes when you are not physically active and a bit more when you are. This is because your muscle burns more energy when you are active and less energy when you are sedentary. The most common mistake that people make is that they continue to eat the same portions of food even on the days when they are not exercising or physically active.

Ideally, the correct thing to do is to cut back on your food portions (carbohydrate, protein and fat sources), and make sure that you have abundant non-starchy leafy green vegetables with each meal. Later, you can gradually increase your food portions slightly when you return to being active. This will ensure that you will burn instead of store most of the calories in your meal. Also be cautious not to over judge your activity level and eat more than your body and muscles can process just because you are engaged in some form of routine exercise or physical activity. It is all about making sure that you eat most of the time the amount of food that your body can efficiently use – always think of demand and supply. Also think of your body as a biological machine that needs the best oil and gasoline to keep the engine working properly.

A simple method to determine your calorie needs is to let your body be your guide. You simply eat until you feel partially full and then stop regardless of whether you finished your food or not. This is a very effective way of controlling your portion and your calories as long as you make healthy choices and eat meals that are high in nutrients and antioxidants and also contain soluble fiber. Again, the key is to get into the habit of eating your meals in courses. The body will take care of the rest.

## Chapter 15

# UDP Meal Plan

In this chapter, you will find a breakdown of the UDP meal plan and an interpretation – including an easy-to-follow 30-day meal plan in Chapter 16. You will also have in your collection delicious and nutritionally balanced recipes, some of which have been submitted by our patients. You will love our recipes for their good taste and simplicity. The menus will indicate a range of serving sizes and portions for a female. However, males can also use the meal plan provided they increase their portion of food slightly (the key is learning to listen to your body, instead of counting calories). At any rate, I urge you to refer to the appropriate serving sizes and portions in the book or on food labels to guide you. My primary intention is to help you develop a reference point. Therefore, the meal plans are only templates that will help you to individualize and tailor your food intake to your level of physical activity. It will require some tinkering until you're satisfied, and remember that nothing is written in stone. Use common sense.

During the first 12 weeks of the UDP program, you are expected to lose on the average about 24-30 pounds on the ordinary bathroom scale. But your true progress using machines that measure body fat will show that most of your weight loss probably came from loss of body fat – this is healthy and a very good thing. However, it's not unusual to also lose a small amount of muscle tissue initially and you shouldn't be worried about it as long as you're eating enough protein and nutritionally balanced meals. On the other hand, if you are actually tailoring your food intake to physical activity level, you will be amazed by your progress and level of energy. For instance, Micheal in eight weeks lost a total of 14 pounds, but his actual weight loss was even more dramatic: he lost 27 pounds of body fat and gained 10 pounds of muscle mass. The gain in muscle mass makes the total weight loss of 14 pounds to be a modest loss. But in actuality it's not. Losing body fat and gaining muscle mass is very positive and encouraging.

You will also have a sense that you are heading in the right direction if the clothes that you were not able to fit into previously begin to fit easily – you may even have to shop for new clothes. You will notice a boost in your energy, concentration, and focus, including control of craving and binges.

After you have celebrated your first 12 weeks of UDP, you should still continue to eat proper meals, exercise regularly and try to keep your stress level under control or as low as possible. Always use the same basic principles that have been successful for you in the past. Remember that you should never diet and, as long as you are eating, make sure every meal is a proper one – that it has adequate antioxidants, nutrients, lean protein, healthy fat and fiber instead of just calories.

Whenever you find yourself dieting for any reason, you are on the wrong path (and it's definitely not UDP). This may cause you to regress – and can happen if you stop including your food template in your major meals. Some signs of regression include neglecting your mid-afternoon snack, eating a large dinner, skipping breakfast, or failing to keep up with your exercises while still eating the same amount of food. Go back to the basics, refresh, and start eating again. Never allow a minor mishap to derail your entire progress. Always remind yourself that this is a lifetime commitment and not a quick fix or fad. Keep in mind that unless you acquire a new way of eating and physical activity habits, losing weight and keeping it off over the long-term is unlikely. Going back to your old bad habits of eating and physical activity, and not completing the transition to a healthier lifestyle is the primary reason most people fail.

If you're female, it is best you start with a roughly 1,300-calorie meal plan per day and for a male about 1,600-calorie meal plan seems appropriate. In addition to cutting back on calories, eat fewer carbohydrates: About 15-35 grams (1-2 servings) whole grains per meal for a sedentary woman and 15-45 grams (1-3 servings) whole grains for a sedentary man. It's very easy to figure the actual amount of food using the serving sizes listed on food labels.

As your activity level increases, your caloric intake, including carbohydrates and other macronutrients will have to be increased appropriately and vice versa. The key is to do this on a meal- per- meal basis and it should be treated as an ongoing process.

Counting calories is not necessary. The ultimate goal is to eat what your body can burn and not what you perceive you need. The simple way to achieve this goal is to eat to slight fullness and stop regardless of the amount still left (see Chapter 14). For instance, when you eat the right amount of food and nutrients that your body needs, you won't feel extremely full and sluggish. Instead, you will feel energized, alert, and satisfied both mentally and physically.

All of this takes time and a bit of patience. It's very helpful to keep a journal of your progress – recording your energy level, sleep patterns, emotions and mood, cravings, and also changes in your physical appearance (skin, hair, nails, distribution of fat, etc). If you are diabetic, you should monitor your blood sugars (fasting and 2 hours after breakfast, lunch, and dinner). If you are eating right, your blood sugar should be normal within a few weeks and that can be very rewarding (fasting 110 or below and the 2 hours after meals less than 150).

Take Rosalyn, for instance (she was introduced briefly in Chapter 5. See Chapter 18 for her testimonial ). She was taking about 130 units of insulin injections daily when I first met her. In spite of this, her blood sugars were 300 mg/dl or more most of the time. In addition to a big appetite, she was constantly hungry and craved sugary food. But all that changed within a few weeks of eating an anti-inflammatory diet that was tailored to her level of activity.

She was sedentary at the start of the program, but gradually she increased her level of physical activity. It didn't take long before she was doing about 10-15 minutes five times a week on the treadmill. It wasn't much, but for Rosalyn this was a monumental step to regaining her energy, health and life.

Amazingly, she lost her craving for sweets in just a few weeks. She had a boost of energy and a sense of empowerment with a new image to show for it. The most profound change, however, is the increased sensitivity of her body to insulin: She now uses only a third of the insulin dose to adequately control her blood sugars, which are normal (FBS below 110 and 2 hours after meals are below 150 mg/dl).

Measure your weight weekly at about the same time of the day, preferably without clothes. Remember that, though your overall weight is important, it's the body fat and muscle that are the most critical and by all means most important. They are intimately linked not only to how good you look and feel, but also to your health. Being able to see rapid transformation in your body fat regardless of your weight should encourage you to stay the course. If you don't have a scale that measures body fat, your waist measurement, and the fitness of your clothes and energy level through the day are good indicators of progress. In other words, don't rely on the bathroom scale alone to follow your progress. In this program, you will lose body fat rapidly while maintaining or developing muscle mass. That's why you should get a good scale that measures body fat and muscle mass. Invest in one and you won't regret it. If you lose muscle initially, don't worry about it. Your body composition will stabilize later as long as you are eating proper meals and being physically active (aerobic exercise is the key to burning fat).

Now let's start with the sample meal plan, but in order to get an individualized food plan specifically designed for your needs you will have to make specific adjustments or visit our UDP center or web site.

## A Breakdown of the UDP Meal Plan

- **Calories:** 1,300 cal (15-65% carb, 20-35% fat and 20-35% protein)
- **Vegetables:** 5-7 servings daily (2½ -3 ½ cups cooked or 5-7 cups raw) or more depending on the caloric level and need. Start your major meals with vegetable soup and non-starchy dark green leafy vegetables (without the fatty and salty dressings). This group is very important in providing an adequate amount of vital antioxidants and nutrients. Naturally, some vegetables will add to your overall carbs, but you shouldn't be too concerned if you choose the non-starchy, low glycemic types. You can ignore their carb contribution. Preparation: raw, steamed, baked, stir-fried, grilled, soup, etc.
- **Fruits:** 1-2 servings daily (1-2 fiber-rich whole fresh fruits or ½-1 cup chopped) as a snack or with your meals, but be careful of carbohydrate and sugar overload. Don't forget to balance the carbohydrate with lean protein or healthy fat (an apple plus ½ cup low-fat cottage cheese, mozzarella string cheese, or boiled egg, etc.).
- **Carbohydrates:** 15% - 65%<br>Sedentary individual (15-25%): 3-5 servings (49-81g/day) whole grains<br>Slightly active (25-35%): 5-7 servings (81-114g/day) whole grains<br>Moderately active (35-45%): 7-9 servings (114-146g/day) whole grains<br>Very active (45-65%): 9-14 servings (146-211g/day) whole grains
- **Protein:** 20-35% or 3-5 servings (65-114 grams) daily. This is the equivalent of about 8-14 ounces of lean proteins, such as fish, chicken, turkey, sirloin, tenderloin, and top shoulder, including beans, soy, eggs, low-fat cheeses, and yogurt. Eight grams of protein is approximately equal to an ounce of fish and lean meat, an ounce

of tuna or cheese, an 8 ounce glass of milk, an egg, a half cup of cooked beans, or one tablespoon of peanut butter or soy protein powder.

- **Fats:** 20-35% or 2-4 servings (28-56 grams) daily – the equivalent of 2-4 tbsp of oil. The fat breakdown is 80% monounsaturated fatty acids from olive oil or canola oil (1-3 tbsp daily) and 20% from polyunsaturated oils, such as flaxseed oil or fish oil and safflower or corn oil in a ratio of 1:1 (such as 2-3 tsp flaxseed oil + 2-3 tsp safflower or corn oil daily). You can take 1 tbsp canola oil if you prefer and it will give you a favorable ratio of 2:1.

## 1600-Calorie Diet

- **Calories:** 1,600 cal (15-65% carb, 20-35% fat, and 20-35% protein)
- **Vegetables:** 5-7 servings daily (2 ½ -3 ½ cups cooked or 5-7 cups raw) or more depending on the caloric level and need. Eat non-starchy vegetables (without the fatty and salty dressings) or light vegetable soups before major meals. Preparation: raw, steamed, baked, grilled, stir-fried, soup, etc.
- **Fruits:** 1-2 servings daily (1-2 fiber-rich whole fresh fruits or ½-1 cup chopped) or more – as a snack or with your meals (but be careful of carbohydrate and sugar overload). Don't forget to balance the carbohydrate with lean protein or healthy fats (such as an apple and 2 tsp peanut butter, low-fat mozzarella string cheese, or boiled egg, etc.).
- **Carbohydrates:** 15-65%

| | |
|---|---|
| Sedentary individual (15-25%): | 4-6 servings (60-100g/day) whole grains |
| Slightly active (25-35%): | 6-9 servings (100-140g/day) whole grains |
| Moderately active (35-45%): | 9-12 servings (140-180g/day) whole grains |
| Very active (45-65%): | 12-17 servings (180-240g/day) whole grains |

- **Protein:** 20-35% or 3-6 servings (80-140 grams) daily. This is the equivalent of about 10-17 ounces of lean meat; such as fish, chicken or turkey breasts, and other lean meats (sirloin, tenderloin, or top shoulder). Other sources of protein include beans, lentils, soy, eggs, milk, yogurt, and low-fat cheeses. Eight grams of protein is approximately equal to an ounce of fish and lean meat, an ounce of tuna or cheese, an 8 ounce glass of milk or an egg, half cup of cooked dry beans, or one tablespoon of peanut butter or soy protein powder.
- **Fats:** 20-35% or 3-5 servings (42-70 grams) daily – the equivalent of 3-5 tbsp of oil. The fat breakdown is 80% monounsaturated fatty acids from olive oil and canola oil (2-4 tbsp daily) and 20% from polyunsaturated oils, such as flax oil or fish oil and safflower or corn oil in a ratio of 1:1 (such as 1 tbsp flaxseed oil + 1 tbsp safflower or corn oil daily). You can take 2 tbsp canola oil if you prefer and it will give you a ratio of 2:1.

## The Basic Nutritional Supplements

- *Omega-3 fatty acids, 1,000 mg (fish oil delivering 200 mg DHA and 300 mg EPA per serving or flaxseed oil) with meals three times a day – recommended for those not eating fatty fish (such as salmon and regular tuna) three or more times a week. Flaxseed oil is another option: 1-2 tbsp daily (add to cereals, rice, vegetables, smoothie, etc). Capsules for those not tolerating the oil: 1,000 mg three capsules three times daily. Recent advancement has been in the development of 100% pure Krill Oil containing a unique blend of Omega-3 and Omega-6 fatty acids, phospholipids, choline, and antioxidants: Vitamin A and E. *Davinci Lab* Neptune Krill Oil (1,000 mg: 150 mg EPA and 90 mg DHA) yielding phospholipids Omega-3 complex that is highly bioavailable and absorbable.

**Omega-3 Fatty Acids or Fish Oil for Special Therapeutic Use:**

- Omega-3 fatty acids or 1,000 mg fish oil: 5-6 grams (5-6 capsules) daily for diabetes, heart disease, high blood pressure, high cholesterol, high triglycerides, low HDL (good) cholesterol, high LDL (bad) cholesterol, and Syndrome X or insulin resistance. Flaxseed oil at doses of 2-4 tbsp daily is also beneficial, but don't take more than 3 tbsp daily if you are trying to lose weight. Flaxseed oil capsules at 1,000 mg, 3 capsules three times daily in combination with fish oil capsules (3-6 grams daily).
- Fish oils at 6-8 grams (6-8 capsules) daily is suggested for inflammatory diseases, such as arthritis, depression, attention deficit disorder, severe mood swings, painful menstruation, elevation of CRP, and IL-6 inflammatory markers. In combination with anti-inflammatory doses of vitamin E at 800-1,200 IU daily.
- Concentrated levels of DHA and EPA are found in some brands of cod liver oil, such as *Nordic Naturals Arctic Cod Liver Oil* (1 tsp delivers 700 mg DHA, 450 mg EPA, 875-1950 IU Vitamin A, 5-40 IU vitamin D, and 8 IU vitamin E). One major concern is vitamin A toxicity. However, acute toxicity usually occurs after an accidental ingestion of large amounts of vitamin A, about 25,000 IU/kg of body weight. Chronic toxicity appears after ingestion of 25,000 IU daily or more over a prolonged period of time. Check your local pharmacy and health food stores for well-tolerated brands of cod liver oil that are inexpensive.
- Multivitamin (without iron) with meals three times a day. See label or below for dosage.
- Multi-mineral (calcium, magnesium, selenium, etc.). See below for dosage.
- *Borage oil capsule or liquid (for PMS and menopausal symptoms, loss of hair and nails, dry skin, etc). See direction on label (For example, each 1,300-1,500 mg capsule yields about 300 mg of Gamma Linolenic Acid (GLA): 1 capsule 1-3 times daily) or about 1,000 mg per day.
- B-complex 75 once a day or Spirulina (for energy, brain stabilization)
- Vitamin E, 400-800 IU/day (antioxidant)
- 1-3 tbsp of wheat germ daily (source of vitamin E and folic acid)
- 1 tsp ground cinnamon daily (sprinkle over cereals, fruits, hot drinks, toasts, and sweet potatoes for control of blood sugar).
- Green tea, caffeinated or de-caffeinated, several cups daily (antioxidants)

- *Soy protein and soy products (optional): Get about 25-30 grams of soy protein daily, which is the equivalent of about three servings of soy. Example of a single serving of soy: 8 oz glass of soymilk; 2 by 2 inch square of tofu (½ inch thick); 1 tbsp of soy protein powder; 1 cup of raw soybeans (called edamame). The health benefits are due largely to the isoflavones. To give you an idea, about ½ cup of tofu has 25 to 35 mg isoflavones; 1 cup of soymilk contains about 30 to 40 mg isoflavones; 1 scoop or 3 tbsp soy protein powder contains about 50 mg isoflavones or more.
- *Spectra Greens *(DaVinci Lab)* is a combination of nutrient rich vegetables, fruits, herbs, Chlorella, soy, digestive enzymes, and probiotic cultures designed to support the body's ability to cleanse, detoxify, and rejuvenate. 1 scoop daily in 8 oz water or juice. It can replace your multivitamin but not mineral supplements.
  *Note: These are optional

### Recommended Dosages of Multivitamin/Mineral Supplement/Day:

Beta-carotene or mixed carotenoids: 15,000-20,000 IU; vitamin E: 400-800 IU in natural form plus mixed tocopherols; vitamin C: 250 mg or 500-1,000 mg if heart disease is present; B6: 50-100 mg; B12: 50-100 mcg; Folic acid: 400 mcg; calcium: 1,000-1,500 mg; vitamin D: 400 IU if not included in calcium supplement; Selenium: 100-200 mcg; magnesium: 500 mg; potassium: 98 mg; coenzyme Q10: 60-120 mg. Check the dosage of other supplements you may be taking to make sure you are not overdosing or not getting adequate amounts. Don't forget to consult with your physician before taking any dietary supplements to prevent interactions with other drugs. Note that most mineral and vitamin supplements only give you about 50-90 mg of potassium per serving, even though your daily requirement is about 4,700 mg daily. This shouldn't be a problem, because potassium is found abundantly in foods, such as oranges, lemons, grapefruit, green leafy vegetables, potatoes, bananas and sunflower seeds.

## SUMMARY Of The UDP Program

1) Healthy weight: Should be based on Body Fat Percentage instead of Body Mass Index (BMI) or a combination of both.
2) Quality of food emphasized over quantity and calories: Foods high in nutrients, antioxidants, and fiber, particularly soluble fiber and also low in sugar, saturated fat, trans-fat, cholesterol, Omega-6, and salt.
3) The Food Template (this is the first rule): Forms the basic foundation of healthy and proper meal plans and should be an integral part of all meals, especially lunch and dinner.
4) Eating in Courses (this is the second rule): Eat your meals in courses to allow your body ample time to prepare for the high-energy foods, such as carbohydrates and starches (side dishes).
5) Carbohydrates: Eat mostly whole grains, or low glycemic high fiber carbohydrates: About 15-35 grams (1-2 servings) whole grains per meal for a sedentary woman and

15-45 grams (1-3 servings) whole grains for a sedentary man. It's very easy to figure the actual amount of food using the serving sizes listed on food labels. This does not include carbohydrates from non-starchy vegetables. Treat carbohydrates and starchy vegetables as side dishes. Limit processed foods and refined carbohydrates, such as cookies and sodas. When indulging, keep portion small. Limit pure sugar to less than 10 grams or 15 grams (about 1-2 tsp or 1-3 tsp for a 1,300 and 1,600 calorie diet, respecticely.) or less per serving.

6) Whole Foods: Choose whole foods over processed ones. Example: fresh fruits over juices or long whole grain brown rice over short grain white rice. Choose minimally refined cereals over quick or instant cooking ones. Limit processed foods, especially those with sweeteners, such as fructose and its derivatives.
7) Eat to fullness and stop regardless of the amount left unconsumed (listen to your body, instead of your eyes).
8) Have 1-2 cups or more of non-starchy dark green leafy vegetables and soups or fiber-rich fruits before lunch and dinner (prepare according to preference). Be creative. For example, eating salads the entire time can be boring, but eating a variety of vegetables prepared in different types of ways can be refreshing and inspiring (For example, "Turn your vegetables into soups").
9) Choose fiber-rich foods that are not sweetened with sugar and contain at least 3 or more grams of fiber per serving. Aim for a total of 7-10 grams of fiber per meal. Eat a variety of foods that are rich in both insoluble and soluble fiber. Soluble fiber should account for close to 25-30% of total fiber (daily requirement 20-35 grams/day). Aim to have about 3-5 grams of soluble fiber as a side dish or with each major meal, especially dinner (oat bran, oats, apples, beans, lentils, chana dal, soybeans, edamame, carrots, broccoli, eggplant, asparagus, Brussel sprouts, okra, blueberries, strawberries, raspberries, cherries, grapefruit slices, kiwifruit, orange slices, fresh peaches with skin, fresh pear with skin, plum, celery, cabbage, bean sprout, French cut green beans, snow peas, split peas, green peas, zucchini, kale, turnip, cactus, dry okra powder, textured vegetable protein, sweet potatoes with skin, etc). You may use soluble fiber supplements if necessary, such as *Benefiber* and *Clearly fiber* and *Beano* to eliminate flatulence.
10) Fats: Minimally processed and high nutrient vegetable oils, such as extra virgin olive and cold-pressed canola oils are preferred as primary cooking oils over highly refined vegetable oils, such as corn and safflower oils. You will need two to four servings (28-56 grams or 2-4 tbsp) per day or 10-19 grams per meal for a sedentary person on a 1,300-calorie diet and three to five servings (42-70 grams or 3-5 tbsp) or 14-23 grams per meal for a sedentary person on a 1,600-calorie diet. Choose foods with 5 grams or less of fat per serving except for fatty fish, such as mackerel, tuna, and salmon. Seafood is the preferred source of fat and protein, followed by beans and lentils, egg whites and so forth: (seafood > beans and lentils, egg whites, skinless chicken and turkey white meat > lean veal > lean beef > lean pork > lean lamb). Choose foods with saturated fat not greater than 3 grams per ounce. Limit the use of foods with trans fat, such as cookies and chips.

11) Protein: Keep protein sources lean and low-fat and eat adequate portion to support an active metabolism. Get about 24-38 grams and 24-48 grams of protein per meal for a 1,300 and 1,600-calorie diets, respectively. To give you an idea, 3 oz fish or lean meat averages about 24 grams protein (salmon, tuna, halibut, chicken breast, turkey breast, lean beef, lean veal, lean pork, lean lamb). Refer to the averages of calories and portion sizes below.
12) Non-starchy vegetables and fruits: Eat about 2 ½ -3 ½ cups cooked or 5-7 cups raw or more of non-starchy dark green leafy and colored vegetables and 1-2 fiber-rich fruits or ½ -1 cup chopped fruit daily, preferably for snacks.
13) Starchy vegetables: Treat as major source of carbohydrates and starches as well as a side dish (potatoes, plantain, sweet potatoes, new potatoes, yam, beans, corn, parsnip, rutabaga, and winter squashes). The same thinking applies to fruits with high carbohydrate and sugar content, such as overripe bananas and plantains, pear, papaya, pineapples, mango, cantaloupe, and nectarines (especially when portion is large).
14) Sodium: Keep daily sodium intake to 2,300 mg or less (the equivalent of about 1 tsp of table salt). For canned foods, select those with salt content less than 800mg per serving or reduce the portion size. Also take into account that most processed and frozen foods, such as meat, seasonings, vegetables, and beans are loaded with salt.
15) Cholesterol: No more than 300 mg of cholesterol daily, the equivalent of one medium whole egg (not more than one yolk a day). A medium egg has about 215-230 mg of cholesterol.
16) Alcohol: Limit beer and alcoholic drinks and, if you do drink, eat before in order to slow down absorption. Weekend social drinking and binges are non-productive and can hinder your progress. In general, it is wise to drink only occasionally and if you choose to drink, keep it to a minimum. Drinking alcohol can sabotage your weight loss effort.
17) Wine: Red or white wine with some dinners is acceptable if you can work it off (2 servings delivers about 400 calories). Red wine has more antioxidants.
18) Coffee: Limit if trying to lose weight (1 cup a day is better than 3-6 cups).
19) Tea: Drink green or black tea regularly (high in antioxidants and can help burn body fat).
20) Water: Drink adequate water – about 6-8 glasses per day or less if eating adequate vegetables and fruits.
21) Stop eating after 8 pm or 3 hours before bedtime. Herbal tea for sleep or relaxation is acceptable.
22) Eat what you can burn (this is the third rule): Eat your calories and carbohydrates in line with your level of physical activity. For example: Eat less when not physically active (cut down food portion by 25-50%) and increase portion slightly when active. At the same time, keep in mind that eating too much of any food, no matter how healthy it is, can cause fat storage and weight gain.
23) Exercise (this is the fourth rule): Aim for moderate intensity aerobic exercises daily (preferably first thing in the morning after a cup of green tea or another choice) for about 30-60 minutes. Aim to burn about 400-500 calories/day (like walking 4 miles in one hour, jogging, treadmill, bicycling, or any other activity

that you enjoy for a total of 1 hour). You can divide your time and do about 30 minutes per session. Start slowly and gradually, but be consistent. Always start and end with some form of flexibility exercises to prevent injury. Also partake in resistance exercise to build and strengthen muscles shortly after dinner (to prevent fat storage). Hint: Aerobic exercises that are done for 30-60 minutes before breakfast seem to help to burn body fat more efficiently and resistance exercise done in the evening helps to burn the dinner you ate as well as strengthen muscle.

24) Relaxation (this is the fifth rule): Get a minimum of 10-30 minutes each day of relaxation – yoga, meditation, self-hypnosis or listening to soothing music and sounds to help reduce stress and cortisol levels (also an important rule). Take time for yourself daily. Chronic stress, depression, sadness, anxiety, and uncontrolled anger can cause the buildup of stubborn and toxic belly fat, as well as suppress the immune system.

## A Glance At Portion Size

Know or measure out your portion sizes before you begin eating, as this will help ensure that you eat within the range that is appropriate for your level of activity. Controlling your portion size is easy if you get familiar with the food serving sizes and averages of fat, protein, carbohydrates, and calories of the common foods you like to eat.

Try to eyeball them until you reach a degree of high confidence. Use the chart below to help you stay within reasonable portion size, as well figure out at a glance the amount of fat, protein, and carbohydrate in a meal. This is particularly handy when eating out. If you don't remember, look them up.

**Averages of Calories and Portion Sizes of Common Foods**

Non-starchy vegetables, raw: 1 cup (baseball size)---25 calories
Non-starchy vegetables, cooked: ½ cup (tennis ball size)---25 calories
Starchy vegetables: ½ cup or 2 oz (potatoes, corn, 19g carb)---100 calories
Fresh fruits: medium or ½ cup (baseball, ½ baseball)---60 calories
Grains: ½ cup (rice, pasta, hot cereal: 25g carb, 4+g fiber)---120 calories
Cold cereals: ½ cup (24g carb, 8g fiber)---80 calories
Cooked beans: ½ cup (7g fiber, 20g carb, 8g protein)---120 calories
Fish, lean: 3 oz (deck of cards; 2g fat, 23g protein)---110 calories
Fatty fish: 3 oz (salmon, tuna; 9g fat, 23g protein)---180 calories
Meat, lean: 3 oz (top round, eye round roast; 4g fat, 26g prot)---150 calories
Meat, fatty: 3 oz (chuck blade, brisket; 11g fat, 26g prot)---210 calories
Poultry, white: 3oz (deck of cards, 24g protein, 2g fat)---120 calories
Poultry, dark: 3 oz (thigh, drumstick; 22g protein, 6g fat)---140 calories
Bread, multigrain: 1 slice (15g carb, 4g fiber)---60 calories
Oat bran/whole-wheat tortilla, *Joseph's:* (11g carb, 6g fiber)---70 calories
Oat bran/whole-wheat pita bread, *Joseph's:*(10g carb, 5g fiber)---60 calories
Bagel: 100% whole-wheat, 1 (23g carb, 7 g fiber)---140 calories
English muffin: 100% whole-wheat, 1 or small (23g carb, 3g fiber)---120 calories
Butter, margarine: 1tsp (size of a stamp, 2g fat)---36 calories
Oil: 1 tbsp (olive, canola, vegetable oils; 14g fat)---120 calories

Cheese, low-fat: 1 oz (a woman's thumb: 1g fat, 5g protein)---40 calories
Cheese, regular: 1 slice or 1 oz (9g fat, 6g protein)---100 calories
Bacon: 3 slices (8g fat, 6g protein)---90 calories
Canadian bacon: 2 slices (3g fat, 10g protein)---69 calories
Ham, lean: 1 slice (1g fat, 5g protein)---30 calories
Nut/seeds: 1 tbsp chopped (4g fat, 2g protein)---47 calories
Nut/seeds: 1 oz (handful; 14-21g fat, 6g protein)---170-204 calories
Egg: 1 large (5g fat, 213 mg cholesterol, 6g protein)---75 calories
Egg white: 3 or ½ cup eggbeaters (12g protein, 0 fat)---60 calories
Milk, skim: 1 cup (0.4g fat, 8g protein, 1g sugar)---85 calories
Sugar: 1 tsp (4g sugar)---16 cal or Splenda: 1 pct (0g sugar)---0 calories
Peanut butter: 1 tbsp (8g fat, 4g protein)---94 calories
Salad dressing: 1-2 tsp olive oil+2 tbsp vinegar or 1 tbsp lemon juice + herbs, spice + black ground pepper to taste (5-10g fat, 1-2g sat)---43-86 calories

## Chapter 16

# 30-Day Meal Plan

- Start your days with a cup of green or black tea or another choice (caffeinated or decaffeinated) with 1-2 tablespoons of lemon juice, apple cider or other vinegar of your choice. You can add low-fat milk, low-fat cream, or Splenda if you like.
- Do at least 30 minutes of aerobic exercise before breakfast (if you're diabetic, make sure your blood sugar is not low before you exercise. Eat something and recheck it before you exercise). The ultimate goal is to reach 60 min daily.
- Women: The food portions in this book are intended for women whose lifestyle is sedentary to slightly active. That implies that your level of activity is so low that you may be burning less than 1,750 calories per week. You recall the magic number that in order to burn a pound of body fat, you need to exercise and burn about 3,500 calories in a week (brisk walking 4 miles an hour seven days a week will get you there, but jogging will get you there faster).
- As you increase your activity level, you may also have to increase your food portion. It is best you do so in small increments. At the same time, don't fail to reduce your portion sizes any time your activity level declines. It is important to make the adjustments on a meal-to-meal basis.
- Men: You can also use this meal plan, but increase your portion sizes slightly. For instance, you may require 1-1.5 cup of *Kashi GOLEAN* cereal and 3-6 ounces of meat initially. Don't forget that the actual amount of food that you eat will depend on your energy need and activity level.
- Reduce your portion sizes and eat less when you are not active. You are very vulnerable at this time; therefore, you should make all effort to eat more foods that deliver nutrients and antioxidants instead of pure energy and calories.
- Food Portions: To control your food portions, you need to become familiar with serving sizes listed on food labels. However, a simple and practical approach is to reduce the amount of food you previously ate by about 25% or even by 50%. Record your mood, energy level, craving, hunger pangs, sleep patterns, satisfaction, and weekly weight loss or gain. This will give you a rough idea whether you are on the right track.
- Liquids: Drink enough liquid (such as water, green tea, black tea, crystal light, skim milk, soymilk, *Mountain Sun* cranberry juice, and other unsweetened juices – apple, grapefruit, and orange juices). If it makes you feel better, you may also have diet sodas a few times a week (maybe once or twice a week. Even diet sodas contain chemicals that may increase the levels of free radicals that trigger inflammation).
- For some, the urge for coffee is so strong that they are unable to go without several cups of coffee daily even with the knowledge that it blocks weight loss. To these

people, my advice is to cut back gradually to fewer cups a day. A single cup of coffee a day may not be that harmful to your weight loss effort. As you cut back on coffee, drink more green tea, both caffeinated and decaffeinated.

- How much you eat at a glance: Non-starchy vegetables – eat abundantly. Fruits – 1-2 daily, preferably for snacks. Cereals – refer to nutritional label. In general, eat the suggested amount of cereal (the serving size) only if you are fairly active. Eat less than the serving size if you are sedentary. For example, the portion size for *Kashi GOLEAN* for a sedentary person is ¾ cup (1.4 oz) and for an active person 1 cup (1.8 oz) or more.
  - Meat and Fish – 3-4 oz per meal (sedentary females) and 3-6 oz per meal (sedentary males).
  - Carbohydrates – multigrain or 100% whole-wheat bread – 1 slice (sedentary individuals) and 1-2 slices (fairly active individuals). Rice and pasta: ½-1 cup cooked (sedentary females) and 1-2 cups (sedentary males).
  - Potatoes – small new potatoes (2-3 small potatoes), sweet potatoes (3-4 oz), white large potatoes (2 –3 oz), and mashed potatoes (½ -1 cup) if you are sedentary.
  - Corn – eat ½-1 cup or one corn on the cob if you are sedentary. Refer to the calorie and portion chart.
  - Get Adequate Fiber In Every Meal: Because you are reducing your caloric intake, you may also be reducing your fiber intake. As a result of this, you may have constipation. But making sure you have adequate fiber in every meal can prevent this. A high-quality fiber source, such as 2-3 dried prunes can be added to breakfast cereals, yogurt, and vegetables. Other readily available sources of high-quality fiber that can be added include oat bran, wheat bran, high fiber cereals like *General Mills* Fiber One, and *Kellogg's* All Bran (1-3 tbsp).

    Start this program on a Sunday to get the optimum benefit, and feel free to make adjustments to meet your needs. Nothing is written in stone. Use your imagination.

*Don't forget to eat your meals in a gentle and polite manner and in courses. Pretend that you are being treated in a luxurious, 5-star hotel and your chef is world-renowned. He is very delighted to please and serve you.*

**Day 1 (1st Sunday)**

**Breakfast---Cold Cereal**

High fiber and low sugar cereal (such as ½ cup Kashi Good Friends, Original; ½ cup Kashi GOLEAN; ¼ cup Kellogg's All-Bran with extra fiber or Fiber One, etc.)
½ cup low-fat or soymilk
2 tbsp ground flaxseeds (*Barlean's Forti-Flax*) + 1-3 tsp flax oil or (1-3 tsp cod liver oil – take separately if cholesterol is high or history of diabetes, arthritis, high blood pressure, or heart disease).

1 tbsp wheat germ
1 tbsp oat bran or wheat bran
1 tsp fresh ground cinnamon
1 tbsp chopped nuts (walnuts, butternut, chestnuts, almonds, or sunflower seeds)
2-3 dried prunes, sliced (if problems with constipation)
¼ cup berries (strawberries, blueberries, etc)
1 tbsp Benefiber or 2 tsp Clearly Fiber (mix into cereal or dissolve in fluid)
¾ scoop (19g) soy protein powder or whey protein (mix into milk and add to cereal)
**Note**: *You can have other protein sources if you don't like soy or whey protein:*
2 boiled eggs (eat only the egg whites or one whole egg + one egg white) or ½ cup eggbeaters or ¼ cup textured vegetable protein:
With any one of these (choose only one): 1 oz tuna, sardines, lean smoked salmon, turkey, or ham (low sodium); or 2 oz veggie soy bacon; one low-fat mozzarella string cheese; ½ cup 1-2% cottage cheese, ½ cup cooked beans, 1 tbsp peanut butter – feel free to alternate choices as you like.
Stats: 392 cal, 31g protein, 43.7g carb, 14g fat, 1g sat, 16g fiber, 352mg sodium, 2mg chol, 1,277mg potassium, 422mg calcium
*Kashi GOLEAN is one of the best cold cereals (1 cup, 30g carb, 13g protein, 10g fiber, 1g soluble fiber, 9g insoluble fiber, 6g sugar)*

**Morning Snack (Optional):**
½ fruit (apple, pear, ½ grapefruit, etc.)
8 oz water or green tea
Stats: 40 cal, 0g protein, 11g carb, 0g fat, 2.5g fiber

**OR**

6 oz low sodium V8 Vegetable Juice or Tomato juice
Stats: 60 cal, 2g protein, 11g carb, 0g fat, 2g, fiber

**Lunch---Andreas Mediterranean Grilled Chicken Salad**

1. Start with lemonade fluid (½ tbsp lemon juice with 4 oz water, green tea, or other fluid)
2. Main course: 3 oz chicken in 14 oz portion Andreas Mediterranean Grilled Chicken Salad (recipe 1)
3. 3 medium strawberries or ¼ cup berries
4. End with 4 oz lemonade fluid
   Stats: 298 cal, 30g protein, 18g carb, 12.6g fat, 2g sat, 6g fiber, 389mg sodium, 96mg chol, 925mg potassium, 113mg calcium

- **Alternatives:**
  - *McDonald's* Grilled Chicken Caesar Salad – omit cheese and croutons and use only ½ pkt Newman's Own Low-fat Balsamic Vinaigrette or Cobb Dressing
  - *Wendy's* Mandarin Chicken Salad (use only ½ pkt Fat Free French Style Dressing) or *Wendy's* Chicken BLT Salad (omit cheese)

- *Burger King* Fire-Grilled Chicken Caesar Salad – ½ pkt Honey Mustard, Fat Free Dressing or ½ pkt Garden Ranch Dressing
- *Subway* Grilled Chicken Breast and Baby Spinach – use ½ pkt *Kraft* Fat Free Italian Dressing

**Mid Afternoon Snack (Must Have):**
½ cup low-fat cottage cheese or 4 oz nonfat low sugar yogurt or plain
1 tsp wheat germ or ground flaxseeds
½ apple
8 oz water or green tea
Stats: 128 cal, 15g protein, 16g carb, 1g fat, 1g fiber

**Dinner (1) Roasted Salmon With Flame-Roasted Vegetable Platter**

1. Start with lemonade fluid (½ tbsp lemon juice with 4 oz water, green tea, or other fluid)
2. Follow with ½ cup Vegetable Broth Soup (recipe 2a)* or non-creamy Lite Soup
3. Follow with 1 cup Flame-Roasted Vegetable Platter (recipe 2b)
4. Main course: 4 oz portion Roasted Salmon (recipe 3)
5. Serve with roasted sweet potato wedges with skin (2 oz, about 14g carb)
6. 1 tbsp Benefiber or 2 tsp Clearly Fiber (mix into soup or fluid)
7. End with 4 oz lemonade fluid or herbal tea
   Stats: 360 cal, 27g protein, 32g carb, 14g fat, 2g sat, 13g fiber, 400mg sod, 62mg chol, 1,378mg potassium, 74mg calcium

* *Preparation is key. For example, make a big batch of your choice of vegetable soup for the week – refrigerate in small containers for convenience*

**OR**

**Dinner (2) Oven Baked Crusted Chicken With Roasted Veggies**

1. Start with lemonade fluid (½ tbsp lemon juice with 4 oz water, green tea, or other fluid)
2. Follow with ½ cup Lite Vegetable Soup (recipe 4a) or 1 cup Lime Seafood Vegetable Soup (recipe 4b)
3. Follow with Spinach, Romaine or Arugula Lettuce Salad (2 cups fresh baby spinach or mixed greens + 2 tomato slices + 1 large red onion slice + ½ cup button mushrooms + 1-2 tsp olive oil + 2 tbsp red wine or balsamic vinegar or lemon juice + salt and black pepper or Mrs. Dash to taste)
4. Main course: 3-4 oz portion Oven Baked Crusted Chicken (recipe 4c)
5. With 1 cup Roasted Veggies (recipe 5)
6. End with 4 oz lemonade fluid or herbal tea
   Stats: 383 cal, 34g protein, 33g carb, 15g fat, 0.5g sat, 9g fiber, 722mg sodium, 65mg chol, 1,713mg potassium, 180mg calcium

   * *Make a big batch for the week – refrigerate in small containers for convenience*

## Day 2 (1st Monday)

**Breakfast---Elizabeth's Favorite Breakfast**

6 oz *Yoplait* Plain Yogurt (0 sugar)
1 tbsp chopped Walnuts, Butternuts, or Almonds
1 tbsp ground flaxseeds (*Barlean's*)
1 tbsp Benefiber or 2 tsp *Davinci Labs* Clearly Fiber
1 boiled egg or egg white
½ cup berries (blueberries, strawberries, etc.) or 1 cup diced melon, ½ cup fresh-diced mango, or ½ cup fresh pineapple chunks
8 oz water, green tea, or coffee

**Instructions:**

1. Combine first three ingredients. Serve with egg and ½ cup berries.
2. Dissolve Benefiber or Clearly Fiber in the yogurt or fluid of your choice and take separately
   Stats: 321 cal, 20g protein, 28g carb, 16g fat, 4g sat, 12g fiber, 194 mg sodium, 206mg chol, 667mg potassium, 356mg calcium

**Morning Snack (Optional):**

1 fruit (apple, pear, plum, etc.) or 2-3 dried prunes
8 oz water or green tea
Stats: 80 cal, 0g protein, 22g carb, 0g fat, 5g fiber

**Lunch---Italian Vegetable Chicken Soup**

1. Start with lemonade fluid (½ tbsp lemon juice with 4 oz water, green tea, or other fluid)
2. Main course: 2 cups Italian Vegetable Chicken Soup (recipe 6)
3. Serve with 3 multigrain or whole-wheat crackers (*Carr's*) or 1 oat bran/whole-wheat tortilla or pita (*Joseph's*) or a high fiber multigrain bread
4. End with 4 oz lemonade fluid
   Stats: 312 cal, 39g protein, 24g carb, 9g fat, 2g sat, 11g fiber, 589mg sodium, 68mg chol, 749mg potassium, 139 mg calcium

**Mid Afternoon Snack (Must Have):**

Mozzarella string cheese, low-fat
½ cup canned peaches in water or 1 medium peach, 10 grapes, or ½ grapefruit
8 oz water or green tea or V-8 juice
Stats: 79 cal, 8.5g protein, 8.5g carb, 1.5g fat, 2g fiber.

**Dinner (1)---Easy Turkey Chili With Garden salad**

1. Start with lemonade fluid (½ tbsp lemon juice with 4 oz water, green tea, or other fluid)
2. Follow with ½ cup Italian Vegetable Soup (recipe 7a) or 1 cup One Pot Vegetable Soup (recipe 7b) or non-creamy Lite Soup

3. Follow with 2 cups Garden salad (1 cup romaine, 1 cup spinach or arugula, 2 tomato slices, 3 cucumber slices, 2 bell pepper strips, oregano leaves, ½ tsp ground cinnamon)
4. Dressing: 1-2 tsp olive oil + 2 tbsp fresh lemon juice, salt, and fresh ground black pepper to taste)
5. Main course: 2 oz meat in 9 oz portion of Easy Turkey Chili (recipe 8)
6. And 1 low-fat mozzarella string cheese or ¼ cup fat free ricotta cheese or ¼ cup low-fat cottage cheese – no salt added
7. End with 4 oz lemonade fluid or herbal tea
   Stats: 367 cal, 30g protein, 30g carb, 15g fat, 4g sat, 11g fiber, 908mg sodium, 64mg chol, 1,391mg potassium, 176mg calcium

**OR**

**Dinner (2)---Golden Baked Fish With Vegetable Pot Soup**

1. Start with lemonade fluid (½ tbsp lemon juice with 4 oz water, green tea, or other fluid)
2. Follow with 1 cup Vegetable Pot Soup (recipe 72) or 1 cup Lime Seafood Vegetable Soup (recipe 4b)
3. Main course: 4 oz portion Golden Baked Fish (recipe 9)
4. Serve with 1 cup Mixed Veggies (recipe 46a)
5. End with 4 oz lemonade fluid or herbal tea
   Stats: 229 cal, 33g protein, 19g carb, 6g fat, 1g sat, 9g fiber, 270mg sodium, 61mg chol, 1,465mg potassium, 143mg calcium

**Day 3 (1stTuesday)**

**Breakfast—Hot Cereal (Oat Bran or 100% Whole Grain Rolled Oats)**

¼ cup (4 tbsp) Oat Bran Hot Cereal (such as *Quaker* Oatmeal 100% Natural Old Fashioned, *Quaker* Oat Bran Hot Cereal, or *Hodgson Mill* Oat Bran Hot Cereal). Also ½ pkt *Quaker* Oatmeal Weight Control, Cinnamon: high total fiber, high soluble fiber, and low sugar cereals. Avoid the instant or 1-minute varieties. Prepare according to instructions (recipe 10) and make sure to add the extra ingredients listed.

½ cup skim, soymilk, or lactose-free milk

2 tbsp ground flaxseeds (*Barlean's*) + 1-3 tsp flax oil or (2-3 tsp cod liver oil – take separately if cholesterol is high or history of diabetes, arthritis, high blood pressure, or heart disease).

1 tsp fresh ground cinnamon

1 tbsp wheat germ

1 tbsp oat bran or wheat bran

1 tbsp chopped or sliced walnuts, butternut, chestnuts, almonds, or sunflower seeds

½ scoop (12.5g) soy protein or whey protein (mix into cereal, milk, or water) or 1 slice lean smoked salmon, turkey or ham; 2-3 oz canned sardine or ¼ cup textured vegetable protein or ½ cup eggbeaters or one whole egg + one egg white or one low-fat mozzarella string cheese or ½ cup 1-2% cottage cheese, etc—feel free to alternate

Accompany with ¼ cup berries (strawberries, blueberries, raspberries)

8 oz water, green tea, or coffee.

1 tbsp Benefiber or 2 tsp Clearly Fiber (mix into milk or fluid).
Stats: 369 cal, 28g protein, 40g carb, 12g fat, 1g sat, 12.5g fiber, 236mg sodium, 3mg chol, 1,227mg potassium, 354mg calcium

Quaker Oatmeal Weight Control can help to lower blood cholesterol and sugar levels (1 pkt or 45g: 160 cal, 29g carb, 6g fiber, 4g soluble fiber, 1g sugar, 7g protein, and 3g fat); Quaker Oatmeal-Old Fashioned (½ cup: 150 cal, 27g carb, 4g fiber, 2g soluble fiber, 0g sugar, 5g protein, 2.5g fat); Quaker Oat Bran Hot Cereal (½ cup: 25g carb, 6g fiber, 3g soluble fiber, 3g insoluble fiber, 1 g sugar, 7g protein, 3g fat); Hodgson Mill Oat Bran Hot Cereal (¼ cup: 120 cal, 23g carb, 6g fiber, 3g soluble fiber, 3g insoluble fiber, 0g sugar, 6g protein, 3g fat).

Soluble fiber slows down food digestion and stomach emptying, which helps to maintain healthy blood sugar and insulin levels and thereby boost metabolism as well as reduce inflammatory compounds that are the root cause of chronic degenerative diseases (such as heart disease, diabetes, arthritis, premature aging, and even obesity).

When you choose cereals, pay attention to the total amount of fiber as well as the soluble fiber. The higher the soluble fiber, the better the cereal in terms of losing weight and improving health (lowers cholesterol, triglycerides, and blood sugar). On the other hand, for regularity, look for cereals with high insoluble fiber. I do not usually recommend the instant cereals due to lack of adequate fiber as a result of over-processing. However, the exception is made for Quaker Instant Oatmeal Weight Control because it has a high amount of the all-important soluble fiber, as well as whole grain rolled oats and probably is low glycemic.

**Morning Snack (Optional):**

4 oz nonfat low sugar yogurt or plain
¼ cup berries (blueberries, strawberries, etc.)
1 tsp ground flaxseeds or wheat germ
8 oz water or green tea
Stats: 105 cal, 5g protein, 18g carb, 1.8g fat, 2g fiber

**Lunch---Tuna Salad Sandwich With Mixed Green Salad**

1. Start with lemonade fluid (½ tbsp lemon juice with 4 oz water, green tea, or other fluid)
2. Follow with 2 cups Mixed Green Salad or Prepackaged Greens (2 cups mixed greens, ¼ green bell peppers, ¼ red bell peppers, 3 tomatoes slices, 3 medium or button mushrooms slices, ¼ cucumber slices, ½ tsp ground cinnamon)
3. Dressing: Olive/vinegar (1 tsp extra virgin oil + 2 tbsp balsamic vinegar or any other vinegar you like); or 2 tbsp lemon juice + salt, herbs, and ground black pepper to taste; or 1-2 tbsp fat free dry *Italian* dressing (see package instructions).
4. Main course: Tuna Salad Sandwich (7 oz portion):
   3 ounces regular tuna in water (drained)
   2 tsp low sodium light mayonnaise
   1 tbsp chopped green onions
   1 tsp chopped celery
   1 slice multigrain bread or 1 oat bran/whole-wheat pita pocket *(Joseph's)*
   3 tomato slices

**Instructions:**

1. Combine first four ingredients.
2. Serve with tomatoes on bread or stuffed into pita pocket.
   Stats: 283 cal, 31g protein, 25g carb, 8.6g fat, 1.5g sat, 11g fiber, 772mg sodium, 39mg chol, 933mg potassium, 97mg calcium

- Alternative: *Subway* Tuna Deli Sandwich

**Mid Afternoon Snack (Must Have):**

1 medium apple, pear, nectarine, or grapefruit
1 boiled egg or mozzarella string cheese, low-fat
Stats: 130 cal, 8g protein, 23g carb, 2.5g fat, 5g fiber

**OR**

4 oz nonfat low sugar yogurt or ½ cup 2% cottage cheese
1 tsp toasted wheat germ or ground flaxseeds
Mozzarella string cheese, low-fat
8 oz water or green tea or V-8 juice
Stats: 118 cal, 13g protein, 13g carb, 2g fat, 0.3g fiber

**Dinner (1)---Greek Chicken Kabobs With Tabouleh Salad**

1. Start with lemonade fluid (½ tbsp lemon juice with 4 oz water, green tea, or other fluid)
2. Follow with 1 cup Broccoli and Dill Weed Soup (recipe 11a), 1 cup Broccoli Soup (recipe 11b), or non-creamy Lite Vegetable Soup
3. Follow with 4 oz portion (3/4 cup) Tabouleh Salad (recipe 12)
4. Main course: 3-4 oz chicken in 6 oz portion Greek Chicken Kabobs (recipe 13)
5. 1 tbsp Benefiber or 2 tsp Clearly Fiber (mix into soup or fluid)
6. End with 4 oz lemonade fluid or herbal tea
   Stats: 381 cal, 34g protein, 31g carb, 15g fat, 3g sat, 13g fiber, 163mg sodium, 73mg chol, 973mg potassium, 181mg calcium

**OR**

**Dinner (2) Steam Roasted Red Snapper With Eggplant and Zucchini**

1. Start with lemonade fluid (½ tbsp lemon juice with 4 oz water, green tea, or other fluid)
2. Follow with 1 cup Lite Vegetable Soup (recipe 4a) or non-creamy Lite Vegetable Soup
3. Follow with 2 cups Garden Salad (recipe 15) or 1 cup Pan-Roasted Lime Broccoli (recipe 14)
4. Main course: 4 oz fish in 10oz portion Steam Roasted Red Snapper (recipe 16)
5. Serve with 1 cup Pan-Roasted Eggplant and Zucchini (recipe 17)
6. End with 4 oz lemonade fluid or herbal tea
   Stats: 331 cal, 34g protein, 32g carb, 10g fat, 3g sat, 12g fiber, 345mg sodium, 44mg chol, 2,158mg potassium, 309mg calcium
   * *You can use fish fillets (such as tilapia, salmon, halibut, sea bass, etc.)*

## Day 4 (1st Wednesday)

**Breakfast---Strawberry Tofu Smoothie**

5 large strawberries or ½ cup berries
½ cup soft tofu
1 tsp lemon juice
1 scoop Soy protein powder or whey protein (25 grams)
1 tbsp ground flaxseed
1 tsp ground cinnamon
¼ cup fresh orange juice
Water – add as needed or ice cubes
1 tbsp Benefiber or 2 tsp Clearly Fiber (mix into orange juice or fluid).

**Instructions:**

1. Blend first six ingredients until smooth. Add water to get desired smoothness
   Stats: 287 cal, 34g protein, 24g carb, 7g fat, 1g sat, 9g fiber, 313mg sodium, 0mg chol, 661mg potassium, 335mg calcium

**Morning Snack (Optional):**

2 tbsp Hummus Tahini (recipe 18a) or Quick salsa (Recipe 18b)
Assorted vegetable sticks (celery stalks, 1/8 medium green bell peppers, 1/8 medium red bell peppers, 1/8 cucumber, 2 baby carrots, 2 cherry tomatoes, 2 celery stalks).
You can also use 3 tbsp nonfat sour cream + ½ tsp dry nonfat *Italian* dressing
8 oz water or green tea
Stats: 61 cal, 3g protein, 13g carb, 0g fat, 3g fiber

**Lunch---Grilled Chicken Sandwich With Vegetable Soup**

1. Start with lemonade fluid (½ tbsp lemon juice with 4 oz water, green tea, or other fluid)
2. Follow with 4 oz Canned *Progresso* Healthy Classic Lentil Soup or non-creamy Lite Vegetable soup
3. Main course: 8 oz portion Grilled Chicken Sandwich
   3 oz grilled or baked chicken or turkey breast (recipe 18c)
   2 slices tomatoes
   3 leaves romaine
   3 dill pickles, slices
   1 tsp Dijon mustard
   1 tsp low sodium lite mayonnaise or mustard
   2 slices multigrain bread or 1 oat bran/whole-wheat tortilla or pita bread (*Joseph's*)

**Instructions:**

1. Assemble sandwich and enjoy
   Stats: 332 cal, 34g protein, 33g carb, 8g fat, 2g sat, 9g fiber, 883mg sod, 82mg chol, 677mg potassium, 90mg calcium

**Mid Afternoon Snack (Must Have):**

1 oz low-fat mozzarella string cheese
10-15 grapes, 1 apple, medium peach, kiwi, tangerine, or 2-3 dried prunes
8 oz water or green tea or V-8 juice
Stats: 148 cal, 9g protein, 22g carb, 5g fat, 5g fiber

**Dinner (1) Spinach and Mushroom Omelet With Asparagus and Celery Soup**

1. Start with lemonade fluid (½ tbsp lemon juice with 4 oz water, green tea, or other fluid)
2. Follow with 1 cup Asparagus and Celery Soup (recipe 19) or non-creamy Lite Vegetable Soup
3. Follow with 2 cups Garden Salad (recipe 15)
4. Main course: 12 oz portion of Spinach and Mushroom Omelet (recipe 20a)
5. End with 4 oz lemonade fluid or herbal tea
   Stats: 324 cal, 30g protein, 35g carb, 9g fat, 2.5g sat, 11g fiber, 927mg sodium, 21mg chol. 1,632mg potassium, 306mg calcium

OR

**Dinner (2) Andreas Chicken With Okra & Pasta**

1 Start with lemonade fluid (½ tbsp lemon juice with 4 oz water, green tea, or other fluid)
2 Follow with 2 cups Mixed Green Salad + 1 tsp extra virgin olive oil + 2 tbsp Red Wine Vinegar or lemon juice with salt and black pepper to taste or Mrs. Dash.
3 Main course: 4 oz chicken in 13 oz portion Andreas Chicken with Okra (recipe 20b)
4 Serve with ½ -1 cup whole-wheat pasta or spaghetti
5 End with 4 oz lemonade fluid or herbal tea
Stats: 431 cal, 32g protein, 33g carb, 21g fat, 3g sat, 9g fiber, 768mg sodium, 77mg chol. 1,122mg potassium, 227mg calcium

## Day 5 (1st Thursday)

**Breakfast---Hot Cereal (Oat Bran or 100% Whole Grain Rolled Oats) see Day 3 Breakfast**

**Morning Snack (Optional):**

4 oz nonfat low sugar yogurt or pudding
¼ cup berries (blueberries, strawberries, etc.)
1 tsp ground flaxseeds or wheat germ
8 oz water or green tea
Stats: 105 cal, 5g protein, 18g carb, 1.8g fat, 2g fiber

**Lunch---Oriental Seafood and Vegetable Soup**

1 Start with lemonade fluid (½ tbsp lemon juice with 4 oz water, green tea, or other fluid)

2 Follow with 2 cups Oriental Seafood and Vegetable Soup (recipe 21)
3 Serve with ½-1 cup cooked Chinese Vermicelli Pasta Noodles (recipe 22); or ½--1 cup cooked Brown rice or *Uncle Ben's* Converted rice (recipe 23).
4 And 1 tbsp Benefiber or 2 tsp Clearly Fiber (mix into soup or fluid)
5 End with 4 oz lemonade fluid
Stats: 296cal, 35g protein, 31g carb, 4g fat, 1g sat, 8g fiber, 383mg sodium, 86mg chol. 752mg potassium, 88mg calcium

**Mid Afternoon Snack (Must Have):**

3-multi grain or whole-wheat crackers (*Carr's*) or equivalent
1 tbsp sugar free preserves or jams
1 oz low-fat mozzarella string cheese
3 strawberries or ¼ cup berries
8 oz water or green tea or V-8 juice
Stats: 116 cal, 9g protein, 16g carb, 2g fat, 2g fiber

**Dinner (1)---Easy Grilled Beef Fajitas and Roasted Veggies**

1. Start with lemonade fluid (½ tbsp lemon juice with 4 oz water, green tea, or other fluid)
2. Follow with 1 cup Vegetable Broth Soup (recipe 2a) or non-creamy Lite Vegetable Soup
3. Follow with 1-2 cups fresh Baby Spinach – 1-2 tbsp lemon juice or vinegar + salt and black pepper or Mrs. Dash to taste
4. Main course: 3 oz meat in 11 oz portion Grilled Beef Fajitas (recipe 24)
5. Serve with 1 cup Roasted Veggies (recipe 5)
6. End with 4 oz lemonade fluid or herbal tea
   Stats: 376 cal, 33g protein, 35g carb, 14g fat, 4g sat, 13g fiber, 542mg sodium, 40mg chol, 1,341mg potassium, 166mg calcium

**OR**

**Dinner (2)---Seared Tuna With Fruit Salsa**

1. Start with lemonade fluid (½ tbsp lemon juice with 4 oz water, green tea, or other fluid)
2. Follow with 1 cup Vegetable Broth Soup (recipe 2a) or non-creamy Lite Vegetable Soup
3. Follow with ½ cup Steamed Broccoli, Spinach or Cabbage – flavored with 1 tsp minced garlic + Mrs. Dash or salt and black pepper to taste
4. Main course: 4 oz fish in 7 oz portion Seared Tuna with Fruit Salsa (recipe 25)
5. Serve with 3 oz portion Cheryl's Comfort Food (recipe 26)
6. End with 4 oz lemonade fluid or herbal tea
7. And 1 tbsp Benefiber or 2 tsp Clearly Fiber (mix into soup or fluid)
   Stats: 269 cal, 29g protein, 35g carb, 2g fat, 0.7g sat, 12 g fiber, 341mg sodium, 53mg chol, 1,057 mg potassium, 132mg calcium

## Day 6 (1st Friday)

**Breakfast (1)---Cold Cereal----see Day 1 breakfast**

**OR**

**Breakfast (2)---Banana-Kiwi Breakfast Smoothie**

Start with 8 oz water, green tea and coffee with 1 tbsp lemon
1/3 small-medium banana, not overripe
½ medium kiwi fruit, peeled
1 tbsp fresh lemon juice
½ cup soft tofu, silk
¼ cup fresh orange juice
1 tbsp ground flaxseeds
1 slice (1 oz) smoked salmon, turkey, or ham (low sodium)
½ cup berries (strawberries, blueberries, blackberries, or raspberries) or melons
¼ cup LoSodium LoFat Cottage Cheese
1 tbsp Benefiber or 2 tsp Davinci Labs Clearly Fiber (mix into cheese or fluid)

**Instructions:**

1. Combine and blend the first six ingredients to make smoothie
2. Follow smoothie with the meat, berries, and cottage cheese
   Stat: 370 cal, 26g protein, 41g carb, 12g fat, 2g sat, 12g fiber, 447md sodium, 24mg chol, 1,623mg potassium, 161mg calcium

**Morning Snack (Optional)**

2 tbsp hummus (recipe 18a)
Vegetable sticks (2 celery stalks, 6 baby carrots, and 2 asparagus spears)
8 oz water or green tea
Stats: 50 cal, 2g protein, 11g carb, 0g fat, 4g fiber

**Lunch---Ham and Cheese Sandwich With Soup**

1. Start with lemonade fluid (½ tbsp lemon juice with 4 oz water, green tea, or other fluid)
2. Follow with 1 cup Lite Vegetable Soup (recipe 14) or 4 oz Canned LoSodium Vegetable Chicken Soup w/ Water
3. Ham and Cheese Sandwich:
   2 oz (2 slices) lean ham, low sodium
   1 oz (1 slice) Swiss cheese, reduced fat, low sodium
   2 tsp low sodium lite mayonnaise
   1 tsp Dijon mustard
   3 leaves, romaine lettuce
   2 tomato slices
   2 slices multigrain bread

**Instructions:**

1. Assemble sandwich and enjoy

Stats: 340 cal, 31g protein, 32g carb, 11g fat, 4g sat, 7g fiber, 985mg sodium, 58mg chol, 595mg potassium, 341mg calcium

- **Alternatives:** *Subway* Ham Deli Sandwich with 2 servings of Veggie Delite Salad. Dressing: ½ pkt *Kraft* Fat Free Italian Dressing

**Mid Afternoon Snack (Must Have):**

½ cup low-fat cottage cheese or (4 oz nonfat low-sugar yogurt or plain)
1 tsp ground flaxseeds or wheat germ
½ tsp ground cinnamon
½ cup berries, ½ (apple, orange, or grapefruit)
8 oz water or green tea or V-8 juice
Stats: 129 cal, 15g protein, 15g carb, 2g fat, 1.3g fiber.

**Dinner---Fresh Mozzarella Pizza With Garden Salad**

1. Start with lemonade fluid (½ tbsp fresh lemon juice with 4 oz water, green tea, or other fluid)
2. Follow with 1 cup Broccoli and Dill Weed Soup (Recipe 11a) or 1 cup Broccoli Soup (recipe 11b) or non-creamy Lite Vegetable Soup
3. Follow with 2 cups Garden Salad (recipe 15)
4. Main course: 6 oz portion Mozzarella Pizza (recipe 27)
5. End with 4 oz lemonade fluid or herbal tea
   Stats: 377 cal, 32g protein, 39g carb, 14g fat, 4g sat, 16g fiber, 854mg sodium, 16mg chol, 1,204mg potassium, 431mg calcium

## Day 7 (1st Saturday)

**Breakfast---Canadian Bacon With Eggs**

2 oz Canadian bacon or 2 strips lean turkey bacon
1 egg plus 2 egg whites or ½ cup eggbeaters scrambled with vegetables (such as ¼ cup chopped spinach, 3 button mushrooms sliced, 1 tbsp chopped red peppers, ¼ medium tomatoes, 1 tbsp chopped onions, etc) with 1 tsp flaxseed oil, olive oil, or 1 tsp Smart Balance with omega plus or *Benecol* or soft margarine
Serve with ¼ cup berries (medium strawberries, blueberries, etc.) and 1 slice multigrain or 100% whole-wheat bread
And ½ cup 1% or skim milk or 6 oz low sodium V-8 juice, tomato juice, or green tea/coffee
1 tbsp Benefiber or 2 tsp Clearly Fiber (mix into juice or fluid)
Stat: 305 cal, 24g protein, 27g carb, 12g fat, 3g sat, 10g fiber, 805mg sodium, 32mg chol, 652mg potassium, 363mg calcium

**Morning Snack (Optional):**

1-cup cherries or watermelon or ½ cup fruit cocktail or pineapple canned in water
Stats: 45 cal, 1g protein, 11g carb, 0g fat, 2g fiber

**Lunch---Grilled Chicken Salad With Cheese**

1. Start with lemonade fluid (½ tbsp fresh lemon juice with 4 oz water, green tea, or other fluid)
2. Follow with ½ cup *Progresso* Healthy Classic Lentil Soup or any light soup
3. Main course: 3-4 oz meat in 13 oz portion Grilled Chicken Salad w/ Cheese (recipe 28)
4. With ¼ cup berries (strawberries, blueberries, etc.) or melons
5. End with 4 oz lemonade fluid
   Stats: 319 cal, 34g protein, 19g carb, 12g fat 2g sat, 7g fiber, 293mg sodium, 73mg chol, 1,018mg potassium, 133mg calcium

**Afternoon Snack (Must Have):**

1 oz low-fat cheese (goat cheese, mozzarella, etc.)
3 multi grain crackers (*Carr's*) or equivalent
2 thin slices apple or cantaloupe
8 oz water or green tea
Stats: 118 cal, 9g protein, 13g carb, 4g fat, 2g fiber

**Dinner (1)---Grilled Beef Tenderloin With Cucumber and Tomato Salad**

1. Start with lemonade fluid (½ tbsp lemon juice with 4 oz water, green tea, or other fluid)
2. Follow with 1 cup Broccoli Soup (recipe 11b) or Lite Vegetable Soup (recipe 4a)
3. Follow with 1 cup Cucumber and Tomato Salad (recipe 29) or 1 cup (3 spears) Pan-Roasted Lime Broccoli (recipe 14)
4. Main course: 3-4 oz portion Grilled Beef Tenderloin with Rosemary (recipe 30)
5. Serve with 1 oat bran/whole-wheat tortilla or a slice of multigrain bread
6. End with 4 oz lemonade fluid or herbal tea
   Stats: 347 cal, 33g protein, 33g carb, 12g fat. 4g sat, 11g fiber, 578mg sodium, 58mg chol, 807mg potassium, 165mg calcium

**OR**

**Dinner (2)---Roasted Salmon With Crunchy Fennel Salad**

1. Start with lemonade fluid (½ tbsp lemon juice with 4 oz water, green tea, coffee, or other fluid)
2. Follow with ½ cup Crunchy Fennel Salad (recipe 31) + with 1 cup Evelyn's Favorite Salad (recipe 32) – mix the two salads together
3. Main course: 4 oz portion Roasted Salmon (recipe 3)
4. Serve with ½ cup Steamed Green Peas and Carrots or Strings Beans
5. End with 4 oz lemonade fluid or herbal tea
6. 1 tbsp Benefiber or 2 tsp Clearly Fiber (dissolve in fluid)
   Stats: 360 cal, 30g protein, 27g carb, 15g fat, 2g sat, 11g fiber, 511mg sodium, 62mg chol, 1,280mg potassium, 100mg calcium

## Day 8 (2nd Sunday)

**Breakfast (1) Smoked Salmon on Toasted Whole-Wheat English Muffin**

Start with lemonade fluid (½ tbsp lemon juice with 4 oz water, green tea, or other fluid)
2 oz (2 slices) smoked salmon (can also use lean low sodium ham or turkey or Canadian bacon)
1 tsp extra virgin olive oil or canola oil
1 tsp shallots, chopped
1 tsp green peppers, chopped
½ 100% whole-wheat English muffin, toasted
½ cup low-fat or 1% cottage cheese
½ cup berries (strawberries, blueberries, blackberries, raspberries)
½ grapefruit
1 cup green tea or coffee
Low-fat cream (optional)
1 pct Splenda or stevia (optional)
1 tbsp Benefiber or 2 tsp Clearly Fiber (mix into cottage cheese or fluid)

**Instruction:**

1. Sauté shallots and peppers in oil until brown; add the salmon. Season to taste.
2. Serve on ½ toasted whole-wheat muffin or ½ 100% whole-wheat bagel (*Thomas*).
3. Combine berries with cottage cheese and enjoy
   Stats: 326 cal, 28g protein, 35g carb, 9.5g fat, 2g sat, 11g fiber, 1052mg sodium, 28mg chol, 564mg potassium, 216mg calcium
   * *Decrease sodium in subsequent meals for the day*

**OR**

**Breakfast (2)---Hot Cereal (Oat Bran or 100% Whole Grain Rolled Oats)----see Day 3 Breakfast**

**Morning Snack (Optional):**

10 grapes, kiwi fruit, peach, tangerine, orange, or ½ cup berries
8 oz water or green tea
Stats: 35 cal, 0.5g protein, 9g carb, 0g fat, 2g fiber

**Lunch---Turkey Ham Sandwich With Garden Salad**

1. Start with lemonade fluid (½ tbsp lemon juice with 4 oz water, green tea, or other fluid)
2. Follow with 2 cups Garden salad (1 cup romaine, 1 cup spinach or arugula, 2 tomato slices, 3 cucumber slices, 2 bell pepper strips, ¼ cup cilantro leaves, and ½ tsp ground cinnamon)
3. Dressing: 1-2 tbsp fresh lemon juice or balsamic vinegar, salt, and fresh ground black pepper to taste)
4. Turkey Ham Sandwich:

2 slices (2 oz) ham (lean, low sodium)
1 slice (1 oz) *Louis Rich* Deli thin smoked turkey breast (lean, low salt)
2 slices tomato
3 lettuce leaves
3 slices dill pickle, low sodium
1 tbsp low sodium lite mayonnaise or 1 tsp mustard

5. 1 oat bran/whole-wheat pita pocket (*Joseph's*) or ½ whole-wheat pita bread
6. ½ cup low sodium canned tomato soup or V-8 juice

**Instructions:**

1. Stuff all ingredients into pita pocket.
2. Enjoy with tomato soup, V-8 juice, or 4 oz lemonade fluid
   Stats: 284 cal, 31g protein, 27g carb, 7.5g fat, 2g sat, 7g fiber, 848mg sodium, 29mg chol, 534mg potassium, 91mg calcium

- **Alternative**: *Subway* Ham Deli Sandwich, Turkey Breast Deli Sandwich or *Subway* Turkey Breast and Ham Salad + ½ pkt *Kraft* Fat Free Italian Dressing

**Afternoon Snack (Must Have):**

1 low-fat mozzarella string cheese or boiled egg
1 fruit (such as apple, pear, nectarine, medium non-overripe banana, small mango, ½ cup papaya, or ½ cup cantaloupe)
8 oz water or green tea or V-8 juice
Stats: 148 cal, 9g protein, 22g carb, 4.6g fat, 5g fiber

**Dinner (1)---Andreas Lemon Chicken in a Pot and Potatoes With Greek Salad**

1. Start with lemonade fluid (½ tbsp lemon juice with 4 oz water, green tea, or other fluid)
2. Follow with 1 cup Vegetable Broth Soup (recipe 2a) or non-creamy Lite Vegetable Soup
3. Follow with 1 cup Andreas Greek Salad (recipe 33)
4. Main course: 3 oz Chicken in 13 oz portion Andreas Lemon Chicken in a Pot with Potatoes (recipe 34a)
5. Serve with 3 small cooked or baked New Potatoes with skin or ½ cup Lentils (34b)
6. 1 tbsp Benefiber or 2 tsp Clearly Fiber (mix into soup or fluid)
7. End with 4 oz lemonade fluid or herbal tea
   Stats: 389 cal, 32g protein, 31g carb, 14g fat, 3g sat, 11g fiber, 816mg sodium, 78mg chol, 733mg potassium, 154mg calcium

**OR**

**Dinner (2)---Pan-Roasted Lemon and Pepper Salmon With Escarole and Beans**

1. Start with lemonade fluid (½ tbsp lemon juice with 4 oz water, green tea, or other fluid)
2. Follow with 1 cup Lime Seafood Vegetable Soup (recipe 9a)
3. Follow with 1 cup Escarole and Beans (recipe 95)

4. Main course: 4 oz portion Pan-Roasted Lemon and Pepper Salmon (recipe 34c)
5. Serve with 1 cup Mashed Cauliflower (recipe 69a)
6. End with 4 oz lemonade fluid or herbal tea
   Stats: 386 cal, 35g protein, 28g carb, 15.5g fat, 2.5g sat, 13g fiber, 442mg sodium, 80mg chol, 1,474mg potassium, 221mg calcium

**Day 9 (2nd Monday)**

**Breakfast---Cold Cereal----see Day 1 Breakfast**

**Morning Snack (Optional):**
½ fruit (grapefruit, apple, pear) or 1 medium peach, tangerine, or 2-3 dried prunes
Stats: 30 cal, 0.5g protein, 8g carb, 0g fat, 3g fiber

**Lunch (1)---Egg Salad Pocket With Mixed Greens**
1. Start with lemonade fluid (½ tbsp lemon juice with 4 oz water, green tea, or other fluid)
2. Follow with 5 oz Canned Fat Free Hearty Lentil w/ Vegetable Soup or 1 cup Lite Vegetable Soup (recipe 4a)
3. Follow with 2 cups plain Mixed Vegetable Greens (such as baby spinach, red leaf lettuce, romaine or arugula, etc.) with 3 slices of tomato and 1-2 tbsp lemon juice or balsamic vinegar + salt and ground black pepper to taste or Mrs. Dash
4. Main course: 8 oz portion Egg Salad Pocket (recipe 35)
5. End with 4 oz lemonade fluid, tea or coffee
   Stats: 335 cal, 24g protein, 33g carb, 12g fat, 4g sat, 14g fiber, 443mg sodium, 378mg chol, 724mg potassium, 175mg calcium

**OR**

**Lunch (2)---Turkey Sandwich With Mixed Greens**
1. Start with lemonade fluid (½ tbsp lemon juice with 4 oz water, green tea, or other fluid)
2. Follow with 4 oz Canned Low Sodium Vegetable Chicken Soup with Water
3. Follow with 2 cups plain Mixed Vegetable Greens (such as baby spinach, red lettuce, romaine, or arugula, etc.) with 3 slices of tomato and 2 tbsp lemon juice or balsamic vinegar + salt and ground black pepper to taste
4. Turkey Sandwich:
   2 slices or 2 oz cooked turkey (low sodium and lean)
   2 tbsp shredded Cheddar cheese, light
   1 tbsp low sodium lite mayonnaise or 1 tsp mustard
   3 slices lettuce leaves (romaine, arugula, or red lettuce)
   2 slices tomatoes
   3 slices dill pickle, low sodium
   2 slices multigrain bread or 1 sourdough bread or multigrain sandwich bun or oat bra/whole wheat pita *(Joseph's)*

**Instructions:**

1. Assemble sandwich and enjoy
2. End with 4 oz lemonade fluid, green tea, or coffee
   Stats: 334 cal, 26g protein, 42g carb, 9g fat, 3g sat, 10g fiber, 976mg sodium, 47mg chol, 939 mg potassium

- **Alternative**: *Subway* Turkey Breast Deli Sandwich

**Afternoon Snack (Must Have):**

4 oz nonfat low-sugar yogurt or (½ cup low-fat cottage cheese)
1 tsp wheat germ or ground flaxseeds
1 slice smoked salmon (or lean and low sodium turkey or ham)
Stats: 102 cal, 10g protein, 12g carb, 1g fat, 0.3g fiber

**Dinner---Grilled Salmon With Spring Salad**

1. Start with lemonade fluid (½ tbsp lemon juice with 4 oz water, green tea, or other fluid)
2. Follow with 1 cup Mushroom Soup (recipe 36) or Lite Vegetable Broth Soup (recipe 2a)
3. Main course: 14 oz portion Grilled Salmon with Spring Salad (recipe 37)
4. Serve with 3 Steamed Asparagus Spears
5. And 1 cup Pan-Roasted Eggplant and Zucchini (recipe 17)
6. End with 4 oz lemonade fluid or herbal tea
   Stats: 381 cal, 32g protein, 24g carb, 18.5g fat, 4g sat, 10g fiber, 503mg sodium, 74mg chol, 1,609mg potassium, 180mg calcium
   * *You can substitute other fish of your choice*

## Day 10 (2nd Tuesday)

**Breakfast (1)---Tofu Omelet**

1. 15 oz portion tofu omelet (recipe 38)
2. 1 oat bran/whole-wheat pita pocket or tortilla (*Joseph's*) or a multigrain bread
3. 4 oz unsweetened grapefruit or apple juice (apple, orange, grapefruit) or V-8 juice
   Stats: 307 cal, 24g protein, 29g carb, 12g fat, 2g sat, 8g fiber, 549mg sodium, 189mg chol, 717mg potassium, 62mg calcium

**OR**

**Breakfast (2)---Cold Cereal----see Day 1 Breakfast**

**Morning Snack (Optional):**

1 low-fat mozzarella string cheese
8 oz water or green tea
Stats: 51 cal, 8g protein, 1g carb, 1.5g fat, 0g fiber

**Lunch---Tuna Caesar Salad**

1. Start with lemonade fluid (½ tbsp lemon juice with 4 oz water, green tea, or other fluid)
2. Follow with 4 oz Canned *Progresso* Healthy Classic Vegetable Soup or your choice of non-creamy soup
3. Tuna Caesar Salad:
   3-4 oz canned regular tuna, packed in water (drained) – do not use light canned tuna
   2 tsp low sodium lite mayonnaise
   2 cups greens (romaine or arugula), shredded
   2 tomato slices
   ¼ medium cucumber, sliced
   1 large red onion slice
   2 tbsp Diet Italian Salad Dressing, *no salt*
   2 tbsp red wine vinegar
   1 tsp extra virgin olive oil
   1 tbsp Parmesan cheese, grated
   1 tbsp fresh parsley, chopped
   Salt and black pepper to taste
   ½ multigrain sandwich bun or 1 oat bran/whole-wheat tortilla or pita (*Joseph's*)

**Instructions:**

1. In a medium bowl, break apart tuna into bite-size pieces and mix with mayonnaise
2. Shred greens and add to salad bowl
3. Add tomatoes, onion and cucumber. Toss gently
4. Sprinkle with parsley and cheese
5. Pour dressing (oil and vinegar or Diet Italian Salad Dressing) over the salad and tuna mixture
6. Serving size is 20 oz portion. Serves 1
   Stats: 352 cal, 31g protein, 34g carb, 10g fat, 3g sat, 8g fiber, 720mg sodium, 43mg chol, 899mg potassium, 137mg calcium

- **Alternative:** *Subway* Tuna Deli Sandwich

**Mid Afternoon Snack (Must Have):**

4 tbsp 2% cottage cheese
5 medium grapes or 8 small ones
1 slice or 1 oz lean smoked salmon, ham, or turkey (low sodium)
3 slices apple or peach
1 slice tomato or 2 cherry tomatoes
8 oz water or green tea or V-8 juice
Stats: 110 cal, 11g protein, 11g carb, 2g fat, 1g fiber

**Dinner (1)---Seasoned Turkey Breast With Three-Bean Salad**

1. Start with lemonade fluid (½ tbsp lemon juice with 4 oz water, green tea, or other fluid)

2. Follow with ½ cup Italian Vegetable Soup (recipe 7) or Lite Escarole Soup (recipe 39a)
3. Follow with ½ cup Three Bean Salad (recipe 40a)
4. Main course: 4 oz portion of Seasoned Turkey Breast cutlets (recipe 40b)
5. Serve with ½ cup Steamed Sugar Snap Peas and Carrots – flavored with 1 tsp minced garlic and Mrs. Dash or salt and black pepper to taste or 1 cup Pan-Roasted Lime Broccoli (recipe 14)
6. 1 tbsp Benefiber or 2 tsp Clearly Fiber (mix into soup or fluid)
7. End with 4 oz lemonade fluid or herbal tea
   Stats: 360 cal, 34g protein, 29g carb, 13.5g fat, 3g sat, 13g fiber 184mg sodium, 68mg chol, 882mg potassium, 200mg calcium

**OR**

**Dinner (2)---Escarole Beans and Grilled Chicken Salad**

1. Start with lemonade fluid (½ tbsp lemon juice with 4 oz water, green tea, or other fluid)
2. Follow with ½ cup *Progresso* Healthy Classics Vegetable Soup or 1 cup Lite Vegetable Broth Soup (recipe 2a) or non-creamy Lite Vegetable Soup
3. Main course: 2-3 oz chicken in 21 oz portion Escarole Beans and Grilled Chicken Salad (recipe 41)
4. End with 4 oz lemonade fluid or herbal tea
   Stats: 365 cal, 31g protein, 35g carb, 12g fat, 2g sat, 15g fiber, 488mg sodium, 55mg chol, 1,459mg potassium, 251mg calcium

## Day 11 (2nd Wednesday)

**Breakfast (1)---Peach Smoothie With Flax**

1 small peach or ½ cup canned peaches, unsweetened, water or light syrup
4 oz non-fat, low sugar yogurt, or low-fat plain yogurt
1 tbsp ground flaxseeds
1 tsp pure vanilla extract
½ tsp ground cinnamon
4 ice cubes or ½ cup cold water
½ cup 2% cottage cheese
1 tbsp Benefiber or 2 tsp Clearly Fiber (mix into cottage cheese or fluid)
½ cup berries

**Instructions:**

1. Place all ingredients except cottage cheese in a blender. Run on high until smooth.
2. Accompany smoothie with ½ cup cottage cheese
3. Add ½ cup berries (strawberries, blueberries, etc.)
4. Serving size is 19 oz portion.

Stats: 345 cal, 26g protein, 39g carb, 9g fat, 2g sat, 11g fiber, 547mg sodium, 12mg chol, 668 mg potassium, 289mg calcium

**OR**

**Breakfast (2)---Cold Cereal---see Day 1 Breakfast**

**Morning Snack (Optional):**
1-cup cantaloupe or papaya cubes
8 oz water or green tea
Stats: 56 cal, 1.4g protein, 13g carb, 0.4g fat, 1g fiber

**Lunch---Ham Sandwich With Sharon's Salad**

1. Start with lemonade fluid (½ tbsp lemon juice with 4 oz water, green tea, or other fluid)
2. Follow with 2 cups Sharon's Salad (1 cup spinach, 1 cup romaine or arugula, ¼ summer squash, 3 raw asparagus spears, ½ medium tomato, ¼ cucumber, 3 button mushrooms, ¼ red bell peppers, ¼ cup chopped cilantro, 1 tsp ground cinnamon
3. Dressing: 1 tsp olive oil + 2 tbsp fresh lemon juice or vinegar, salt, and black pepper to taste
4. Main course: ½ Ham Sandwich (2 oz lean ham, 2 tsp low sodium lite mayonnaise and 1 tsp mustard on a slice of multigrain bread)
5. End with 4 oz lemonade fluid or herbal tea
6. Feel free to use any lean, low sodium sliced meat (roast beef, turkey, etc.)
   Stats: 261 cal, 20g protein, 26g carb, 10g fat, 3g sat, 8g fiber, 788mg sodium, 96mg chol, 1,148mg potassium, 124mg calcium

- **Alternative:** *Subway* Ham Deli Sandwich or *Subway* Ham Salad with 6 grams of fat or less. Use ½ pkt *Kraft* Fat Free Italian Dressing

**Mid Afternoon Snack (Must Have):**
4 oz or ½ cup low-fat cottage cheese or 4 oz non-fat low sugar yogurt or plain
1 tsp toasted wheat germ or ground flaxseeds
½ cup berries
8 oz water or green tea or V-8 juice
Stats: 139 cal, 13g protein, 16g carb, 2g fat, 1g fiber

**Dinner (1)---Grilled Shrimp Kabobs With Tomato Basil Salad**

1. Start with lemonade fluid (½ tbsp lemon juice with 4 oz water, green tea, or other fluid)
2. Follow with 1 cup Lite Vegetable Broth Soup (recipe 2a) or non-creamy Lite Vegetable Soup
3. Follow with 1 cup Tomato Basil Salad (recipe 42a) or 1 cup Tomato Cucumber Fennel Salad (recipe 42b)
4. Main course: 5 oz portion Grilled Shrimp Kabobs (recipe 43)
5. Serve with 1 cup Steamed Spinach, Broccoli, or Cabbage – flavored with 1 tsp minced garlic and Mrs. Dash or salt and black pepper to taste
6. End with 4 oz lemonade fluid or herbal tea
7. And 1 tbsp Benefiber or 2 tsp Clearly Fiber (mix into soup or fluid)
   Stats: 340 cal, 33g protein, 27g carb, 13g fat, 2g sat, 14g fiber, 337mg sodium, 172mg chol, 1,722mg potassium, 469mg calcium

**OR**

**Dinner (2)---Lemon Salmon in Foil With Roasted Veggies**

1. Start with lemonade fluid (½ tbsp lemon juice with 4 oz water, green tea, or other fluid)
2. Follow with ½ cup Lite Vegetable Soup (recipe 4a) or non-creamy Lite soup
3. Follow with 1 cup Roasted Veggies (recipe 5)
4. Main course: 3-4 oz fish in 10 oz portion Lemon Salmon in Foil (recipe 44)
5. Serve with 3 Steamed Asparagus Spears
6. End with 4 oz lemonade fluid or herbal tea
   Stats: 344 cal, 29g protein, 29g carb, 14g fat, 2g sat, 11g fiber, 206mg sodium, 61mg chol, 1,826mg potassium, 160mg calcium

## Day 12 (2nd Thursday)

**Breakfast (1)---Boiled Egg With Toast**

1. 1 boiled egg, 2 egg whites, or ½ cup eggbeaters
2. 2 slices multigrain bread or 1 oat bran/whole-wheat flour tortilla (*Joseph's*)
3. 2 tsp smooth peanut butter or 1 tsp omega butter (recipe 45a)
4. ½ cup berries (strawberries, blueberries, raspberries, etc) or ½ cup cantaloupe cubes
5. ½ cup 1% or skim milk or 4 oz unsweetened juice (apple, grapefruit, orange, *Mountain Sun* cranberry)
6. 1 tbsp Benefiber or 2 tsp Clearly Fiber (mix into milk or fluid)
   Stats: 298 cal, 17g protein, 34g carb, 13g fat, 3g sat, 10g fiber, 402mg sodium, 196mg chol, 519mg potassium, 348mg calcium

**OR**

**Breakfast (2)---Hot Cereal (Oat Bran or 100% Whole Grain Rolled Oats)----see Day 3 Breakfast**

**Morning Snack (Optional):**

½ fruit (grapefruit, apple, pear) or 1 medium peach, tangerine, or 2-3 dried prunes
8 oz water or green tea
Stats: 30 cal, 0.5g protein, 8g carb, 0g fat, 3g fiber

**Lunch---Tuna With Green Salad**

1. Start with lemonade fluid (½ tbsp lemon juice with 4 oz water, green tea, or other fluid)
2. Tuna with Green Salad:
   4 oz can regular white tuna, packed in water (drained)
   2 tsp low sodium light mayonnaise
   1 cup chopped greens (romaine, arugula, or red lettuce, etc)
   1-cup spinach, chopped
   3 tomato slices
   6 seedless grapes

¼ medium cucumber, sliced
¼ red medium bell pepper cut in strips
¼ green medium bell pepper cut in strips
3 red onion slices
1 tbsp wheat germ
1 tsp ground cinnamon
1 tsp olive oil
2 tbsp lemon juice, red wine, or any other vinegar

**Instructions:**

1. Combine drained tuna with mayonnaise.
2. Serve on top of salad.
3. End with lemonade fluid or green tea
   Stats: 350 cal, 34g protein, 33g carb, 10.5g fat, 2g sat, 8g fiber, 517mg sodium, 51mg chol, 1,356 mg potassium, 177 mg calcium

**Afternoon Snack (Must Have):**

½ cup low-fat cottage cheese or non-fat low sugar yogurt or plain
1 tsp ground flaxseeds or wheat germ
½ tsp fresh ground cinnamon + ¼ tsp nutmeg
8 oz water or green tea or V-8 juice.
Stats: 107 cal, 15g protein, 5g carb, 3g fat, 1.3g fiber

**Dinner (1)---Ginger Chicken With Garlic and Steamed Broccoli**

1. Start with lemonade fluid (½ tbsp lemon juice with 4 oz water, green tea, or other fluid)
2. Follow with ½ cup Lite Escarole Soup (recipe 39a) or ½ cup Mushroom Soup (recipe 36) or Lite Vegetable Soup (recipe 4a) or non-creamy Lite Vegetable Soup
3. Follow with 2 cups Garden Salad (recipe 15)
4. Main course: 4 oz portion Ginger Chicken with Garlic (recipe 45b)
5. Serve with ¼ cup or 4 tbsp cooked Uncle Ben's Converted rice or Brown rice (recipe 23) with 1 cup Steamed Broccoli or Spinach tossed or mixed into rice
6. End with 4 oz lemonade fluid or herb tea
   Stats: 339 cal, 36g protein, 35g carb, 7.5g fat, 1g sat, 11g fiber, 234mg sodium, 73mg chol, 1,451mg potassium, 209mg calcium

**OR**

**Dinner (2)---Baked Tuna Fillet With New Potatoes and Sautéed Spinach**

1. Start with lemonade fluid (½ tbsp lemon juice with 4 oz water, green tea, or other fluid)
2. Follow with ½ cup Lite Vegetable Broth Soup (recipe 2a) or non-creamy Lite Vegetable Soup
3. Follow with ½ cup Mixed Vegetables (recipe 46a)
4. Main course: 4 oz fish in 12 oz portion Baked Tuna Fillet with New Potatoes (recipe 47)

5. Serve with 3 New Potatoes with skin
6. And with 2 cups Sautéed Spinach with Roasted Red Peppers (recipe 46b)
7. 1 tbsp Benefiber or 2 tsp Clearly Fiber (mix into soup or fluid).
8. End with 4 oz lemonade fluid or herbal tea
   Stats: 372 cal, 34g protein, 33g carb, 13g fat, 1.5g sat, 13g fiber, 681mg sodium, 53mg chol, 1,569mg potassium, 233mg calcium

## Day 13 (2nd Friday)

**Breakfast---Open-Faced Breakfast Sandwich**

1 slice high fiber multigrain bread or 1 oat bran/whole-wheat flour tortilla (*Joseph's*)
2 oz lean ham or smoked salmon, low sodium
1 oz low-fat cheese (provolone, cheddar, Swiss, goat cheese, etc.)
3 tomato slices
3 pieces large romaine

**Instructions:**

1. On bread, add ham and cheese. Broil until cheese melts
2. Top with tomato and lettuce
3. Serve with ½ glass skim, soymilk, 4 oz tomato juice, or V-8 juice (low sodium)
4. And ½ cup berries
   Stats: 268 cal, 29g protein, 25g carb, 7.6g fat, 2.5g sat, 7g fiber, 862mg sodium, 33mg chol, 692mg potassium, 377mg calcium

**Morning Snack (Optional):**

6 baby carrots
2 celery sticks
2 asparagus spears
2 tbsp hummus or Quick Salsa Dip (recipes 18a and 18b)
8 oz water or green tea
Stats: 50 cal, 2g protein, 11g carb, 0g fat, 4g fiber

**Lunch---Grilled Chicken Salad With Almonds**

1. Start with lemonade fluid (½ tbsp lemon juice with 4 oz water, green tea, or other fluid)
2. Main course: 4 oz chicken in 17 oz portion Grilled Chicken Salad with Almonds (recipe 48)
3. Follow with fruit (such as ½ apple, 1 medium peach, ½ pear, ½ grapefruit, or 10 grapes)
4. End with 4 oz lemonade fluid
   Stats: 325 cal, 27g protein, 25g carb, 14g fat, 2g sat, 8g fiber, 77mg sodium, 63mg chol, 1,008mg potassium, 141mg calcium

- **Alternatives:** see Day 1 Lunch Mediterranean Greek Chicken Salad

**Afternoon Snack (Must Have):**

3 multigrain crackers or 2 whole grain crackers (*Carr's*)
1 slice (1oz) smoked salmon, lean ham or turkey (low sodium)
1 tbsp low-fat cream cheese
3 tbsp low-fat cottage cheese
1 tomato slice
8 oz water or green tea
Stats: 115 cal, 13g protein, 12g carb, 2g fat, 1g fiber.

**OR**

**Karen's Tortilla Toast:**

½ oat bran/whole-wheat tortilla (*Joseph's*) or ½ whole-wheat pita – toasted until it puffs up and becomes soft or crunchy
1.5 oz white tuna or salmon canned in water, drained
1 slice large red onion, divide into 4 halves
4 slice lemon wedge
8 oz water or green tea
(Divide the toasted tortilla into four halves and spread equal amount of the other ingredients. Serve with lemon wedges)
Stats: 106 cal, 14g protein, 9g carb, 2g fat, 4g fiber

**Dinner---Sautéed Scallops With Fresh Tomato Cucumber Salad**

1. Start with lemonade fluid (½ tbsp lemon juice with 4 oz water, green tea, or other fluid)
2. Follow with 1 cup Lite Vegetable Soup (recipe 4a) or Lite Escarole Soup (39a)
3. Follow with 1 cup Fresh Cucumber Tomato Salad (recipe 49)
4. Main course: 6 each in 4 oz portion Sautéed Scallops (recipe 50)
5. Serve with 1 cup Steamed Broccoli, Spinach, Cabbage, or Asparagus (seasoned with 1 tsp minced garlic, salt, and black pepper to taste or Mrs. Dash
6. End with 4 oz lemonade water, green tea, or herbal tea, etc.
   Stats: 372cal, 34g protein, 35g carb, 12g fat, 2g sat, 10g fiber, 487mg sodium, 62mg chol, 1,627mg potassium, 175mg calcium

## Day 14 (2nd Saturday)

**Breakfast---Southwestern Scrambled Eggs**

Southwestern scrambled eggs or eggbeaters (recipe 51)
1 slice Multi grain bread or 1 oat bran/whole-wheat pita or tortilla (*Joseph's*)
½ cup cubed melons (cantaloupe, honeydew, etc.) or ½ cup pineapple or papaya
3 strawberries or ¼ berries
1 cup green tea or coffee
Light cream and Splenda or stevia (optional)
Stats: 317 cal, 30g protein, 31g carb, 10g fat, 2g sat, 9g fiber, 903mg sodium, 200 mg chol, 518mg potassium, 45mg calcium

**Morning Snack (Optional):**

1 Blue cheese stuffed tomato (recipe 52a)
8 oz water or green tea
Stats: 97 cal, 3g protein, 11g carb, 5g fat, 2g sat, 2g fiber

**Lunch (1)---Turkey Wrap With Tossed Salad**

1. Start with lemonade fluid (½ tbsp lemon juice with 4 oz water, green tea, or other Fluid)
2. Follow with 2 cups Mixed Greens Salad (2 cups fresh mixed greens or prepackaged greens, ¼ red bell pepper cut in strips, ¼ green bell pepper cut in strips, 3 medium or button mushrooms thinly sliced, 4 cherry tomatoes, ¼ medium cucumber – sliced and cut in half and salt and black pepper to taste).
3. Dressing: Olive/vinegar (1-2 tsp extra virgin oil + 2 tbsp balsamic vinegar or any other vinegar you like); or 2 tbsp lemon juice + salt, herbs, and ground black pepper to taste; or 1-2 tbsp fat free dry *Italian* dressing (see package instructions).
4. Main course: 4 oz meat in 6 oz Turkey Wrap (recipe 52b)
5. Follow with 3 oz portion Blueberry Yogurt Sorbet (recipe 53)
6. End with 4 oz lemonade fluid
   Stats: 343 cal, 24g protein, 38g carb, 15g fat, 2g sat, 13 g fiber, 923mg sodium, 26mg chol, 1,092mg potassium, 238mg calcium

**OR**

**Lunch (2)---Mixed Fruit Salad (Recipe 54)**

½ cup berries (strawberries, blueberries, etc.)
¼ cup grapes, seedless
1 cup melon chunks (cantaloupe, honeydew, etc.)
½ tbsp chopped almonds
½ tbsp chopped walnuts
½ tbsp sunflower seeds
1 cup 2% fat cottage cheese
1 tbsp ground flaxseed or wheat germ (add to cottage cheese)
1 oz lean ham, turkey, smoked salmon or low-fat mozzarella string cheese

**Instruction:**

1. Combine fruit and nuts.
2. Serve along with cottage cheese, lean ham, turkey, or smoked salmon
3. End with 4 oz lemonade fluid or green tea
4. And 1 tbsp Benefiber or 2 tsp Clearly Fiber (mix into cottage cheese or fluid)
5. Serving size is 10 oz portion (1 cup). Serves 2. For snack use ½ cup
   Stats: 282 cal, 21g protein, 26g carb, 11g fat, 2,5g sat, 11g fiber, 604mg sodium, 17 mg chol, 862mg potassium, 237mg calcium

**Afternoon Snack (Must Have):**

3 tbsp low-fat cottage cheese or plain yogurt
5 medium grapes

1 oz low sodium, low-fat ham, or smoked salmon
2 thin apple slices or cantaloupe
8 oz water or green tea or V-8 juice
Stats: 87 cal, 9g protein, 11g carb, 1.5g fat, 1g fiber

**OR**

**Karen's Peanut Butter Tortilla Toast:**
½ oat bran/whole-wheat tortilla or 1 multigrain bread – toasted until it puffs up soft or becomes crunchy
½ tbsp peanut butter or omega butter (recipe 45a)
1 tsp reduced sugar preserves/jam
(Divide tortilla into four halves and spread equal amount peanut butter and jam)
8 oz water or green tea or V-8 juice
Stats: 94 cal, 6g protein, 10g carb, 4.8g fat, 4g fiber

**Dinner (1)---Roasted Chicken With Flame-Roasted Vegetable Platter**

1. Start with lemonade fluid (½ tbsp lemon juice with 4 oz water, green tea, or other fluid)
2. Follow with 1 cup Vegetable Broth Soup (recipe 2a) or non-creamy Lite Soup
3. Follow with 1 cup Mixed Veggies (recipe 46a)
4. Main course: 4 oz portion Roasted Chicken or Turkey Breast (recipe 55)
5. Serve with 1 cup Flame-Roasted Vegetable Platter (recipe 2b)
6. End with 4 oz lemonade fluid or herb tea
   Stats: 362 cal, 33g protein, 29g carb, 14.6g fat, 2g sat, 11g fiber, 411mg sodium, 81mg chol, 1,410mg potassium, 139mg calcium

**OR**

**Dinner (2)---Lemon Salmon With Roasted Sweet Potatoes and Steamed Vegetables**

1. Start with lemonade fluid (½ tbsp lemon juice with 4 oz water, green tea, or other fluid)
2. Follow with ½ cup Lite Vegetable Soup (recipe 4a) or non-creamy Lite Soup
3. Follow with 1 cup Baby Spinach Salad, Romaine, Arugula, or Boston Lettuce + 1-2 tbsp lemon juice or vinegar + salt and black pepper to taste or Mrs. Dash
4. Main course: 3-4 oz serving in 7 oz portion Lemon Salmon in Foil (recipe 44)
5. Serve with ½ cup Steamed Broccoli, Cabbage, Brussels Sprouts, or Asparagus
6. 3-4 oz Baked Sweet Potato with skin or serve with Baked Sweet Potato Mash (3-4 oz about ½ cup) seasoned with ground cinnamon, nutmeg, Splenda, and *I Can't Believe It's Not Butter* (recipe 26)
7. End with 4 oz lemonade fluid or herb tea
   Stats: 365 cal, 30g protein, 36g carb, 11.5g fat, 2g sat, 8g fiber, 123mg sodium, 1mg chol, 995mg potassium, 264mg calcium

## Day 15 (3rd Sunday)

**Breakfast (1)---Smoked Salmon on Toasted Whole-Wheat English Muffin**

2 oz (2 slices) smoked salmon
1 tsp extra virgin olive oil or canola oil
1 tsp shallots, chopped
1 tsp green peppers, chopped
½ whole-wheat English muffin, toasted
½ cup 2% cottage cheese
½ cup berries (strawberries, blueberries, raspberries)
¼ grapefruit
1 cup green tea or coffee
Low-fat cream (optional)
1 pct Splenda or Stevia (optional)
1 tbsp Benefiber or 2 tsp Davinci Lab Clearly Fiber (mix into cottage cheese or fluid)

**Instructions:**

1. Sauté shallots and peppers in oil until brown; add the salmon. Season to taste
2. Serve on toasted whole-wheat muffin
3. Combine berries with cottage cheese and enjoy
   Stats: 326 cal, 28g protein, 35g carb, 9.5g fat, 2g sat, 7g fiber, 1,052mg sodium, 28mg chol, 565mg potassium, 216mg calcium
   * *Even though the salt content is high, this should not be problem because this is not a meal you eat every day. However,* reduce *sodium in subsequent meals.*

**OR**

**Breakfast (2)---Hot Cereal (Oat Bran or 100% Whole Grain Rolled Oats)----see Day 3 Breakfast**

**Morning Snack (Optional):**

½ cup berries, cube cantaloupe or pineapple chunks canned in water
Stats: 41 cal, 0.5g protein, 10g carb, 0.3g fat, 1g fiber

**OR**

½ medium banana (not overripe) or ½ apple
2 tsp peanut butter or almond butter
Stats: 110 cal, 3g protein, 14g carb, 5.6g fat, 2g fiber

**Lunch (1)---Zucchini Soup and Flax Caesar Salad**

1. Start with lemonade fluid (½ tbsp lemon juice with 4 oz water, green tea, or other fluid)
2. Follow with ½ cup Zucchini Soup (recipe 56) or 4 oz canned *Progresso* Healthy Classic Vegetable Soup
3. Main course: 1 cup Flax Caesar Salad (recipe 57)
4. Serve with 3 oz grilled/baked Seasoned Turkey or Chicken Breast (recipe 40) or 3 oz lean sliced ham, turkey, smoked salmon etc. (low sodium)

5. And ½ cup fruit cocktail in water or ½ cup cubed/diced melon (cantaloupe, honeydew, watermelon, etc)
6. End with 4 oz lemonade fluid

Stats: 360 cal, 33g protein, 24g carb, 17g fat, 1g sat, 8g fiber, 467mg sodium, 72mg chol, 885mg potassium, 115mg calcium

OR

**Lunch (2)---Escarole Beans and Grilled Chicken Salad**

1. Start with lemonade fluid (½ tbsp lemon juice with 4 oz water, green tea, or other fluid)
2. Follow with ½ cup canned *Progresso* Healthy Classic Vegetable Soup or non-creamy Lite Soup
3. Main course: 2 ½ cups Escarole Beans and Grilled Chicken Salad (recipe 41)
4. With ½ cup fruit cocktail or pineapple packed in water or ½ cup diced/cubed melon (cantaloupe, watermelon, honeydew, etc.) or ½ cup berries
5. End with 4 oz lemonade fluid or green tea

Stats: 365 cal, 31g protein, 35g carb, 12g fat, 2g sat, 15g fiber, 488mg sodium, 55mg chol, 1,459mg potassium, 251mg calcium

**Afternoon Snack (Must Have):**

2 oz canned regular tuna in water or oil, drained
1 tsp soy sauce, low sodium
1 tbsp toasted sesame seeds or ground flaxseeds
1 tbsp Quick Salsa (recipe 18b) or a good commercial brand
(Mix in a bowl and grill in a pan)
Serve with:
3 Roasted vegetable or multigrain crackers (*Carr's*) or equivalent
3 cucumber slices
3 cherry tomatoes
8 oz water or green tea
Stats: 144 cal, 16g protein, 7g carb, 6g fat, 3g fiber.

**OR**

1 fruit (apple, pear, nectarine, etc.) or ½ cup berries or 2-3 dried prunes
1 string cheese (mozzarella) or boiled egg
8 oz water or green tea
Stats: 130 cal, 8g protein, 23g carb, 2.5g fat, 5g fiber

**OR**

Granny smith apple with cheddar (Recipe 58)
8 oz water or green tea
Stats: 197 cal, 17g protein, 24g carb, 5g fat, 5g fiber

**Dinner (1)---Spinach Ham Quiche With Mushroom Shrimp Soup**

1. Start with lemonade fluid (½ tbsp lemon juice with 4 oz water, green tea, or other fluid)

2. Follow with 1 cup Mushroom Shrimp Soup (recipe 36) or Lite Escarole Soup (recipe 39a)
3. Follow with 2 cups Garden Salad (recipe 15)
4. Main course: 4 oz portion (1 slice) Spinach Ham Quiche (recipe 59 or 60)
5. And ½ cup low-fat Cottage Cheese + 1 tsp wheat germ + ½ tsp ground cinnamon or ¼ cup Fat Free Ricotta cheese
6. 1 tbsp Benefiber or 2 tsp Clearly Fiber (mix into cottage cheese, soup, or fluid)
7. 8 oz wine (170 cal, 4 g carb – optional*)
8. End with 4 oz lemonade fluid or herbal tea
   Stat: 350 cal, 32g protein, 25g carb, 14g fat, 3g sat, 10g fiber, 872mg sodium, 58mg chol, 919mg potassium, 252 mg calcium
   * *Malt Beverages (12 oz, 32 cal, 5g carb); Gin, Brandy, Rum, Vodka, Whiskey (4 fl oz, 257 cal, 0g carb); Beer (12 oz, 148 cal, 13g carb); Beer, Lite (12 oz, 100 cal, 5g carb); Bloody Mary (5 oz, 116 cal, 5g carb); Screwdriver (7 oz, 174 cal, 18g carb); Cordials and Liqueurs (1 oz, 34 cal, 12g carb)*; Wine, red or white (8 fl oz, 170 cal, 4g carb). *Add their contribution to your meal plan any time you indulge! Moderate to heavy alcoholic consumption on a regular basis regardless of good intentions can cause fat storage and sabotage weight loss!*

**OR**

**Dinner (2)---Baked Salmon With Fennel and Goat Cheese**

1. Start with lemonade fluid (½ tbsp lemon juice with 4 oz water, green tea, or other fluid)
2. Follow with ½ cup Lite Vegetable Soup (recipe 4a) or non-creamy Lite Soup
3. Follow with 2 cups Garden Salad (recipe 15) + 2 tbsp lemon juice or vinegar + salt and black pepper or Mrs. Dash
4. Main course: 3-4 oz fish in 9 oz Baked Salmon with Beets and Goat Cheese (recipe 61)
5. Serve with 1 cup Steamed Mixed Veggies (recipe 46a)
6. End with 4 oz lemonade fluid or herbal tea
   Stats: 346 cal, 32.5g protein, 31.5g carb, 11g fat, 3g sat, 14g fiber, 413mg sodium, 67mg chol, 1,955mg potassium, 241mg calcium

## Day 16 (3rd Monday)

**Breakfast (1)---Cold Cereal---see Day 1 Breakfast**

**OR**

**Breakfast (2)---Elizabeth's Favorite Breakfast**

6 oz *Yoplait* Plain Yogurt (0 sugar)
1 tbsp chopped walnuts, butternuts, or almonds
1 tbsp ground flaxseeds (*Barlean's*)
1 tbsp Benefiber or 2 tsp *Davinci Labs* Clearly Fiber
1 boiled egg or 2 egg whites

½ cup berries (blueberries, strawberries, etc.) or 1 cup diced/cubed melon or ½ cup fresh-diced mango, or ½ cup fresh pineapple chunks
8 oz water, green tea, or coffee

**Instructions:**

1. Combine all ingredients. Serve with egg and ½ cup berries.
2. Dissolve Benefiber or Clearly Fiber in yogurt or fluid

Stats: 320 cal, 20g protein, 28g carb, 16g fat, 4g sat, 10g fiber, 194 mg sodium, 206mg chol, 667mg potassium, 356mg calcium

**Morning Snack (Optional):**

1 apple, pear, nectarine, orange, or grapefruit
8 oz water or green tea or V-8 juice
Stats: 80 cal, 0g protein, 22g carb, 0g fat, 5g fiber

**Lunch---Grilled Chicken Sandwich With Vegetable Chicken Soup**

1. Start with lemonade fluid (½ tbsp lemon juice with 4 oz water, green tea, or other fluid)
2. Follow with 1 cup Vegetable Broth Soup (recipe 2a) or 4 oz Canned Low Sodium Vegetable Chicken Soup with Water
3. Main course: 3-4 oz chicken in 8 oz portion Grilled Chicken Sandwich (recipe 18c) 3 oz grilled or baked chicken or turkey breast + 2 slices tomatoes + 3 leaves romaine + 3 dill pickles, slices + 1 tsp Dijon mustard + 1 tsp low sodium lite mayonnaise or mustard
4. With 1 oat bran/whole-wheat tortilla or pita (*Joseph's*) or 2 high fiber multigrain slices
5. Assemble sandwich and enjoy
6. End with 4 oz lemonade fluid
   Stats: 326 cal, 39g protein, 24g carb, 9g fat, 3g sat, 7g fiber, 881mg sodium, 77mg chol, 439mg potassium, 71mg calcium

- **Alternatives:** see Day 1 Lunch Mediterranean Greek Chicken Salad

**Afternoon Snack (Must Have):**

½ cup low-fat cottage cheese or (4 oz nonfat low sugar yogurt or plain yogurt)
½ cup slices of peach canned in water or lite syrup
8 oz water or green tea or V-8 juice
Stats: 135 cal, 15g protein, 15g carb, 2.5g fat, 1g fiber

**Dinner---Baked Spaghetti Squash With Meatballs and Spinach Salad**

1 Start with lemonade fluid (½ tbsp lemon juice with 4 oz water, green tea, or other fluid)
2 Follow with ½ cup Lite Vegetable Soup (recipe 4a) or non-creamy Lite Soup
3 Follow with 1 cup Spinach Salad (1 cup baby spinach + 2 slices tomato + 3 slices cucumber + 3 button mushrooms slices + 1-2 tbsp lemon juice or vinegar + salt and black pepper or Mrs. Dash to taste

4 Main course: 13 oz (about 2 cups) Baked Spaghetti Squash with Meatballs (recipe 62)
5 Serve with ½ cup seasonal steamed non-starchy vegetables (such as broccoli, cauliflower, asparagus, Brussels sprouts, collards, mustard greens, eggplant, zucchini, summer squash, etc.)
6 End with 4 oz lemonade fluid or herbal tea
Stats: 349 cal, 35g protein, 32g carb, 10.5g fat, 3g sat, 8g fiber, 701mg sodium, 92mg chol, 1,224mg potassium, 218mg calcium

## Day 17 (3rd Tuesday)

**Breakfast (1)---Cold Cereal---see Day 1 Breakfast**

**Morning Snack (Optional):**
½ medium banana (not overripe), apple, pear, nectarine, or grapefruit
8 oz water or green tea
Stats: 54 cal, 1g protein, 14g carb, 0g fat, 1.4g fiber

**Lunch---Turkey Sandwich With Lite Vegetable Soup**

1. Start with lemonade fluid (½ tbsp lemon juice with 4 oz water, green tea, or other fluid)
2. Follow with 1 cup Lite Vegetable Soup (recipe 4a) or 4oz Canned LoSodium Vegetable Chicken Soup with Water
3. Turkey Sandwich:
   2 –3 oz cooked turkey (low sodium and lean)
   2 tbsp shredded Cheddar cheese, light
   1 tbsp low sodium lite mayonnaise or 1 tsp mustard
   3 slices lettuce leaves (romaine or arugula, or red leaf lettuce)
   2 slices tomatoes
   3 slices dill pickle, low sodium
   2 slices multigrain bread or 1 sourdough bread or multigrain sandwich bun

**Instructions:**

1. Assemble sandwich and enjoy
2. End with 4 oz lemonade fluid or green tea or coffee
   Stats: 303 cal, 25g protein, 36g carb, 7g fat, 3g sat, 7g fiber, 943mg sodium, 47mg chol, 457 mg potassium, 173mg calcium

- **Alternative:** *Subway* Turkey Breast Deli Sandwich

**Afternoon Snack (Must Have):**
½ cup low-fat cottage cheese or 4 oz non-fat low sugar yogurt or plain yogurt
1 tsp ground flaxseeds or wheat germ
½ cup berries
8 oz water or green tea or V-8 juice
Stats: 131 cal, 12g protein, 14g carb, 2g fat, 1g fiber

**OR**

**Easy Granola Mix**

½ cup All-bran cereal or crunchy cereal
½ cup dried cherries or prunes
1 tbsp almonds, chopped
1 tbsp walnuts, chopped
2 tbsp sunflower seeds or ground flaxseeds
8 oz water or green tea

**Instructions:**

1. Combine and store in airtight container
2. Serving size is 1 tbsp (1 oz). Serves 5
3. Serve with ¼ cup or 4 tbsp low-fat cottage cheese, 3 tbsp fat free ricotta cheese, or one mozzarella string cheese stick
   Stats: 139 cal, 9.5g protein, 19g carb, 4g fat, 4g fiber

**Dinner---Veggie Marinara With Sauteed Turkey Breast**

1. Start with lemonade fluid (½ tbsp lemon juice with 4 oz water, green tea, or other fluid)
2. Follow with ½ cup Vegetable Broth Soup (recipe 2a) or non-creamy Lite Soup
3. Follow with 5 oz portion Grilled Eggplant with Mozzarella (recipe 63)
4. Main course: 10 oz portion (slightly over 1 cup) Veggie Marinara (recipe 64)
5. Serve with 4 oz portion Sauteed Turkey Breast (recipe 40)
6. End with 4 oz lemonade fluid or herbal tea

Stats: 373 cal, 33g protein, 31g carb, 14g fat, 2g sat, 9g fiber, 242mg sodium, 64mg chol, 999mg potassium, 154mg calcium

## Day 18 (3rd Wednesday)

**Breakfast---Grilled Cheese Sandwich**

2 slices high fiber multi grain bread or 100% whole grain or wheat bread
1 slice low-fat cheese (lite provolone cheese, goat cheese, etc)
1 oz Canadian bacon, turkey bacon, or veggie bacon
1 oz low sodium lean ham, smoked salmon, or roasted turkey breast (low sodium)
4 oz low sodium canned sodium tomato soup or V-8 Juice, low sodium
¼ cup berries (blueberries, strawberries, etc.) or ½ cup melons (cantaloupe, honeydew)
8 oz water, green tea, or coffee

**Instructions:**

1. Grill sandwich in a nonstick pan sprayed with canola or olive cooking spray.
2. Eat with berries or melons
   Stats: 311 cal, 25g protein, 35g carb, 9g fat, 3g sat, 7g fiber, 1,054mg sodium*, 54mg chol, 421mg potassium, 303mg calcium
   * *Reduce sodium in subsequent meals for the day*

**Morning Snack (Optional):**

½ apple or pear
1 boiled egg
8 oz water or green tea
Stats: 108 cal, 5.5g protein, 11g carb, 4.6g fat, 2.5g fiber

**Lunch---Grilled Tuna Pita Pocket With Oriental Blend Vegetables**

1. Start with lemonade fluid (½ tbsp lemon juice with 4 oz water, green tea, or other fluid)
2. Follow with 1 cup Oriental Blend Vegetables (recipe 65) or 2 cups spinach or romaine + 1-2 tbsp lemon juice or vinegar + salt and black pepper to taste or Mrs. Dash
3. Main course: 3 oz tuna in 7 oz portion Grilled Tuna Pita Pocket (recipe 66)
4. 1 tbsp Benefiber or 2 tsp Clearly Fiber (dissolve in fluid)
5. End with 4 oz lemonade fluid

Stats: 367 cal, 33g protein, 25g carb, 13g fat, 4g sat, 10g fiber, 679mg sodium, 59mg chol, 314mg potassium, 276mg calcium

**Afternoon Snack (Must Have):**

1 apple, pear, peach, orange, or nectarine
1 low-fat mozzarella string cheese or boiled egg
8 oz water or green tea
Stats: 148 cal, 9g protein, 22g carb, 4.6g fat, 5g fiber

**OR**

**Quick Soy Smoothie**

½ scoop (12.5 grams protein) soy or whey protein
½ cup 2% cold milk
¼ cup cold water
1 tbsp ground flaxseeds

**Instructions:** Mix well and enjoy with ¼ cup berries or melons

Stats: 162 cal, 18g protein, 13g carb, 4.8g fat, 3g fiber

**Dinner (1)---Tofu-Turkey Meatloaf With Mashed Cauliflower**

1. Start with lemonade fluid (½ tbsp lemon juice with 4 oz water, green tea, or other fluid)
2. Follow with 1 cup Tofu Vegetable Soup (recipe 67a) or 1 cup Greek Style Lemon Soup (recipe 67b)
3. Follow with ½-1 cup Steamed Spinach, Broccoli, or 2/3 cup Sugar Snap Peas or 1 cup Steamed Napa Cabbage (recipe 86)
4. Main course: 5 oz portion Tofu-Turkey Meatloaf (recipe 68) with 1 cup Mashed Cauliflower (recipe 69a)
5. End with 4 oz lemonade fluid or herbal tea
6. 1 tbsp Benefiber or 2 tsp Clearly Fiber (dissolve in soup or fluid)

Stats: 332 cal, 26g protein, 28g carb, 14g fat, 2g sat, 11g fiber, 563mg sodium, 47mg chol, 1,355mg potassium, 240mg calcium

**OR**

**Dinner (2)---Citrus Marinated Skinless Chicken Breast Skewers**

1. Start with lemonade fluid (½ tbsp lemon juice with 4 oz water, green tea, or other fluid)
2. Follow with 1 cup Vegetable Broth Soup (recipe 2a)
3. Main course: 4 oz chicken in 8 oz Citrus Marinated Skinless Chicken Breast Skewers (recipe 69b)
4. Serve with 1 cup Zesty Tabouleh Salad (recipe 12)
5. 1 tbsp Benefiber or 2 tsp Clearly Fiber (dissolve in soup or fluid)
6. End with 4 oz lemonade fluid or herbal tea

   Stats: 452 cal, 30g protein, 31g carb, 22g fat, 4.6g sat, 12g fiber, 788mg sodium, 68mg chol, 833mg potassium, 127mg calcium

## Day 19 (3rd Thursday)

**Breakfast---Hot Cereal (Oat Bran or 100% Whole Grain Rolled Oats)----see Day 3 Breakfast**

**Morning Snack (Optional):**

1 low-fat mozzarella string cheese
½ cup peaches in water canned, or 10 grapes, ½ medium grapefruit, or 2-3 dried prunes
8 oz water or green tea
Stats: 79 cal, 8.5g protein, 8g carb, 1.5g fat, 2g fiber

**Lunch (1)—Tuna Pasta Salad With Fresh Cucumber Tomato Salad**

1. Start with lemonade fluid (½ tbsp lemon juice with 4 oz water, green tea, or other fluid)
2. Follow with 1 ¼ cup Basic Cucumber Tomato Salad (recipe 70)
3. Main course: 3 oz tuna in 9 oz portion Tuna Pasta Salad (recipe 71)
4. End with 4 oz lemonade fluid

   Stats: 328 cal, 28g protein, 37g carb, 10g fat, 2g sat, 7g fiber, 603mg sodium, 41mg chol, 1,011mg potassium, 111mg calcium

**OR**

**Lunch (2)---Ham Sandwich With Sharon's Salad**

1. Start with lemonade fluid (½ tbsp lemon juice with 4 oz water, green tea, or other fluid)
2. Follow with 2 cups Sharon's Salad (1 cup spinach, 1 cup romaine or arugula, ¼ summer squash, 3 raw asparagus spears, ½ medium tomato, ¼ cucumber, 3 button mushrooms, ¼ red bell pepper, ¼ cup chopped cilantro, 1 tsp ground cinnamon
3. Dressing: 1-2 tsp olive oil + 1-2 tbsp fresh lemon juice or vinegar + salt and black pepper or Mrs. Dash to taste

4. Main course: ½ Ham Sandwich (2-3 oz lean ham, 2 tsp low sodium lite mayonnaise + 1 tsp mustard on a slice of multigrain bread)
5. End with 4 oz lemonade fluid or herbal tea
   Stats: 261 cal, 20g protein, 26g carb, 10g fat, 3g sat, 8g fiber, 788mg sodium, 96mg chol, 1,148mg potassium, 124mg calcium
   *Feel free to use any lean, low sodium sliced meat (roast beef, turkey, etc.)*

- **Alternative**: *Subway* Ham Deli Sandwich or *Subway* Ham Salad with 6 grams of fat or less

**Afternoon Snack (Must Have):**

½ cup low-fat cottage cheese or 4 oz nonfat low sugar yogurt or plain yogurt
1 tsp wheat germ or ground flaxseeds
8 oz water or green tea or V-8 juice
Stats: 89 cal, 15g protein, 5g carb, 2g fat, 0.3g fiber

**Dinner (1)---Chicken Picata Platter With Steamed Broccoli**

1. Start with lemonade fluid (½ tbsp lemon juice with 4 oz water, green tea, or other fluid)
2. Follow with 1 cup Lite Vegetable Soup (recipe 4a) or 1 cup Vegetable Pot Soup (recipe 72) or UDP Signature Soup (recipe 73)
3. Follow with 1 cup Fresh Green Salad (baby spinach, romaine, arugula, or mixed greens; Mrs. Dash or salt and black pepper for flavor)
4. Dressing: 1-2 tbsp fresh lemon juice or balsamic vinegar or other choices
5. Main course: 4 oz chicken in 6 oz portion Chicken Picata Platter (recipe 74)
6. Serve with 1 cup steamed broccoli, asparagus spears, eggplant, cabbage or kale + 1 tsp minced garlic + seasoning with Mrs. Dash or salt and black pepper
7. End with 4 oz lemonade fluid or herbal tea
   Stats: 342 cal, 37g protein, 35g carb, 11g fat, 2g sat, 12g fiber, 312mg sodium, 64mg chol, 1428mg potassium, 160mg calcium

**OR**

**Dinner (2)---Zesty Gazpacho With Seafood and Toasted Tortilla**

1. Start with lemonade fluid (½ tbsp lemon juice with 4 oz water, green tea, or other fluid)
2. Follow with 1 cup Lite Vegetable Soup or Canned low Sodium/Low-fat Soup
3. Follow with 2 cups Garden Salad (recipe 15)
4. Main Course: 3-4 oz Seafood in 15 oz portion (2 cups) Zesty Gazpacho with Seafood (recipe 75a)
5. Serve with toasted 1 oat bran/whole-wheat tortilla or multigrain bread
6. End with 4 oz lemonade fluid or herbal tea
   Stats: Stats: 382 cal, 34g protein, 38g carb, 13g fat, 1g sat, 13g fiber, 729mg sodium, 137mg chol, 1,131mg potassium, 194mg calcium

## Day 20 (3rd Friday)

**Breakfast (1)---Cold Cereal---see Day 1 Breakfast**

**Morning Snack (Optional):**

4 oz nonfat low sugar yogurt or pudding
1 tsp wheat germ or ground flaxseeds
8 oz water or green tea
Stats: 69 cal, 5g protein, 12g carb, 0.3g fat, 0.3g fiber

**OR**

½ medium banana, not overripe
15 dry roasted peanuts or 1.5 tsp peanut butter
8 oz water or green tea
Stats: 102 cal, 3g protein, 15g carb, 4g fat, 2g fiber

**Lunch---Andreas Mediterranean Grilled Chicken Salad**

1. Start with lemonade fluid (½ tbsp lemon juice with 4 oz water, green tea, or other fluid)
2. Main course: 4 oz chicken meat in 15 oz portion Andreas Mediterranean Grilled Chicken Salad (recipe 1)
3. With 3 medium strawberries, ¼ cup berries or ¼ cup melons
4. End with 4 oz lemonade fluid
   Stats: 345 cal, 38g protein, 18g carb, 14g fat, 2g sat, 6g fiber, 410mg sodium, 96mg chol, 998mg potassium, 117mg calcium

- **Alternatives:** see Day 1 Lunch Mediterranean Greek Chicken Salad

**Afternoon Snack (Must Have):**

1 apple, pear, 1-cup cantaloupe, or 1-cup fruit cocktail canned in water
1 low-fat mozzarella string cheese or 1 tsp peanut butter
8 oz water or green tea or V-8 juice
Stats: 130 cal, 9g protein, 23g carb, 2.5g fat, 5g fiber

**Dinner ---Grilled Tuna Steaks With Couscous Salad and Steamed Spinach**

1. Start with lemonade fluid (½ tbsp lemon juice with 4 oz water, green tea, or other fluid)
2. Follow with 1 cup Vegetable Pot Soup (recipe 72) or 1 cup Lite Vegetable Soup (recipe 4a)
3. Follow with 1 cup Steamed Spinach, Broccoli, Cabbage, or Turnip Greens – steam gently and add 1 tsp minced garlic + salt and black pepper or Mrs. Dash to taste
4. Main course: 4 oz portion Grilled Tuna Steaks (recipe 75b)
5. Serve with 3 oz portion Couscous Salad (recipe 76) or ½ cup String Beans Casserole (recipe 77) or 3 cups non-starchy dark leafy green vegetable salad (such as romaine, arugula, etc)
6. End with 4 oz lemonade fluid or herbal tea
   Stats: 328 cal, 38g protein, 27g carb, 9g fat, 2g sat, 10g fiber, 299mg sodium, 45mg chol, 1,692mg, potassium, 252mg calcium

## Day 21(3rd Saturday)

**Breakfast (1)---Tina's Favorite Breakfast**

1 high fiber multigrain, oat bran or 100% whole-grain or wheat bread, toasted
2 slices (2 oz) smoked salmon, lean ham, or turkey
1 oz Veggie Soy Canadian bacon or lean low sodium Canadian bacon
2 tomato slices
1 boiled egg
¼ cup berries or melon (cantaloupe and honeydew, etc.)
3 asparagus spears, raw
1 tbsp Benefiber or 2 tsp Clearly Fiber (mix into juice or fluid)

**Instructions:**

1. Serve toasted bread with smoked salmon, bacon, eggs, tomato slices, and asparagus
2. With 4 oz low sodium tomato juice, V-8 juice, skim milk, or unsweetened grapefruit juice
   Stats: 270 cal, 26g protein, 25g carb, 8g fat, 2g sat, 8g fiber, 852mg sodium, 202mg chol, 500mg potassium, 93mg calcium.

**OR**

**Breakfast (2)---Hot Cereal (Oat Bran or 100% Whole Grain Rolled Oats)---see Day 3 Breakfast**

**Morning Snack (Optional):**

1 Blue cheese stuffed cherry tomato (recipe 52a)
8 oz water or green tea
Stats: 67 cal, 2g protein, 7g carb, 5g fat, 1g fiber

**Lunch---Chickpea and Tuna Salad**

1. Start with lemonade fluid (½ tbsp lemon juice with 4 oz water, green tea, or other fluid)
2. 2 cups Mixed Green Salad + 1 tsp extra virgin olive oil + 2 tbsp Red Wine Vinegar or lemon juice with salt and black pepper to taste or Mrs. Dash.
3. Main course: 1 cup portion Chickpea and Tuna Salad (recipe 78)
4. Serve with ½ Grilled or Toasted high fiber whole-wheat Pita Bread
5. End with 4 oz lemonade fluid
   Stats: 364 cal, 30g protein, 30g carb, 14g fat, 2g sat, 8g fiber, 673mg sodium, 26mg chol, 727mg potassium, 106mg calcium

**Afternoon Snack (Must Have):**

(Raspberries and Strawberries Smoothie)
6 frozen raspberries
8 frozen strawberries
1 cup 2% milk or soymilk
1 pct Splenda or stevia
¾ scoop soy protein or whey protein
1 tsp flaxseed oil or 1 tbsp ground flaxseeds

**Instructions:**

1. Blend until smooth
2. Serving size is 1 cup. Serves 2
   Stats: 129 cal, 14g protein, 14g carb, 2.5g fat, 2.4g fiber

**OR**

**Sauteed Garlic Shrimp** (recipe 105)

Serve with a slice of toasted high fiber multigrain bread
8 oz water or green tea or V-8 juice
Stats: 92 cal, 7g protein, 13g carb, 2g fat, 3g fiber, 49 mg chol

**Dinner (1)---Baked Chicken With Sun Dried Tomatoes and Feta Cheese**

1. Start with lemonade fluid (½ tbsp lemon juice with 4 oz water, green tea, or other fluid)
2. Follow with ½-1 cup Lite Vegetable Soup (recipe 4a), ½-1 cup Vegetable Pot Soup (recipe 72), or 1 cup Lime Vegetable Soup (recipe 4b)
3. Follow with 1 cup raw or ½ cup steamed Broccoli florets, Romaine lettuce, or Cabbage with salt and black pepper or Mrs. Dash for flavor
4. Main course: 6 oz portion Baked Chicken with Sun Dried Tomatoes (recipe 79)
5. Serve with Baked Sweet Potato Mash (3-4oz) seasoned with 1 tsp fresh ground cinnamon, ½ tsp nutmeg, ½ pkt Splenda, and 1 tsp *I Can't Believe It's Not Butter* (recipe 26 or Cheryl's Comfort Food)
6. 1 tbsp Benefiber or 2 tsp Clearly Fiber (mix into mash potato, soup, or fluid)
7. End with 4 oz lemonade fluid or herbal tea
   Stats: 386 cal, 38g protein, 36g carb, 10g fat, 2g sat, 8g fiber, 394mg sodium, 87mg chol, 1,384mg potassium, 174mg calcium

**OR**

**Dinner (2)---Pan-Roasted Lemon Pepper Salmon With Spinach**

1. Start with lemonade fluid (½ tbsp lemon juice with 4 oz water, green tea, or other fluid)
2. Follow with ½-1 cup Lite Vegetable Soup (recipe 4a) or ½-1 cup Vegetable Pot Soup (recipe 72) or non-creamy Lite Soup
3. Follow with 1 cup Roasted Asparagus and Zucchini (recipe 80)
4. Main course: 4 oz fish in 8 oz portion Pan-Roasted Lemon Pepper Salmon with Spinach (recipe 81)
5. Serve with Rice and Broccoli (1 cup Steamed Broccoli tossed into ¼ cup or 4 tbsp cooked Brown Rice or *Uncle Ben's* Converted Rice (recipe 23) or ¼ cup (4 tbsp) cooked canned Red Kidney, Black or White Beans, or ½ cup cooked Chinese vermicelli pasta noodles (recipe 22)
6. End with 4 oz lemonade fluid or herbal tea
   Stats: 399 cal, 34g protein 38g carb, 14g fat, 2g sat, 11g fiber, 602mg sodium, 62mg chol, 2,310mg potassium, 342mg calcium
   * *Beans and lentils are high in fiber, especially soluble fiber (Navy beans: ½ cup cooked delivers 148 cal, 27g carb, 10g protein, 7g fiber and 4g soluble*

*fiber; Lima beans: ½ cup cooked delivers 95 cal, 18g carb, 6g protein, 6g fiber, and 2g soluble fiber). 1-2 tbsp added to your salad, vegetables, or rice could help to increase fiber without adding extra carbohydrate. Chana dal (a lentil) can help to give you a better control of your blood sugar and insulin (look for it in Indian, Mediterranean, or Middle Eastern stores).*

## Day 22 (4th Sunday)

**Breakfast---Scrambled Eggs and Turkey**

½ cup eggbeaters or 1 whole egg + 2 egg whites
½ tbsp chopped onion
1 tbsp low sodium low-fat *Colby* shredded cheese
2 slices (2oz) 97% fat free oven roasted turkey breast, low-fat, low sodium ham, or 2 oz Canadian bacon – cut into small pieces
3 thin slices tomato
½ 100% whole-wheat bagel (*Thomas's*)
Cooking spray, canola or olive oil
1 tbsp Benefiber or 2 tsp Clearly Fiber (mix into fluid)

**Instructions:**

1. Combine eggs, turkey, or ham pieces and onion in a bowl
2. Scramble eggs in a non-stick pan sprayed with canola spray
3. Top with cheese
4. Serve on ½ 100% whole-wheat bagel with tomato slices
5. With 4 oz unsweetened juice (grapefruit, apple, orange, or *Mountain Sun* cranberry juice, or skim milk)
   Stats: 242 cal, 25g protein, 33g carb, 3g fat, 0g sat, 8g fiber, 743mg sodium, 16mg chol, 728mg potassium, 211mg calcium
   * *Use eggbeaters or Omega-3 enriched eggs if you are concerned about your cholesterol.*

**Morning Snack (Optional):**

3 tbsp low-fat cottage cheese, 4 oz nonfat low sugar yogurt, or plain yogurt
5 grapes
¼ cup cubed melons (cantaloupe, honeydew, etc.)
1 oz low sodium and low-fat ham, turkey, or smoked salmon
8 oz water or green tea
Stats: 87 cal, 9g protein, 11g carb, 1.5g fat, 1g fiber

**Lunch (1)---Andreas Greek Salad With Baked Chicken Thighs**

1. Start with lemonade fluid (½ tbsp lemon juice with 4 oz water, green tea, or other fluid)
2. Follow with 1 cup Andreas Greek Salad (recipe 33)

3. Main course: 4 oz (1 thigh) Baked Chicken Thigh with Fennel (recipe 82) or use left over from your dinner
4. And 4 oz (snack size) Mixed Berry Sorbet (recipe 53)
5. 1 tbsp Benefiber or 2 tsp Clearly Fiber (mix into fluid)
6. End with 4 oz lemonade fluid or herbal tea
   Stats: 381 cal, 29g protein, 25g carb, 19g fat, 4g sat, 10g fiber, 371mg sodium, 15mg chol, 871mg potassium, 296mg calcium

**OR**

**Lunch (2)---Ground Turkey Meatloaf Wrap**

1. Start with lemonade fluid (½ tbsp lemon juice with 4 oz water, green tea, or other fluid)
2. Follow with 1 cup Lite Escarole Soup (recipe 39a) or Lite Vegetable Soup (recipe 4a) or Chicken Noodle Soup (recipe 83)
3. Follow with 2 cups Spinach, Romaine, Red Leaf Lettuce, or Arugula Salad + 1-2 tbsp lemon juice or vinegar + salt and black pepper or Mrs. Dash for flavor or Romaine Radish Salad (recipe 85)
4. Main course: 3-4 oz meat in 8 oz portion Ground Turkey Meatloaf Wrap (recipe 84)
5. End with 4 oz lemonade fluid or herbal tea
   Stats: 358 cal, 35g protein, 22g carb, 14.5g fat, 5g sat, 11g fiber, 658mg sodium, 167mg chol, 1,117mg potassium, 494mg calcium

**Afternoon Snack (Must Have):**

1 tsp sunflower seeds
1 tsp ground flaxseeds
1 tsp chopped walnuts or almonds
¼ cup peach slices canned or ¼ peach chopped
3 strawberries, sliced, or ¼ cup berries
4 grapes
1 tbsp lemon juice
2 tbsp low-fat cottage cheese or yogurt

**Instructions:**

1. Combine all the ingredients and serve
   Stats: 132 cal, 6g protein, 17g carb, 5g fat, 3g fiber

**OR**

**Berry and Yogurt Sorbet (Recipe 107):**

Stats: 89 cal, 4g protein, 10.5g carb, 4g fat, 1g fiber

**Dinner (1)---Grilled Salmon With Grilled Eggplant**

1. Start with lemonade fluid (½ tbsp lemon juice with 4 oz water, green tea, or other fluid)
2. Follow with ½-1 cup Lite Vegetable Soup (recipe 4a) or ½-1 cup Greek Style Lemon Soup (recipe 67b) or 1 cup Lime Vegetable Soup (recipe 4b)

3. Follow with ½-1 cup Steamed Spinach, Broccoli, Kale, Cabbage, or Escarole + seasoning with 1 tsp minced garlic and Mrs. Dash or salt and pepper to taste
4. Main course: 4 oz salmon in 14 oz portion Grilled Salmon with Vegetables (recipe 37)
5. Serve with 5 oz portion Grilled Eggplant with Mozzarella (recipe 63)
6. End with 4 oz lemonade fluid (water, green tea, or herbal tea)
   Stats: 380 cal, 33g protein, 30g carb, 15g fat, 3g sat, 12g fiber, 543mg sodium, 73mg chol, 1,827mg potassium, 218mg calcium

**OR**

**Dinner (2)---Oven Baked Crusted Chicken With Italian Style Peas and Mushrooms**

1. Start with lemonade fluid (½ tbsp lemon juice with 4 oz water, green tea, or other fluid)
2. Follow with ½-1 cup Lite Vegetable Soup (recipe 4a) or non-creamy Lite Soup
3. Follow with 2-3 cups Garden Salad (recipe 15) or Romaine Radish Salad (recipe 85)
4. Main course: 3-4 oz Oven Baked Crusted Chicken (recipe 4c)
5. Serve with 1 cup Italian Style Peas and Mushrooms Sauté (recipe 87) or 1 cup String Beans Casserole (recipe 77)
6. End with 4 oz lemonade fluid (water, green tea, or herbal tea)
   Stats: 292 mg cal, 33g protein, 28g carb, 6g fat, 1g sat, 9g fiber, 850mg sodium, 65mg chol, 972mg potassium, 135mg calcium

## Day 23 (4th Monday)

**Breakfast---Cold Cereal---see Day 1 Breakfast**

**Morning Snack (Optional):**

1 low-fat mozzarella string cheese or boiled egg
8 oz water or green tea
Stats: 51 cal, 8g protein, 1g carb, 3.5g fat, 1g sat, 0g fiber

**Lunch---Grilled Chicken Sandwich With Soup**

1. Start with lemonade fluid (½ tbsp lemon juice with 4 oz water, green tea, or otherfluid)
2. Follow with 1 cup Vegetable Broth (recipe 2a) or 4 oz Canned Low Sodium Vegetable Chicken Soup with Water
3. Main course: 3 oz chicken in 8 oz portion Grilled Chicken Sandwich (recipe 18c) 3 oz grilled or baked chicken or turkey breast + 2 slices tomatoes + 3 leaves romaine + 3 dill pickle slices + 1 tsp Dijon mustard + 1 tsp low sodium lite mayonnaise or mustard
4. With 1 oat bran/whole-wheat tortillas or pita (*Joseph's*) or a high fiber multigrain or 100% whole grain slice
5. End with 4 oz lemonade fluid

6. 1 tbsp Benefiber or 2 tsp Clearly Fiber (mix into soup or fluid)
   Stats: 257 cal, 35g protein, 16g carb, 7g fat, 2g sat, 10g fiber, 874mg sodium, 77mg chol, 615mg potassium,

- **Alternatives:** see Day 1 Lunch Mediterranean Greek Chicken Salad

**Afternoon Snack (Must Have):**

½ cup low-fat cottage cheese (4 oz low-fat, low sugar yogurt, or plain yogurt)
1 tsp ground flaxseeds or wheat germ
¼ tsp ground cinnamon
½ cup berries (blueberries, raspberries, strawberries, etc.)
8 oz water or green tea or V-8 juice
Stats: 130 cal, 15g protein, 15g carb, 2g fat, 1g fiber

**Dinner---Spinach and Feta Wrap With Mixed Vegetables**

1. Start with lemonade fluid (½ tbsp lemon juice with 4 oz water, green tea, or other fluid)
2. Follow with 1 cup Vegetable Broth Soup (recipe 2a) or ½ cup Greek Style Lemon Soup (recipe 67b) or non-creamy Lite Soup
3. Follow with 1 cup Mixed Veggies, Steamed (recipe 46a)
4. Main course: 3-4 oz chicken breast in 9 oz portion Spinach and Feta Wrap (recipe 88)
5. Serve with 1 oat bran/whole-wheat tortilla or pita bread (*Joseph's*) or a slice of high fiber multigrain bread or 100% whole grain /wheat
6. And ½ cup berries (strawberries, raspberries, blueberries, etc.) or ½ cup melon (cantaloupe, honeydew, watermelon, etc.)
7. End with 4 oz lemonade or herbal tea
   Stats: 324 cal, 34g protein, 28g carb, 12g fat, 1.5g sat, 13g fiber, 652mg sodium, 51mg chol, 1,157mg potassium, 163mg calcium

## Day 24 (4th Tuesday)

**Breakfast (1)---Easy Peach Smoothie**

1 small peach or ¼ cup canned peaches in light syrup, unsweetened
4 oz plain yogurt (*Yoplait*)
½ cup skim milk or soymilk
1 tbsp ground flaxseeds
1 tsp vanilla extract
½-1 pack Splenda or Stevia (optional)
4 ice cubes or ½ cup cold water
½ cup eggbeaters or 2 boiled whole eggs (eat one whole egg + egg white separately)
1 tbsp Benefiber or 2 tsp Clearly Fiber (dissolve in smoothie or fluid)

**Instructions:**

1. Combine all ingredients in a blender and mix until smooth

2. Accompany with eggs (eggbeaters can be added directly to smoothie)
3. And ½ cup (strawberries, blueberries, or raspberries) or ½ cup melon (cantaloupe, honeydew, watermelon, etc.)
   Stats: 308 cal, 21g protein, 36g carb, 9g fat, 2g sat, 10g fiber, 269g sodium, 18mg chol, 1,422mg potassium, 543mg calcium

**OR**

**Breakfast (2)---Hot Cereal (Oat Bran or 100% Whole Grain Rolled Oats)—see Day 3 Breakfast**

**Morning Snack (Optional):**

2 tbsp Hummus (recipe 18a)
Vegetable sticks (2 celery stalks, 6 baby carrots, and 2 asparagus spears)
8 oz water or green tea
Stats: 50 cal, 2g protein, 11g carb, 0g fat, 4g fiber

**OR**

3 multigrain or whole-wheat crackers (*Carr's*) or equivalent
2 tsp smooth peanut butter
8 oz water or green tea
Stats: 93 cal, 4g protein, 9g carb, 5g fat, 2g fiber

**Lunch (1)---Roast Beef Pocket Sandwich With French Cut Green Beans**

1. Start with lemonade fluid (½ tbsp lemon juice with 4 oz water, green tea, or other fluid)
2. Follow with 1 cup Steamed French Cut Green Beans
3. Main course: 8 oz portion Roast Beef Pocket Sandwich (recipe 89)
4. End with 4 oz lemonade fluid
   Stats: 312 cal, 36g protein, 22g carb, 10g fat, 4g sat, 9g fiber, 626mg sodium, 80mg chol, 709mg potassium, 136mg calcium

- **Alternatives:** *Subway* 6" Roast Beef Sandwich or *Subway* Roast Beef Deli Sandwich

**OR**

**Lunch (2)---Ham Sandwich With Sharon's Salad**

1. Start with lemonade fluid (½ tbsp lemon juice with 4 oz water, green tea, or other fluid)
2. Follow with 2 cups Sharon's Salad (1 cup spinach, 1 cup romaine or arugula, ¼ summer squash, 3 raw asparagus spears, ½ medium tomato, ¼ cucumber, 3 button mushrooms, ¼ red bell peppers, ¼ cup chopped cilantro, 1 tsp ground cinnamon)
3. Dressing: 1-2 tsp olive oil + 1-2 tbsp fresh lemon juice or vinegar + salt and black pepper to taste
4. Main course: ½ Ham Sandwich (2 oz lean ham, 2 tsp low sodium lite mayonnaise + 1 tsp mustard on a slice of high fiber multigrain bread)
5. End with 4 oz lemonade fluid or herbal tea

Stats: 261 cal, 20g protein, 26g carb, 10g fat, 3g sat, 8g fiber, 788mg sodium, 96mg chol, 1,148mg potassium, 124mg calcium

* *Feel free to use any lean, low sodium sliced meat (roast beef, turkey, etc.)*

- **Alternative**: *Subway* Ham Deli Sandwich or *Subway* Ham Salad with 6 grams of fat or less. Use ½ pkt *Kraft* Fat Free Italian Dressing

**Mid Afternoon Snack (Must Have):**

½ cup low-fat cottage cheese or 4 oz low-fat, low sugar yogurt or plain
1 tsp ground flaxseeds or wheat germ
½ cup berries (blueberries, raspberries, strawberries, etc.) or ½ cup melon (cantaloupe, honeydew, watermelon, etc.)
8 oz water or green tea or V-8 juice
Stats: 130 cal, 15g protein, 15g carb, 2g fat, 1g fiber

**Dinner (1)---Seafood Picata Platter With String Beans Casserole**

1. Start with lemonade fluid (½ tbsp lemon juice with 4 oz water, green tea, or other fluid)
2. Follow with ½-1 cup Vegetable Broth Soup (recipe 2a) or ½-1 cup Vegetable Pot Soup (recipe 72) or ½-1 cup Greek Style Lemon Soup (recipe 67b) or non-creamy Lite Soup
3. Follow with 1 cup Mixed Veggies (recipe 46a)
4. Main course: 4 oz shrimp and scallop in 7 oz portion Seafood Picata Platter (recipe 90)
5. Serve with ½ cup String Beans Casserole (recipe 77) or 1 cup portion Steamed Green Peas and Carrots
6. End with 4 oz lemonade fluid or herbal tea
   Stats: 331 cal, 33g protein, 36g carb, 10g fat, 1g sat, 13g fiber, 468mg sodium, 106mg chol, 1,111mg potassium, 171mg calcium

**OR**

**Dinner (2)---Oven Baked Crusted Chicken With Mashed Cauliflower**

1. Start with lemonade fluid (½ tbsp lemon juice with 4 oz water, green tea, or other fluid)
2. Follow with 1 cup Lite Vegetable Soup (recipe 4a) or 1 cup Lite Escarole Soup (recipe 39a) or non-creamy Lite Soup
3. Follow with 1 cup Roasted Veggies (recipe 5)
4. Main course: 3-4 oz portion Oven Baked Crusted Chicken (recipe 4c)
5. Serve with 1 cup Mashed Cauliflower (recipe 69a)
6. End with 4 oz lemonade fluid or herbal tea
   Stats: 318 cal, 34g protein, 32g carb, 7g fat, 1g sat, 10g fiber, 728mg sodium, 66mg chol, 1,103mg potassium, 134mg calcium

## Day 25 (4th Wednesday)

**Breakfast (1)---Simple Breakfast**

1. ¾ cup low-fat cottage cheese or ½ cup eggbeaters (prepared with cooking spray)
2. ½ cup canned peaches (packed in water or light syrup) or ½ cup berries or ½ cup fruit cocktail in water or ½ cup diced mango or pineapple chunks canned in water
3. 2 slices (2oz) low, low sodium oven roasted turkey breast, 2 oz low sodium Canadian bacon, 1 *Morningstar* breakfast patty, or 2 oz smoked salmon
4. 3 multigrain crackers (*Carr's*) or equivalent or a slice of high fiber multigrain bread
5. 6 oz tomato juice (low sodium) or V-8 juice
6. 1 tbsp Benefiber or 2 tsp Clearly Fiber (mix with cottage cheese or dissolve in fluid)
   Stats: 260 cal, 28g protein, 35g carb, 3g fat, 2g sat, 6g fiber, 895mg sodium, 31mg chol, 287mg potassium, 186mg calcium

**OR**

**Breakfast (2)---Cold Cereal---see Day 1 Breakfast**

**Morning Snack (Optional):**

1 fruit (10 grapes, ½ grapefruit, ½ apple, medium peach, or medium kiwi)
1 low-fat mozzarella string cheese
8 oz water or green tea
Stats: 87 cal, 9g protein, 11g carb, 1.5g fat, 2g fiber

**Lunch---Sharon's Lunch (Seasonal Vegetables With Baked Chicken)**

1. Start with lemonade fluid (½ tbsp lemon juice with 4 oz water, green tea, or other fluid)
2. Follow with 1 cup Lite Vegetable Soup (recipe 4a) or 4 oz canned Low Sodium Vegetable Soup with Water or ¼ cup Sugar Snap Peas with Lemon Basil (recipe 91)
3. Main course: 3-4 oz baked or grilled chicken breast in 14 oz portion of Fresh Seasonal Vegetables (recipe 92)
4. Serve with 3 multigrain crackers (*Carr's*) or Fat free whole-wheat crackers – Organic or equivalent
5. End with 4 oz lemonade fluid
   Stats: 332 cal, 34g protein, 31g carb, 8g fat, 1g sat, 10g fiber, 246mg sodium, 66mg chol, 1,388mg potassium, 163mg calcium
   * *You can use leftover meat from your dinner*

**Mid Afternoon Snack (Must Have):**

1 low-fat mozzarella string cheese or boiled egg
1 apple, pear, nectarine, small mango, or ½ grapefruit
Stats: 130 cal, 9g protein, 23g carb, 3.5g fat, 5g fiber

**Dinner (1)---Beef Mushroom Stir-Fry With Chinese Vermicelli Pasta Noodles**

1. Start with lemonade fluid (½ tbsp lemon juice with 4 oz water, green tea, or other fluid)

2. Follow with ½-1 cup Lite Vegetable Soup (recipe 4a), 1 cup Chicken Noodle Soup (recipe 83), or non-creamy Lite Soup
3. Follow with 1-3 cups Baby Spinach, Broccoli, Cabbage, Cauliflower, or Romaine + 1-2 tbsp lemon juice or vinegar + salt and black pepper or Mrs. Dash to taste
4. Main course: 4 oz meat in 12 oz portion Beef and Mushroom Stir Fry (recipe 93)
5. Serve with ½ cup al dente cooked Chinese vermicelli pasta noodles (recipe 22) or ½ cup cooked rice, such as brown rice or *Uncle Ben's* converted rice (recipe 23) or 1 cup String Beans Casserole (recipe 77)
6. 1 tbsp Benefiber or 2 tsp Clearly Fiber (dissolve in soup or fluid)
7. End with 4 oz lemonade fluid or herbal tea
   Stats: 401 cal, 32g protein, 32 carb, 16g fat, 5g sat, 10g fiber, 305mg sodium, 43mg chol, 1,373mg potassium, 192mg calcium

**OR**

**Dinner (2)---Garlic and Herb Crusted Salmon With Escarole and Beans**

1. Start with lemonade fluid (½ tbsp lemon juice with 4 oz water, green tea, or other fluid)
2. Follow with ½-1 cup Lite Vegetable Soup (recipe 4a) or non-creamy Lite Soup
3. Follow with 1 cup Steamed Broccoli, Spinach, or Cabbage – seasoned with 1 tsp minced garlic + salt and black pepper or Mrs. Dash to taste
4. Main course: 6 oz portion Garlic and Herb Crusted Salmon (recipe 94)
5. Serve with 1 cup Escarole and Beans (recipe 95)
6. End with 4 oz lemonade fluid or herbal tea
   Stats: 392 cal, 35g protein, 30g carb, 11g fat, 1 g sat, 15g fiber, 524mg sodium, 63mg chol, 1,736mg potassium, 249mg calcium

## Day 26 (4thThursday)

**Breakfast (2)---Hot Cereal (Oat Bran or 100% Whole Grain Rolled Oats)---see Day 3 Breakfast**

**Morning Snack (Optional):**

8 oz low sodium V8 Vegetable Juice or Tomato Juice
Stats: 60 cal, 2g protein, 11g carb, 0g fat, 2g fiber

**OR**

8 oz water or green tea
Stat: 0 calories

**Lunch (1)---Beef and Mushroom Stir Fry Pocket**

1. Start with lemonade fluid (½ tbsp lemon juice with 4 oz water, green tea, or other fluid)
2. Follow with 1 cup Steamed Spinach or Broccoli – seasoned with 1 tsp minced garlic + salt and black pepper or Mrs. Dash to taste
3. Main course: Use the left over from yesterday's dinner – 6 oz portion of Beef and Mushroom Stir Fry or half of your dinner (recipe 93)

4. Stuffed into oat bran/whole-wheat tortilla or pita bread (*Joseph's*) or ½ whole-wheat pita bread
5. And ½ cup canned peaches packed in water, 1 medium peach, kiwi, or ½ cup melons (cantaloupe, honeydew, etc.)
6. End with 4 oz lemonade fluid
   Stats: 248 cal, 22g protein, 25g carb, 9g fat, 2.5g sat, 12g fiber, 446mg sodium, 21mg chol, 1,479mg, potassium, 278mg calcium

- **Alternatives:** *Subway* Roast Beef Deli Sandwich, or 6" roast Beef Sandwich with Veggie Delite Salad (2 servings). Dressing: ½ pkt *Kraft* Fat Free Italian Dressing.

**OR**

**Lunch (2)---Andreas Mediterranean Grilled Chicken Salad**

1. Start with lemonade fluid (½ tbsp lemon juice with 4 oz water, green tea, or other fluid)
2. Main course: 4 oz chicken breast in 15 oz portion Andreas Mediterranean Grilled Chicken Salad (recipe 1)
3. With 3 medium strawberries or ¼ cup berries or ½ cup melons
4. 1 tbsp Benefiber or 2 tsp Clearly Fiber (dissolve in fluid)
5. End with 4 oz lemonade fluid
   Stats: 345 cal, 38g protein, 18g carb, 14g fat, 2g sat, 11g fiber, 410mg sodium, 96mg chol, 998mg potassium, 117mg calcium

- **Alternatives:** see Day 1 Lunch Mediterranean Greek Chicken Salad

**Afternoon Snack (Must Have):**

(Salsa Topped Veggie Burger Wraps)
1 (67g) Morning star veggie patty
Or veggie soy burger patty or Turkey Burgers (low-fat)
1 tbsp Quick salsa (recipe 18b) or organic mild salsa
2 large Romaine lettuce leaves
8 oz water or 6 oz tomato juice/V-8 juice (low sodium)

**Instructions:**

1. Cook patty per package instructions
2. Place on lettuce leaves and top with salsa. Fold and enjoy
   Stats: 102 cal, 12g protein, 13g carb, 0g fat, 3g fiber

**Dinner (1)---Poached Haddock With Mashed Celeriac and Turnip**

1. Start with lemonade fluid (½ tbsp lemon juice with 4 oz water, green tea, or other fluid)
2. Follow with ½-1 cup Vegetable Broth Soup (recipe 2a) or non-creamy Lite Soup
3. Follow with 5 Steamed or Grilled Asparagus Spears
4. Main course: 4 oz fish in 12 oz portion Poached Haddock Fillets (recipe 96)
5. Serve with 1 cup Mashed Celeriac (recipe 97)
6. End with 4 oz lemonade fluid or herbal tea
   Stats: 364 cal, 28g protein, 34g carb, 12g fat, 1.5g sat, 10g fiber, 528mg sodium, 65mg chol, 1,668mg potassium, 210mg calcium

**OR**

**Dinner (2)---Chicken Picata Platter With Roasted Veggies**

1. Start with lemonade fluid (½ tbsp lemon juice with 4 oz water, green tea, or other fluid)
2. Follow with ½-1 cup Vegetable Broth Soup (recipe 2a) or non-creamy Lite Soup
3. Follow with ½-1 cup Steamed Spinach, Broccoli, or Cabbage – flavored with 1 tsp minced garlic + salt and black pepper or Mrs. Dash
4. Main course: 4 oz chicken in 6 oz portion Chicken Picata Platter (recipe 74)
5. Serve with 1 cup Roasted Veggies (recipe 5)
6. End with 4 oz lemonade fluid or herbal tea
   Stats: 341 cal, 33g protein, 34g carb, 12.5g fat, 2g sat, 12g fiber, 251mg sodium, 64mg chol, 1,281mg potassium, 147mg calcium

## Day 27 (4th Friday)

**Breakfast ---Cold Cereal---see Day 1 Breakfast**

**Morning Snack (Optional):**

8 oz low sodium V8 Vegetable Juice or Tomato Juice
Stats: 60cal, 2g protein, 11g carb, 0g fat, 2g fiber

**OR**

½ apple, pear, or grapefruit +8 oz water or green tea
Stats: 40 cal, 0g protein, 11g carb, 0g fat, 2.5g fiber

**Lunch (1)---Turkey Sandwich With Leafy Dark Green Vegetables**

1. Start with lemonade fluid (½ tbsp lemon juice with 4 oz water, green tea, or other fluid)
2. Follow with 2 cups Leafy Dark Greens Vegetables (such as baby spinach, romaine or arugula, etc.) with 3 slices of tomato + 2 tbsp lemon juice or balsamic vinegar + salt and ground black pepper or Mrs. Dash to taste
3. Turkey Sandwich:
   2 -3slices (2-3oz) cooked turkey (low sodium and lean)
   2 tbsp shredded Cheddar cheese, light
   1 tbsp low sodium lite mayonnaise or 1 tsp mustard
   3 slices lettuce leaves (romaine, arugula, or red lettuce)
   2 slices tomatoes
   3 slices dill pickle, low sodium
   2 slices multigrain bread, 1 sourdough bread, or multigrain sandwich bun

**Instructions:**

1. Assemble sandwich and enjoy
2. Serve with 4 oz tomato soup, *Campbell* (low sodium) or V-8 juice
   Stats: 255 cal, 21g protein, 33g carb, 7g fat, 3g sat, 10g fiber, 931mg sodium, 39mg chol, 765 mg potassium, x mg calcium

- **Alternative**: *Subway* Turkey Breast Deli Sandwich

**OR**

**Lunch (2)---Turkey Wrap With Cucumber Tomato Fennel Salad**

1 Start with lemonade fluid (½ tbsp lemon juice with 4 oz water, green tea, or other fluid)
2 Follow with 1 cup Tomato Cucumber Fennel Salad (recipe 42b) or 1 cup Cucumber Tomato Salad (recipe 98)
3 Main course: 5 oz portion Turkey Wrap (recipe 52b)
4 End with 4 oz lemonade fluid
Stats: 348 cal, 16g protein, 37g carb, 17g fat, 2.7g sat, 8g fiber, 791mg sodium, 22mg chol, 933mg potassium, 85mg calcium

**Afternoon Snack (Must Have):**

½ cup 2% cottage cheese
1 tsp wheat germ or ground flaxseeds
½ cup berries (blueberries, raspberries, strawberries, etc.) or ½ cup melons
8 oz water or green tea or V-8 juice
Stats: 130 cal, 15g protein, 15g carb, 2g fat, 1g fiber

**OR**

4 oz nonfat low-sugar yogurt, plain or (½ cup low-fat low sugar pudding)
1 tsp toasted wheat germ or ground flaxseeds
1 slice (1 oz) smoked salmon (or lean and low sodium turkey or ham)
8 oz water or green tea or V-8 juice
Stats: 102 cal, 10g protein, 12g carb, 1g fat, 0.3g fiber

**Dinner---Grilled Salmon With Mixed Greens and Grilled Eggplant**

1. Start with lemonade fluid (½ tbsp lemon juice with 4 oz water, green tea, or other fluid)
2. Follow with 1 cup Broccoli and Dill Weed Soup (recipe 11a) or 1 cup Greek Style Lemon Soup (recipe 67b)
3. Main course: 4 oz salmon in 14 oz portion of Grilled Salmon with Mixed Greens (recipe 37)
4. Serve with ½ cup Grilled Eggplant (recipe 99a)
5. End with 4 oz lemonade fluid, green tea, or herbal tea
   Stats: 423 cal, 38g protein, 35g carb, 18g fat, 3g sat, 13g fiber, 537mg sodium, 72mg chol, 1,967mg, potassium, 415mg calcium

## Day 28 (4th Saturday)

**Breakfast (1)---Smoked Salmon on Toasted Whole-Wheat English Muffin**

2 oz (2 slices) smoked salmon
1 tsp extra virgin olive oil or canola oil
1 tsp shallots, chopped
1 tsp green peppers, chopped

½ 100% whole-wheat English muffin, toasted
½ cup low-fat cottage cheese or ricotta cheese
½ cup berries (strawberries, blueberries, raspberries)
¼ grapefruit
1 cup green tea or coffee
Low-fat cream (optional)
1 pct Splenda or stevia (optional)
1 tbsp Benefiber or 2 tsp Davinci Lab Clearly Fiber (mix into cottage cheese or fluid)

**Instruction:**

1. Sauté shallots and peppers in oil until brown; add the salmon. Season to taste
2. Serve on toasted whole-wheat muffin
3. Combine berries with cottage cheese and enjoy
   Stats: 326 cal, 28g protein, 35g carb, 9.5g fat, 2g sat, 8g fiber, 1,052mg sodium*, 28mg chol, 565mg potassium, 216mg calcium
   * *Reduce sodium in subsequent meals in order to lower your total intake for the day*

**OR**

**Breakfast (2)---Hot Cereal (Oat Bran or 100% Whole Grain Rolled Oats)---see Day 3 Breakfast**

**Morning Snack (Optional):**
1 fruit (apple, plum, orange, grapefruit, etc.)
Stats: 80 cal, 0g protein, 22g carb, 0g fat, 5g fiber

**Lunch---Eggplant and Cheese Wrap**

1. Start with lemonade fluid (½ tbsp lemon juice with 4 oz water, green tea, or other fluid)
2. Follow with ½-1 cup Steamed Broccoli, Asparagus, Brussels Sprouts, or Cabbage
3. Main course: 14 oz portion Eggplant and Cheese Wrap (recipe 99b)
4. Serve with ½ cup low sodium low-fat Cottage Cheese + ½ tsp ground cinnamon + ¼ tsp nutmeg or 4 oz non-fat low sugar Yogurt + ¼ cup berries (blueberries, strawberries, blackberries, etc.) or ¼ cup melons
5. End with 4 oz lemonade fluid, green tea, or herbal tea
   Stats: 278 cal, 30g protein, 29g carb, 7g fat, 3g sat, 11g fiber, 541mg sodium, 15mg chol, 1,243mg potassium, 542mg calcium

**Afternoon Snack (Must Have):**
1 tbsp low-fat cream cheese or nonfat sour cream
3 multigrain crackers or 2 whole-wheat crackers (*Carr's*) or equivalent
1 slice (1 oz) smoked salmon or lean ham or turkey (low sodium)
1 slice tomato
3 tbsp low-fat cottage cheese
8 oz water or green tea or V-8 juice
Stats: 115 cal, 13g protein, 12g carb, 1.8g fat, 1.4g fiber

**OR**

4 oz or ½ cup Blueberry and Yogurt Sorbet (recipe 107)
Stats: 89 cal, 4g protein, 10.5g carb, 3.7g fat, 1g fiber

**Dinner (1)---Garlic Tilapia With String Beans Casserole**

1 Start with lemonade fluid (½ tbsp lemon juice with 4 oz water, green tea, or other fluid)
2 Follow with 1 cup Lite Vegetable Soup (recipe 4a) or 1 cup Lite Escarole Soup (recipe 39a) or ½ cup Greek Style Lemon Soup (recipe 67b)
3 Follow with 1 cup Steamed Spinach, Broccoli, Cabbage, or Asparagus with 1 tsp minced garlic + salt and black pepper or Mrs. Dash to taste
4 Main course: 4 oz fish in 7 oz portion Sauteed Garlic Tilapia or Halibut, Catfish or Salmon (recipe 100)
5 Serve with ½ cup String Beans Casserole (recipe 77) or 1 cup French Cut Green Beans or Sugar Snap Peas
6 End with 4 oz lemonade fluid or herbal tea
Stats: 379 cal, 36g protein, 35g carb, 12g fat, 1g sat, 11g fiber, 582mg sodium, 51mg chol, 1847mg, potassium, 223mg calcium

**OR**

**Dinner (2)---Rosemary Apple Baked Pork Tenderloin With Turnip and Carrots**

1. Start with lemonade fluid (½ tbsp lemon juice with 4 oz water, green tea, or other fluid)
2. Follow with ½ cup Lite Vegetable Soup (recipe 4a) or non-creamy Lite Soup
3. Follow with 1 cup Mixed Veggies (recipe 46a)
4. Main course: 3-4 oz meat in 9 oz portion Rosemary Apple Baked Pork Tenderloin (recipe 101)
5. Serve with 1 cup Steamed Spinach, Broccoli, Brussels Sprouts, or Cabbage + seasoning with 1 tsp minced garlic and Mrs. Dash or salt and black pepper to taste
6. End with 4 oz lemonade fluid or herbal tea
Stats: 325 cal, 37g protein, 33g carb, 8g fat, 2g sat, 14g fiber, 350mg sodium, 69mg chol, 2,104mg potassium, 293mg calcium

## Day 29 (5th Sunday)

**Breakfast ---Open-Faced Breakfast Sandwich**

1 slice multigrain bread or 1 oat bran/whole-wheat flour tortilla (*Joseph's*) or ½ 100% whole-wheat pita
2 oz lean ham, turkey, or smoked salmon
1 oz low-fat, low sodium shredded cheese (mozzarella, provolone, cheddar, Swiss, etc.)
2 slices tomato
3 piece romaine leaves, large
½ cup low-fat milk or soymilk
½ cup berries (strawberries, blueberries, raspberries) or ½ cup melon (cantaloupe, honeydew, etc.)
1 tbsp Benefiber or 2 tsp Clearly Fiber (dissolve in fluid)

**Instructions:**

1. On toasted bread, add ham and cheese
2. Broil until cheese melts
3. Top with tomato and lettuce
4. Serve with ½ glass of skim milk, soymilk, or 6 oz tomato juice or V-8 juice (low sodium)
5. And ½ cup berries or cubed melons
   Stats: 282 cal, 29g protein, 29g carb, 8g fat, 3g sat, 12 g fiber, 878mg sodium, 33mg chol, 707mg potassium, 377mg calcium

**Morning Snack (Optional):**

1 fruit (apple, peach, etc.)
8 oz water or green tea
Stats: 80 cal, 0g protein, 22g carb, 0g fat, 5g fiber

**Lunch (1)---Avocado Salad With Lime Chicken**

1. Start with lemonade fluid (½ tbsp lemon juice with 4 oz water, green tea, or other fluid)
2. Follow with 1 cup Vegetable Sticks with Dip (½ red bell pepper cut in strips, ¼ cucumber cut in strips, 5 baby carrots cut in halves, and 5 cherry tomatoes).
3. Dressing: Add 1 tbsp nonfat sour cream to 1 tbsp nonfat dry Italian dressing or use 2 tbsp Quick salsa or a good commercial brand
4. Main course: 4 oz chicken in 10 oz portion Avocado Salad with Lime Chicken (recipe 102)
5. End with 4 oz lemonade fluid or 4 oz unsweetened apple or grapefruit juice
6. 1 tbsp Benefiber or 2 tsp Clearly Fiber (dissolve in fluid)
   Stats: 331 cal, 29g protein, 25g carb, 14g fat, 3g sat, 10g fiber, 96g sodium, 63mg chol, 1134mg potassium, 40mg calcium

**OR**

**Lunch (2)---Sushi Tuna Tortilla With Vegetables Stir-Fry**

1. Start with lemonade fluid (½ tbsp lemon juice with 4 oz water, green tea, or other fluid)
2. Follow with 1 cup Vegetable Broth (recipe 2a) or non-creamy Lite Soup
3. Main course: 3-4 oz fish in 8 oz portion (4 rolls) Sushi Tuna Tortilla (recipe 103)
4. Serve with 1 cup Vegetables Stir-Fry (recipe 104) or 1 cup *Cascadian Farm,* Organic, Chinese Stir Fry Premium Vegetable Blend or equivalent
5. End with 4 oz lemonade fluid
   Stats: 373 cal, 39g protein, 26g carb, 14g fat, 3g sat, 10g fiber, 968mg sodium, 41mg chol, 923mg potassium, 105mg calcium
   * *You can substitute any other white fish (cod, tilapia, etc.)*

**Mid Afternoon Snack (Must Have):**

3 precooked shrimps or 1 slice lean ham, turkey, or smoked salmon
3 tbsp seafood cocktail sauce or Quick Salsa (recipe 18b)

3 Roasted Vegetable Crackers *(Carr's)* or equivalent
3 celery sticks or asparagus spears
3 lemon slices

**Instructions:**

1. Place sauce or salsa and shrimp on the crackers
2. Top with celery or asparagus and lemon slices
3. 8 oz water or green tea

Stats: 135 cal, 12g protein, 22g carb, 0.7g fat, 5g fiber

**Dinner** (1)---**Tofu Steak Sauté With Steamed Snap Peas and Carrots**

1. Start with lemonade fluid (½ tbsp lemon juice with 4 oz water, green tea, or other fluid)
2. Follow with ½ cup canned Egg Drop Soup or ½ cup Chicken Noodle Soup (recipe 83) or non-creamy Lite Soup
3. Follow with 1 cup raw cabbage, broccoli, or steamed French cut green beans
4. Main course: 4 oz tofu in 15 oz portion Tofu Steak Sauté (recipe 106)
5. Serve with ½ cup steamed sugar snap peas and carrots seasoned with 1 tsp minced garlic and Mrs. Dash
6. And ½ cup berries (strawberries, blueberries, etc) or ½ cup snack size Sorbet (Blueberry and Yogurt Sorbet – recipe 107; Sweet Fruit Sorbet – recipe 108; Chocolate Pineapple Sorbet – recipe 109)
7. End with 4 oz lemonade fluid or herbal tea

Stats: 367 cal, 27g protein, 42g carb, 13g fat, 3g sat, 12.5g fiber, 805mg sodium, 51mg chol, 1,186mg potassium, 357mg calcium

**OR**

**Dinner (2)---Baked Sirloin Steak With Tomato Cucumber Salad**

1. Start with lemonade fluid (½ tbsp lemon juice with 4 oz water, green tea, or other fluid)
2. Follow with 5 oz Canned Fat Free Hearty Lentil with Vegetable Soup or non-creamy Lite Vegetable Soup
3. Follow with ½-1 cup Basic Tomato Cucumber Salad garnished with fresh basil and thyme leaves + 1-2 tbsp red wine vinegar or apple cider vinegar + salt and black pepper to taste or Mrs. Dash (recipe 70)
4. Main course: 4 oz portion Baked Sirloin Steak (recipe 110)
5. Serve with 1 cup steamed green peas and carrots or 1 cup Lemon String Beans (recipe 111)
6. End with 4 oz lemonade fluid or herbal tea

Stats: 334 cal, 38g protein, 30g carb, 7 g fat, 2g sat, 16.5g fiber, 297mg sodium, 69mg chol, 1, 108mg potassium, 153mg calcium

## Day 30 (5th Monday): Sharon's Day:

**Breakfast (1)---Sharon's Favorite Breakfast (Seasonal Veggies With Smoked Salmon)**

¼ raw summer squash, sliced
3 raw asparagus spears
1 cup raw spinach
½ ripe tomato, sliced
½ cup romaine lettuce
½ apple sliced
2 tbsp 2% cottage cheese
1 tsp fresh ground cinnamon (mix into cheese or sprinkle into salad)
2 oz smoked salmon or lean ham or turkey (low sodium)
3 multigrain crackers (*Carr's*) or equivalent
1 tsp extra virgin olive oil + 2 tbsp red wine or balsamic vinegar or lemon juice
1 tbsp Benefiber or 2 tsp Clearly fiber (dissolve in fluid)
Salt and black pepper to taste

**Instructions:**

1. Assemble the first seven ingredients and dress with oil and vinegar
2. Serve with meat and crackers
   Stats: 291 cal, 22g protein, 34g carb, 9g fat, 2g sat, 11g fiber, 776mg sodium, 21mg chol, 1,054mg potassium, 145mg calcium

**OR**

**Breakfast (2)---Hot Cereal (Oat Bran or 100% Whole Grain Rolled Oats)----see Day 3 Breakfast**

**Morning Snack (Optional):**

½ cup steamed edamame (raw soybeans, frozen or fresh)
85 cal, 9g protein, 7g carb, 4.6g fat, 1g fiber

**OR**

1 apple, pear, nectarine, etc.
8 oz water or green tea
Stats: 80 cal, 0g protein, 22g carb, 0g fat, 5g fiber

**Lunch (1)---Sharon's Favorite Lunch (Seasonal Vegetables With Grilled Chicken)**

1. Start with lemonade fluid (½ tbsp lemon juice with 4 oz water, green tea, or other fluid)
2. Sharon's Salad with Grilled Chicken:
   ¼ raw summer squash, sliced
   3 raw asparagus spears
   1 cup raw spinach
   ½ ripe tomato, sliced
   ½ cup romaine lettuce or arugula
   ½ orange, medium
   ¼ cup eggplant, boiled

3 oz grilled, roasted, or baked chicken or turkey breast
3 multigrain crackers *(Carr's)* or equivalent or 1 multigrain bread
1-2 tsp extra virgin olive oil + 2 tbsp red wine or balsamic vinegar or lemon juice
1 tbsp Benefiber or 2 tsp Clearly Fiber (dissolve in fluid)
Salt and black pepper to taste

**Instructions:**

1. Assemble the first seven ingredients and dress with oil and vinegar
2. Serve with meat and crackers
   Stats: 319 cal, 31g protein, 28g carb, 12g fat, 1g sat, 12g fiber, 146mg sodium, 64mg chol, 1,120mg potassium, 121 mg calcium

**OR**

**Lunch (2)---Veggie Burger**

Start with lemonade fluid (½ tbsp lemon juice with 4 oz water, green tea, or other fluid)
1 *Morning Star Farm* (67g) Garden Veggie Burger or Veggie Soy Burger Patty or Turkey Burgers (low-fat)
1 (1 oz) whole-wheat hamburger roll or multigrain sandwich bun or oat bran/whole wheat tortilla or pita *(Joseph's)*
2 tbsp Quick salsa (recipe 18b) or commercial salsa with low-fat and sodium
2-3 Romaine lettuce leaves

**Instructions:**

1. Prepare patty according to package instructions
2. Serve on roll with lettuce and topped with salsa
3. End with 4 oz lemonade fluid or 6 oz tomato or V-8 juice
   Stats: 270 cal, 19g protein, 36g carb, 5.5g fat, 1g sat, 6g fiber, 855mg sodium, 2mg chol, 198mg potassium, 54mg calcium

**Afternoon Snack (Must Have):**

(Sharon's Tuna and Yogurt Snack)
1.5 oz white tuna in water or oil, canned, and drained
¼ cup (4 tbsp) Low-fat Plain Yogurt
½ tbsp sliced or chopped walnut or almonds
¼ medium apple
8 oz water or green tea or V-8 juice
Stats: 128 cal, 14g protein, 10g carb, 3.6 g fat, 2g fiber

**OR**

**Crunchy Mix:**

2 tbsp cereal (Special K, Fiber one, Toasted Honey Crunch, etc)
¼ cup berries or peach
4 oz low-fat plain yogurt
1 tsp dried cranberries
1 tsp ground flaxseeds
8 oz water or green tea
Stats: 139 cal, 8g protein, 19g carb, 4g fat, 2g fiber

**Dinner---Sharon's Favorite Dinner (Seasonal Vegetables With Roasted Salmon)**

1. Start with lemonade fluid (½ tbsp lemon juice with 4 oz water, green tea, or other fluid)
2. Follow with 1 cup Lite Vegetable Soup (recipe 4a) or 4 oz canned LoSodium Vegetable Chicken Soup with Water or 4 oz canned *Progresso* Healthy Classic Lentil Soup
3. Sharon's Salad with Roasted Salmon:
   ¼ raw summer squash, sliced
   3 raw asparagus spears
   1 cup raw spinach
   ½ ripe medium tomato, sliced
   ½ cup romaine lettuce, or arugula
   ¼ cup or 4 tbsp black beans, red beans, or white beans, canned
   3-4 oz Roasted, Grilled, or Baked Salmon (recipe 3), Sea Bass,
   1 tsp olive oil + 2 tbsp balsamic vinegar or lemon juice
   1 tbsp Benefiber or 2 tsp Clearly fiber (dissolve in fluid)
   Salt and black pepper to taste

**Instructions:**

1. Assemble the first seven ingredients and dress with oil and vinegar
2. Serve with fish – broken up into bite size pieces
   Stats: 347 cal, 28g protein, 27g carb, 16g fat, 3g sat, 14g fiber, 204mg sodium, 52mg chol, 1,499mg potassium, 97 mg calcium

# Chapter 17

# Recipes

### The Making of the Meal Plan and Recipes

The whole philosophy of the UDP Program is based on helping people to make the transition from eating poorly and inactivity to a better way of eating and physical activity habits over the long-term. This requires learning better ways of food preparation using the choice of foods and ingredients that they are familiar with and like. It also requires the use of a wide variety of flavors, spices and seasoning to make food more satisfying—so that there is no feeling of dieting (dieters don't stay on a program for any length of time). Perhaps, one of the most important aspects of this program is the fact that instead of giving our patients' ready-made generic recipes and meal plans, we encourage them to provide us with their own choice of recipes and preferred meal plans. The idea behind this approach is to empower each person to individualize and personalize the program into a format that he or she can adhere to over the long-term. This approach makes changing bad eating and physical activity habits more likely to succeed permanently.

Our patient population is quite diverse, so you will see a reflection of this in the recipes, meal plans as well, and you will benefit tremendously from this experiment. As you go through these recipes, keep in mind that they are not written in stones---and you too will benefit greatly by making modifications to meet your own needs (this also applies to the meal plans in Chapter 16).

This chapter won't be complete without mentioning some kind and devoted people whose resources have been invaluable to this experiment. Rosemary, a mortgage broker, sat in our office one morning and wrote from memory eight favorite family recipes. They are very simple and fun to create and you will enjoy them too. Karen, a schoolteacher, took time from her busy schedule to help us transform family recipes into delicious and healthy ones.

Diane, the owner of the famous Andreas restaurant in East Providence, gladly shared some wonderful Greek recipes with us. Taking time off her busy schedule to personally oversee the preparation of the recipes, making sure that they represented the quality that she would deliver at home. Andreas's restaurant serves some of the best dishes in town, and is perfectly located near Brown University. Elizabeth shared with us some tasty and delicious recipes that were passed on to her by her mother and grandmother. Because she is a diabetic, cooking meals that are delicious, but healthy is a major concern and we helped her reached that goal.

Sharon, a corporate executive had a very busy and stressful lifestyle, but that didn't stop her from giving us the time. As you go through the 30-day meal plan, pay close attention to day 30, which has being dedicated to Sharon. Eating an anti-inflammatory diet on a regular basis has helped her reduced her total cholesterol to normal readings as well as increase HDL (good) cholesterol to protective levels without prescribed medications, including a boost of energy. These are just few of the many people who contributed recipes to the UDP program and we are greatly indebted to them. Let's begin the journey.

**Andreas Mediterranean Grilled Chicken Salad (Recipe 1)**

4 oz boneless, skinless chicken breast, grilled, or roasted
2 cups mixed salad greens
1 medium plum tomato
2 small red onion slices
¼ small orange sliced
***For the dressing:***
1 tbsp fresh orange juice
1 tbsp fresh lemon juice
1 tsp Olive oil
1/8 tsp salt
¼ tsp pepper
½ tsp Oregano
1 tsp linseed/flaxseed oil

**Instructions:**

1. Arrange the sliced chicken, onions, tomato, and orange over the salad greens
2. Combine the orange juice, lemon juice, oregano, olive oil, salt, and pepper in a small bowl and dress the salad. Serve with 3 medium strawberries
3. Serving size is 15 oz portion. Serves 1
   Stats: 298 cal, 30g protein, 18g carb, 12.6g fat, 2g sat, 6g fiber, 389mg sodium, 72mg chol, 925mg potassium, 113mg calcium

*Andreas Restaurant*

**Vegetable Broth Soup (recipe 2a)**

1 medium yellow onion
1 medium red onion
2 tsp minced garlic
5 whole carrots
¼ cup scallion (bulbs and greens)
4 celery stalks
2 tsp dried parsley
2 tsp dried thyme
8 cups water
Salt and black pepper to taste

**Instructions:**

1. Chop all vegetables roughly and add to pot containing 8 cups water. Add dried herbs.
2. Bring to low boil and cook for about 1-1.5 hours or until vegetables are tender
3. Garnish with bay leaf, fresh chopped parsley and lemon wedges
4. Serving size is 1 cup. Serves 12

Stats: 25 cal, 1g protein, 6g carb, 0g fat, 0g sat, 2g fiber, 28mg sodium, 0mg chol, 176mg potassium, 26mg calcium

**Flame-Roasted Vegetable Platter (Recipe 2b)**

1 red bell pepper
1 green bell pepper
1 red onion
1 medium zucchini
1 bunch asparagus
1 small sized eggplant
2 Portobello mushrooms
¼ cup olive oil
2 tbsp soy sauce, low sodium
2 tbsp balsamic vinegar
1 tsp black pepper
1 tsp finely minced garlic
1 tsp brown sugar
½ tsp dry thyme
½ tsp dry basil

**Instructions:**

1. Cut the bell peppers into lengthwise strips about one inch wide. Omit the seeds
2. Peel the onion, cut into ¼ inch rounds
3. Remove the stem on the zucchini and cut into ¼ inch rounds
4. Trim the woody ends from the asparagus spears
5. Remove the stem from the eggplant. Peel if desired, although the skin is high in antioxidants
6. Remove the mushroom stem and gently brush away debris. Washing is not recommended since it will waterlog the mushroom and dilute the flavor
7. In a small mixing bowl, combine the olive oil, soy sauce, vinegar, black pepper, garlic, thyme, basil, and brown sugar. Mix well
8. Place the vegetables on a charbroiler grill and brush with the oil mix. Turn the vegetables as needed and continue to brush with oil mix until the vegetables have cooked as desired
9. Optional – Toss the vegetables in the oil mix and spread over a cookie sheet. Roast in 400-degree oven until cooked as desired
10. Serving size is about 1 cup or 9 oz portions. Serves 5
11. Vegetables can be used for sandwiches

Stats: 121 cal, 3g protein, 16g carb, 6g fat, 0.8g sat, 5g fiber, 222mg sodium, 0mg chol, 528mg potassium, 34mg calcium

**Roasted Salmon (Recipe 3)**

1 lb. (16 oz) roasted salmon
1 tsp Lemon pepper

1 tsp Garlic powder
1 tsp extra virgin olive oil
Black or crushed red pepper

**Instructions:**

1. Season salmon with lemon pepper, garlic powder, and pepper
2. Drizzle with olive oil
3. Roast in 400° F oven on non-stick baking sheet 15-20 minutes or until fish is flaky and translucent
4. Serve with lemon wedges
5. Serving size is 3.5-4 oz Serves 4
   Stats: 175 cal, 23g protein, 1g carb, 8g fat, 1g sat, 0g fiber, 159mg sodium, 62mg chol, 565mg potassium, 15mg calcium

*Rosemary*

**Lite Vegetable Soup (Recipe 4a)**

16 oz diced tomatoes, canned
24 oz low sodium chicken broth
1 cup summer squash, chopped
1 cup zucchini, chopped
½ cup sliced mushrooms
1 cup green snap or soybeans (edamame)
2 cups celery, chopped
1 cup asparagus, chopped
Salt and black pepper or Mrs. Dash to taste

**Instructions:**

1. Combine all the ingredients in a pot and cook over medium-high heat until vegetables are tender
2. Add salt and black pepper to taste
3. Serving size is 1 cup. Serves 8
   Stats: 44 cal, 3g protein, 7g carb, 0.8g fat, 0.3g sat, 2g fiber, 99mg sodium, 2mg chol, 268mg potassium, 42mg calcium

*Cheryl*

**Lime Seafood Vegetable Soup (Recipe 4b)**

10 medium shrimps, cut into two (or 3 oz sea bass, cod, scrod, clams, crab, lobster, etc)
3 Lemon grass stem, mashed
4 Lime leaves, whole
2 cup fresh basil leaves, chopped (or chopped bok choy, romaine lettuce, or escarole)
3 tbsp Lime juice
Lemon wedges from 1 lemon
1.5 cup canned straw mushrooms or substitutes (cremini, Italian, oyster, or button mushrooms)
5 cups water or low sodium chicken broth

1 cup dry or a pkt of vermicelli pasta noodles (optional)
1 whole lime zest
Salt and black pepper or Mrs. Dash Lemon Pepper Seasoning to taste

**Instructions:**

1. In a pot, bring chicken broth or water to a boil
2. Add greens, lime leaves, scallions, mushrooms, lime juice, and lemon grass stems
3. Boil 10-15 minutes over medium high heat
4. Add shrimp and cook for 4-5 minutes or until done
5. Season with salt and pepper to taste
6. Serve with lemon wedges
7. Serving size is 1 cup. Serves 5
   Stats: 28 cal, 3.5g protein, 3g carb, 0.4g fat, 0g sat, 1g fiber, 28 mg sodium, 18 mg chol, 216mg potassium, 46mg calcium

**Instructions for Vermicelli:**

1. Bring 1 cup water to a boil. Add 1 cup or a pkt of vermicelli pasta noodles and turn off the heat
2. Let sit covered for 4-6 minutes and then drain
3. Place ½ cup vermicelli in each bowl and top with 1 cup soup
4. Serving size is 1 cup. Serves 5
   Stats: 127 cal, 7g protein, 23g carb, 0.9g fat, 0g sat, 2.4g fiber, 29mg sodium, 18mg chol, 238mg potassium, 51mg calcium

**Oven-Baked Crusted Chicken (Recipe 4c)**

4- (3-4 ounces) chicken breast
1-cup Kellogg's corn flakes crumbs or ½ cup rice flour or oat bran
1 tsp garlic powder
1 tsp dry rosemary
1 tsp dry sage
Salt and pepper to taste

**Instructions:**

1. Preheat oven to 425 degrees
2. Line baking pan with tin foil or baking sheet
3. Spray baking foil with cooking spray lightly
4. Combine the seasonings and herbs (garlic powder, herbs, salt pepper, and corn flakes) – mix well
5. Place the corn flakes and herb mixture on a baking sheet
6. Roll and rub chicken with the mixture (you can spray the chicken lightly to coat the mixture on the chicken if desired)
7. Place chicken in a baking pan
8. Bake at 425 degrees for 45 minutes
9. Serving size is 3-4 oz portion. serves 4.

Stats: 153 cal, 26g protein, 6.5g carb, 2g fat, 0.5g sat, 0.4g fiber, 571mg sodium, 64mg chol, 224mg potassium, 20mg calcium

*Karen*

**Roasted Veggies (Recipe 5)**

1 red bell pepper
1 green bell pepper
1 ½ red onion
1 zucchini
1 bunch asparagus
1 small-medium sized eggplant
½ Tbsp extra virgin olive oil
Garlic, salt and pepper to taste

**Instructions:**

1. Chop veggies into large cubes or slices, add to bowl- toss with ½ tbsp olive oil and add garlic, salt, and pepper to taste. You may add herbs (thyme, rosemary, basil, etc.) to taste
2. Spread veggies on baking sheet and roast at 450° F for 20-25 minutes
3. Serving size is 1 cup. Serves 5

Stats: 71 cal, 2g protein, 13.5g carb, 1.8g fat, 0.2g sat, 5g fiber, 6mg sodium, 0mg chol, 419mg potassium, 24mg calcium

*Rosemary*

**Italian Vegetable Chicken Soup (Recipe 6)**

2 tbsp olive oil
1 clove garlic, chopped
1 small onion, chopped
1 chopped skinless chicken breast (12-16 oz.)
3 diced celery stalks
2 zucchini, sliced in ½ inch chunks
1 small red bell pepper, chopped
½ head cabbage, chopped
2 cans chicken broth, low sodium
1 8 oz can diced tomatoes
1 cup cooked kidney beans
1 cup chopped tomato
1 cup water
8 tbsp low-fat shredded Parmesan or Romano cheese
Salt and pepper to taste

**Instructions:**

1. Heat a small soup pot to high heat
2. Add the olive oil
3. Add the chopped chicken meat and brown

4. Add the raw vegetables and cook these until they are translucent
5. Add the broth, water, tomatoes and kidney beans and bring to a simmer
6. Cook for 20 minutes, until vegetables are cooked thoroughly but are still firm
7. Season with salt and pepper
8. Serve hot with 1 tbsp shredded Parmesan cheese per serving
9. Serving size is 2 cups. Serves 8
   Stats: 242 cal, 31.8g protein, 13 g carb, 7g fat, 2g sat, 5g fiber, 209mg sodium, 68 mg chol, 749mg potassium, 139 mg calcium
   ***Note***: *that this is a whole meal. However, 1 cup portion can be used to accompany other meals.*

*Jane*

**Italian Vegetable Soup (Recipe 7a)**

4 cups water or low sodium chicken broth
1 medium onion, chopped
1 can (14.5 oz) stewed tomatoes, no salt added, undrained
1 medium rib celery, thinly sliced
½ large red bell pepper, chopped
½ large green bell pepper, chopped
1 can (15.5 oz) navy or kidney beans, no salt added
1 cup button mushrooms, sliced
½ cup spinach leaves
1 tbsp balsamic vinegar or lemon juice
1.5 tbsp dried and crumbled bail
2 tbsp extra virgin olive oil
½ cup vermicelli noodles or other thin pasta, broken into thirds
Salt and black pepper to taste or Mrs. Dash

**Instructions:**

1. Heat a large pot over medium-high heat
2. Add the olive oil
3. Cook the peppers, onions, and celery until the onions begin to turn lightly brown, stirring occasionally
4. Add the water, mushrooms, beans, undrained tomatoes, and basil.
5. Increase the heat to high and bring to a boil
6. Stir in the vermicelli and reduce the heat and simmer covered for about 3-4 minutes
7. Stir in the spinach, vinegar, and seasoning and cook for about 1 minute or until spinach is tender, but still firm
8. Serving size is 1 cup. Serves 4.
   Stats: 108 cal, 5g protein, 16g carb, 3g fat, 0.4g sat, 5g fiber, 150mg sodium, 0mg chol, 247mg potassium, 56mg calcium

**One Pot Vegetable Soup (Recipe 7b)**

2 broccoli stalks, sliced
¼ red bell pepper, sliced
1 tsp minced garlic
1 chicken bouillon, dry, low sodium or Mrs. Dash
1 Chinese eggplant or ½ medium eggplant, chopped
½ cup white beans, Cannellini
2 cups water
Red pepper flakes
1 small onion
4 medium-large shrimp, shelled/deveined, cut
3 oz turkey meatballs (recipe 84)
1 tsp olive oil
Salt and pepper to taste

**Instructions:**

1. In a pot, add oil over medium high heat. Add onions, broccoli stalks, red peppers, and meatballs and cook until onions are brown lightly
2. Add all remaining ingredients except shrimp and bring to a boil
3. Cook 10-20 minutes. Reduce heat and add shrimp and cook until shrimp is done
4. Salt and pepper, red pepper flakes to taste. Sprinkle with lemon juice if desired
5. Serving size is 1 cup. Serves 6
   Stats: 95 cal, 7g protein, 11g carb, 3g fat, 0.8g sat, 4g fiber, 278mg sodium, 19mg chol, 348mg potassium, 45mg calcium

*Penny*

**Easy Turkey Chili (Recipe 8)**

1 pound lean ground turkey
1 (8) ounce can of red kidney beans, drained
1 (8) ounce can of diced tomatoes
1 (6) ounce can of tomato paste
1 small onion, chopped
1 small green pepper, chopped
1 cup water
1 tsp chili powder
1 tsp salt

**Instruction:**

1. In a skillet, brown the ground turkey, onion and peppers until cooked
2. Add remaining ingredients and mix thoroughly
3. Let simmer for 30 minutes
4. Serving size is 1 cup. Serves 4
   Stats:187 cal, 17g protein, 16 carb, 6.7g fat, 1.7g sat, 5g fiber, 575mg sodium, 60mg chol, 587mg potassium, 50mg calcium

**Golden Baked Fish (Recipe 9)**

2 lbs. white fish fillets (haddock or cod)
1/8 tsp black pepper
1 egg white
¼ cup light mayonnaise
¼ tsp dill weed (dry or fresh)
½ tsp grated onion
1 tsp canola oil

**Instructions:**

1. Preheat oven to 425 degrees
2. Grease 13x 9" baking dish with 1 tsp canola oil
3. Sprinkle pepper over fish
4. Beat egg white until stiff peaks form (salt optional)
5. Fold in mayonnaise, dill and onion. Spoon over fish
6. Bake uncovered for 15-20 minutes or until topping is puffed and golden and fish flakes easily with a fork
7. Garnish with dill (fresh)
8. Serving size is 5 oz portion. Serves 7
   Stats: 123 cal, 24g protein, 0.6g carb, 2g fat, 0.7g sat, 0g fiber, 101 mg sodium, 59mg chol, 551 mg potassium, 21mg calcium

*Elizabeth*

**Hot Cereal Breakfast (Recipe 10)**

¼ cup Old Fashion Oats, *Quaker* Oat bran, original, Oatmeal, old fashioned or ½ pkt Quaker Oatmeal Weight Control (these cereals have high total fiber, high soluble fiber, and low sugar. They can help to reduce cholesterol and blood sugar and thereby reduce the risk of heart disease and diabetes). Avoid the instant or 1-minute varieties, even of the same brand.
1 cup water
1 tsp salt (optional)
½ scoop soy protein powder or whey protein (12.5 g) or ¼ cup textured vegetable protein
½ cup skim milk or soymilk
1 tbsp flaxseed oil or extra virgin olive oil or simply take 2-3 tsp cod liver/fish oil separately
2 tbsp ground flaxseeds
1 tbsp chopped nuts (such as almonds and walnuts, etc)
1 tbsp wheat germ
1 tbsp oat bran or wheat bran
1 tsp ground cinnamon
2-3 dried prunes, sliced (for constipation)
¼ cup berries (strawberries, blueberries, raspberries, etc.)
8 oz water, green tea, or coffee

1 tbsp Benefiber or 2 tsp *Davinci Lab* Clearly Fiber (mix well in fluid and use separately)

**Instructions:** See direction on package.

**Microwave Direction**

1. Combine water, oats, wheat germ and salt in a microwave bowl. Mix well
2. Add sliced prunes (about 2-3 – for constipation; optional)
3. Microwave on medium 3-4 minutes
4. Remove from microwave, stir in protein powder
5. Add flaxseed, oil, cinnamon, and milk
6. Top with berries and nuts
7. Add additional milk to get the desired consistency

**Stove Top Direction**

1. Bring water and salt to a boil
2. Add oats and wheat germ and reduce heat to medium
3. Sprinkle or stir in soy protein powder, making sure it's well dissolved
4. Cook about 3- 7 minutes, stirring constantly
5. Stir in prunes and cinnamon
6. Transfer to bowl and stir in flaxseeds and flax oil
7. Top with berries and nuts and serve with milk
8. Add more milk to get the consistency desired
   Stats: 369 cal, 28g protein, 40g carb, 12g fat, 1g sat, 12.5g fiber, 236mg sodium, 3mg chol, 1,227mg potassium, 354mg calcium

**Broccoli and Dill Weed Soup (Recipe 11a)**

1-cup low sodium or chicken broth
1-cup water
2 broccoli stalks, cut
1 carrot, cut
1 tbsp minced garlic
2 tbsp celery seed
½ red bell pepper, sliced
1 tbsp scallion, cut (bulb and greens)
3 cups chopped cabbage
3 tbsp fresh Dill Weed
Salt, fresh ground pepper and herbs to taste

**Instructions:**

1. Bring water and broth to boil
2. Add the first nine ingredients and cook covered over reduced heat until vegetables are done
3. Add dill and simmer for about 5 minutes covered. Season to taste

4. Serving size is 1 ¼ cup (10 oz). Serves 4
   Stats: 74 cal, 5g protein, 13g carb, 1.7g fat, 0.2 sat, 5g fiber, 81mg sodium, 1mg chol, 558mg potassium, 137mg calcium

**Broccoli Soup (Recipe 11b)**

4 cups broccoli
2 cups low sodium vegetable or chicken broth
½ red bell pepper, chopped
1 medium red onion, chopped
2-celery stalks cut in large pieces
1 cup 1% milk
1 tbsp finely minced garlic
1 tsp ginger powder or fresh minced ginger
Salt, fresh ground pepper, and cumin to taste

**Instructions:**

1. In a blender, puree the broccoli, pepper, onion and celery covered with the broth
2. Add additional water to get the desired consistency
3. Serve warm or cold after flavoring with ginger, salt, black pepper, or cumin
4. You can also garnish with lemon slice
5. Serving size is 1 cup. Serves 5
   Stats: 72 cal, 5.5g protein, 10g carb, 1.8g fat, 0.9g sat, 1.6g fiber, 101mg sodium, 5mg chol, 393mg potassium, 114mg calcium

**Broccoli and Celery Soup (Recipe 11c)**

4 cups broccoli florets, chopped
2 celery stalks, cut in ½ inch chunks
1 tbsp chopped garlic
3 cups water or low sodium chicken broth
1 low sodium bullion cube if not using chicken broth
Salt and pepper to taste

**Instructions:**

1. Bring water or broth to a boil and add bullion
2. Add celery, broccoli, and garlic
3. Simmer over medium heat until tender. Don't over cook
4. Serving size is 1 cup. Serves 5
   Stats: 28 cal, 2g protein, 5g carb, 0.3g fat, 0 sat, 1g fiber, 156mg sodium, 0mg chol, 306mg potassium, 50mg calcium

*Penny*

**Zesty Tabouleh Salad (Recipe 12)**

1 cup dry Bulgur wheat (or cracked wheat)
1 cup chicken broth (low-fat and low sodium)
¼ cup Red bell peppers, chopped

¼ cup tomatoes, diced
½ cup scallions (bulbs and greens), chopped
1 cup fresh Parsley, chopped
¼ cup fresh lemon juice
2 tbsp extra virgin olive oil
1.5 cup boiling hot water
Salt and fresh ground pepper to taste

**Instructions:**

1. Cover the bulgur wheat with hot water and broth
2. Soak for about 2 hours in the refrigerator tightly covered with a plastic wrap to reconstitute the bulgur
3. Drain excess water and squeeze reconstituted bulgur wheat
4. Chop all the vegetables very fine and mix with bulgur wheat
5. Pour olive oil and lemon juice dressing over bulgur mixture and refrigerate
6. Let stand for about 2 hours before serving. Refrigerate the rest--the taste and flavor are greatly enhanced
7. Serving size is 4 oz (1 cup). Serves 8
   Stats: 104 cal, 3g protein, 16g carb, 4g fat, 0.6g sat, 3g fiber,24 mg sodium, 0mg chol, 161mg potassium, 25mg calcium

**Greek Chicken Kabobs (Recipe 13)**

18 oz boneless, skinless chicken breast, cut into small pieces (1-inch chunks)
2 cloves garlic
2 tbsp lemon juice
3 tbsp olive oil
1 tbs. oregano
1 tbs. fresh chopped mint
½ tsp each of black pepper and salt
1 large red bell pepper, cut into 1-inch chunks
1 large yellow bell pepper, cut into 1-inch chunks
1 medium red onion, cut into 1-inch chunks

**Instructions:**

1. In a plastic bag or large bowl, combine chicken, garlic, lemon juice, olive oil, oregano, mint, salt, and pepper
2. Let marinate in refrigerator for a minimum of 30 minutes
3. Heat grill pan or prepare grill
4. Alternate vegetables and chicken onto metal skewers. If using wooden skewers, let soak about an hour in water
5. Grill over medium-high heat until chicken is done, about 10-12 minutes
6. Serving size is about 1 cup or 6 oz portion size. Kabobs serve 6
   Stats: 228 cal, 27g protein, 6g carb, 10g fat, 1.8g sat, 1.4g fiber, 64mg sodium, 72mg chol, 295mg potassium, 25mg calcium

**Pan-Roasted Lime Broccoli (Recipe 14)**

1.5-2 heads broccoli, florets, and stem, cut
1 lime
2 tsp canola oil
1 tsp *I Can't Believe It's Not Butter*
1 tsp minced garlic
Red pepper flakes
Salt and pepper to taste

**Instructions:**

1. Pre-heat oven broiler
2. In a skillet, mix the broccoli pieces with the butter, garlic, and red pepper flakes
3. Sprinkle with oil and broil 3-4 minutes
4. Squeeze on lime juice and season with salt and black pepper to taste
5. Serving size is 1 cup. Serves 3
   Stats: 64 cal, 4g protein, 9g carb, 2.5g fat,0.2 g sat, 5g fiber, 43mg sodium, 0mg chol, 347mg potassium, 89mg calcium

*Penny*

**Garden Salad (Recipe 15)**

1 cup romaine lettuce, chopped
1 cup spinach, chopped
2 tomato slices
3 cucumber slices
2 bell pepper strips
2 red radish, sliced
2 oregano leaves or ¼ cup chopped cilantro
1 tsp ground cinnamon
1 tbsp fresh lemon juice
Salt and fresh ground pepper to taste

**Instructions:**

1. Toss all ingredients
2. Add ground cinnamon
3. Drizzle lemon juice
4. Add salt and black pepper to taste
5. Serving size is 6 oz. Serves 1
   Stats: 40 cal, 2.5g protein, 9g carb, 0.5g fat, 0g sat, 4g fiber, 34mg sodium, 0mg chol, 516mg potassium, 88mg calcium

**Steamed Roasted Red Snapper (Recipe 16)**

1 whole snapper, scored (1 lb)
2 garlic cloves, chopped,
6 cups baby spinach (Swiss chard, escarole or kale)
1 cup low sodium chicken broth

1 lemon, cut into fourths
1 red or yellow bell pepper, strips
1 medium onion, sliced
2 tbsp chopped basil leaves
2 tsp canola oil
Salt and pepper to taste

**Instructions:**

1. Preheat oven to 425 degrees
2. Lay out parchment cooking paper or tin foil in a baking pan or sheet to make a loose packet around the fish
3. Season the cleaned fish with salt and pepper inside and out
4. Stuff fish inside with some of the garlic, bell pepper and onion slices
5. Place spinach on tin foil and top with seasoned fish in the middle
6. Sprinkle fish with remaining garlic, bell pepper, onion, and canola oil
7. Pour broth around fish and fold the foil unto it self and seal into a package or fold the edges and pinch tightly to seal
8. Place the foil package on a heavy baking sheet
9. Bake until the spinach wilts and the fish is flaky or cooked through, about 20 min
10. Transfer the package to a wide shallow bowl and cool for about 5 minutes
11. Squeeze lemon juice over the fish and sprinkle with basil and oregano or other herbs before serving
12. Serving size is 4 oz fish in 10 oz portion. Serves 4
    Stats: 167 cal, 25g protein, 7g carb, 4.5g fat, 0.6g sat, 2g fiber, 161mg sodium, 39mg chol, 998mg potassium, 141mg calcium
    *You can use other fish (tilapia, sea bass, salmon etc)*

**Pan-Roasted Eggplant and Zucchini (Recipe 17)**

1 whole eggplant
1 zucchini or summer squash
1 tbsp extra virgin oil
½ tbsp red wine vinegar
4 tbsp shredded Parmesan cheese
2 tsp minced garlic

**Instructions:**

1. Cut eggplant into ½ - inch thick slices
2. Cut zucchini into ½ -inch thick diagonally
3. Season eggplant and zucchini with salt and pepper to taste
4. Pre-heat broiler
5. In a pan or skillet, heat oil and sauté zucchini for about 1 minute
6. Add eggplant and sauté for 4-5 minutes or vegetables are tender
7. Sprinkle with cheese and stir in minced garlic and vinegar
8. Place under the broiler for 1-2 minutes or until cheese melts and golden in color
9. Serve immediately
10. Serving size is 1 cup or 6oz. Serves 4

Stats: 80 cal, 3g protein, 9g carb, 4.5g fat, 1g sat, 4g fiber, 50mg sodium, 3mg chol, 376mg potassium, 38mg calcium

**Hummus (Recipe 18a)**

2 cups cooked garbanzo beans
2 cups cooked navy beans
3 garlic cloves
¼ cup fresh lemon juice
1 tbsp sesame butter (Tahini)
½ tsp ground cumin
½ tsp ground coriander
¼ cup extra virgin olive oil
Salt to taste

**Instructions:**

1. Place all ingredients in a food processor and puree to a medium smooth consistency
2. Serve as desired. Serving size 2 tbsp. Serves 25

   Stats: 60 cal, 2g protein, 7g carb, 2.9g fat, 0.4g sat, 2g fiber, 64mg sodium, 0mg chol, 55mg potassium, 21mg calcium

   *Hummus may be served with pita bread, crackers or as a vegetable dip*

**Quick Salsa (Recipe 18b)**

1 15 oz can stewed tomatoes, coarsely chopped
2 tbsp fresh cilantro, chopped
2 tbsp scallions, chopped
2 tsp pickled jalapeno slices, chopped
1 tbsp fresh basil, chopped (or ½ tsp dry)
¼ tsp dry oregano
¼ tsp garlic powder
¼ tsp salt
¼ tsp black pepper

**Instructions:**

1. Place the entire contents of the can of stewed tomatoes in a blender or food processor and pulse to coarsely chopped (can be chopped by hand)
2. Transfer the tomatoes to a small bowl and add the remaining ingredients
3. Stir to thoroughly blend all of the ingredients
4. Let stand in the refrigerator for one hour prior to serving to meld the flavors of all the ingredients
5. Store in the refrigerator in a covered container for up to one week
6. Serving size is 2 tbsp. Serves 7

   Stats: 19 cal, 0.5g protein, 4g carb, 0g fat, 0g sat, 1g fiber, 91 mg sodium, 0mg chol, 86mg potassium, 23mg calcium

**Grilled Chicken (Recipe 18c)**

1 tsp olive or canola oil or cooking spray
½ tsp garlic powder
½ tsp onion powder
Chopped fresh rosemary or other herbs
Ms Dash seasoning or Seasoning salt and pepper to taste
Skinless, boneless chicken or turkey breast (12-16 oz)

**Instructions:**

1. Rub chicken breast cutlets with salt, onion powder, garlic powder, and chopped fresh rosemary or other herbs. You can also use Ms Dash or Seasoning Salt. Rub the chicken with the oil
2. Grill on a grill pan or open grill
3. Serving size is 3 –4 oz portion. Serves 4
   Stats: 152 cal, 26g protein, 0.5g carb, 4g fat, 0.9g sat, 0g fiber, 63mg sodium, 72mg chol, 224mg potassium, 14mg calcium

**Grilled Chicken Sandwich (Recipe 18d)**

3–4 oz grilled or baked chicken or turkey breast (recipe 18c)
2 slices tomatoes
3 romaine leaves
3 dill pickles, slices
Dijon mustard, yellow mustard or 1 tbsp low sodium lite mayonnaise
2 slices multigrain bread or 1 oat bran/whole-wheat tortilla or pita bread (*Joseph's*)

**Instructions:**

1. Assemble sandwich and enjoy
   Stats: 280 cal, 32g protein, 25g carb, 7g fat, 2g sat, 7g fiber, 700mg sodium, 82mg cholesterol, 519mg potassium, 71mg calcium

**Asparagus and Celery Soup (Recipe 19)**

2.5 cups (12 oz) asparagus (wash and snap off tough ends)
3 medium celery stalks, chopped
1 cup low sodium chicken broth
1 cup water or 1% milk
½ medium onion, chopped
1 tbsp minced garlic
1 red bell pepper cut in large pieces
1 tsp canola oil
Salt and fresh ground pepper to taste

**Instructions:**

1. Sauté onion, bell pepper and garlic in oil
2. Add asparagus, celery, including leaves, and broth
3. Cook covered over medium heat until the vegetables are done
4. Add 1% or skim milk and puree the vegetables
5. Salt, ground pepper to taste

6. Serving size is a little over 1 cup. Serves 4
   Stats: 82.5 cal, 6g protein, 11g carb, 2.5g fat, 0.6g sat, 2g fiber, 88mg sodium, 5mg chol, 469mg potassium, 111mg calcium

**Spinach and Mushroom Omelet (Recipe 20a)**

½ cup eggbeaters or 1 whole egg + 2 egg whites
1 tsp water
2 cups chopped spinach
¼ cup sliced button mushrooms
¼ cup slices of zucchini
2 tbsp chopped tomatoes
1 tbsp chopped onions
1 tbsp green bell peppers, chopped
1 tbsp red bell peppers, chopped
1 tbsp (1 oz) Cheddar cheese, diced
1 slice (1 oz) low sodium, lean ham, chopped
Canola or olive oil cooking spray
Salt and ground black pepper to taste

**Instructions:**

1. Heat a small non-stick pan to medium-high heat. Add oil or spray lightly with cooking spray
2. Add the vegetables and sauté for 3 minutes or until the onions become translucent and the vegetables tender
3. Add the eggs and ham. Reduce the heat to medium and cook until the eggs have become firm
4. Season with salt and pepper to taste
5. Add the cheese and gently flip the omelet and remove from the heat. It will finish cooking with the pan's residual heat
6. Serve hot
7. Serving size is 1.5 cup or 12 oz portion. Serves 1
   Stats: 198 cal, 23g protein, 11g carb, 7g fat, 1.5g sat, 3g fiber, 734mg sodium, 17mg chol, 875mg potassium, 148mg calcium

**Andreas Chicken With Okra (Recipe 20b)**

1 whole quartered chicken
1.5 lbs frozen okra, chopped
½ cup cider vinegar (place the okra in the vinegar and set aside for 1 hour before cooking. This is only if you want to reduce the sliminess)
¼ cup extra virgin olive oil
2 tbsp tomato paste
1medium can crushed tomato (approx 13oz)
1 yellow onion, medium
4 garlic cloves, coarsely chopped
1 each bay leaf

1 tbsp dried whole thyme
1 cup green olives
½ cup water
Salt and fresh ground pepper

**Instructions:**

1. Remove the skin and fat from the chicken
2. Quarter the chicken, separating the drumsticks, thighs, breasts, and wings
3. Cut the breasts in half cross-wise, with a heavy knife
4. Season the quartered chicken with thyme, salt, and pepper
5. Heat a braising pan to medium-high heat
6. Brown the chicken on all sides
7. Brown the garlic and onions when the chicken has browned half way
8. Add the remaining ingredients and gently combine (tomato paste, okra, crushed tomatoes, olives, bay leaf, water, salt, and black pepper)
9. Bring to a simmer and reduce heat to low
10. Cook for an additional 15 minutes
11. Serving size is 4 oz chicken in 13 oz portion. Serve with fresh pepper over ½ cup cooked whole-wheat pasta or vermicelli. Serves 6
    Stats: 312 cal, 27g protein, 17g carb, 15.9g fat, 2g sat, 5.4g fiber, 735mg sodium, 77mg chol, 754mg potassium, 158mg calcium

*This chicken recipe can be used for rice pilaf (without the crushed tomato) or with potatoes or macaroni. For macaroni, prepare, drain, and then place in a platter. Sprinkle with grated cheese, tossing it to make sure it's coated well with the cheese. Pour juice from the chicken over the macaroni and serve.*

*Andreas Restaurant*

**Oriental Seafood and Vegetable Soup (Recipe 21)**

2 (14 oz) cans low sodium chicken broth
½ cup water
1 scallion, chopped
½ cup sliced mushrooms
1 (4 oz) can sliced water chestnuts, drained
½ cup celery
1 cup sliced Bok choy
1 (8 oz) can sliced bamboo shoots, drained
½ tbsp lite soy sauce, low sodium
½ cup snow peas
6 oz large scallops or 12 oz cod fillet, cut into 1-inch pieces
3 oz medium shrimp, shelled, and deveined
2 cups Chinese vermicelli noodles dry, broken into thirds
Salt and pepper to taste

**Instructions:**

1. Combine the chicken broth, water, soy sauce, bamboo shoots, mushrooms, and water chestnuts in a pot
2. Bring to a boil and then reduce heat to medium high
3. Add snow peas and Bok choy. Cook 4-6 minutes
4. Add fish, shrimp, and vermicelli noodles. Cook until opaque, about 3-5 min
5. Serve soup with vermicelli and top with scallions
6. Serving size is 2.5 cups. Soup makes 4 servings
   Stats: 296 cal, 35g protein, 31g carb, 4g fat, 1g sat, 4.5g fiber, 383mg sodium, 86mg chol, 752mg potassium, 88 mg calcium
   *If you prefer, you can cook the vermicelli separately, al dente (recipe 22). Add ½-1 cup cooked vermicelli to 2 cups soup.*

**Chinese Vermicelli Pasta Noodles (Recipe 22)**

1-cup water
1-cup vermicelli noodles (dry, broken into thirds)

**Instructions (1):**

1. Bring 1 cup water to a boil. Add 1 cup or a pkt of vermicelli pasta noodles and turn off the heat
2. Let sit covered for 4-6 minutes and then drain
3. Place ½ cup vermicelli (20g carb) in each bowl and top with soup

**Instructions (2):**

1. Bring water to a boil.
2. Add Vermicelli and cook 3-5 minutes stirring occasionally (al dente 3-5 min).
3. Serving size is ½ cup. Serves 5
   Stats: 99 cal, 3g protein, 20g carb, 0.5g fat, 0g sat, 1g fiber, 1mg sodium, 0mg chol, 22mg potassium, 5mg calcium

**Long Grain White or Brown Rice (Recipe 23)**

1 cup brown rice, long grain or Uncle Ben's Converted rice
2 1/3 -cups water or low sodium chicken broth
10 whole okra (optional)
Salt and seasoning to taste

**Instructions:**

1. Bring water or broth to a boil
2. Add rice and cover with a lid
3. Reduce heat
4. Add okra and stir occasionally
5. Simmer over low heat for about 20 minutes
6. Remove from heat. Let stand until all water is absorbed; about 5 minutes
7. Serving size is ½ cup. Serves 7
   Stats: 117 cal, 3g protein, 24g carb, 0.9g fat, 0g sat, 2g fiber, 69mg sodium, 0mg chol, 127mg potassium, 26mg calcium

**Easy Grilled Beef Fajitas With Mixed Grilled Vegetables (Recipe 24)**

6-8 oz Beef Flank steak or Chicken breast, boneless, skinless
1 small sweet green bell pepper cut in strips
1 small sweet red bell pepper cut in strips
1 small yellow onion, sliced
1 medium tomato, chopped
2 tbsp sour cream, fat free
2 tbsp light cheddar cheese, shredded
2 tsp canola oil
2 oat bran /whole-wheat tortillas or 1 whole-wheat pita bread (½ each per person)

**Instructions:**

1. Cut lean flank steak into small strips
2. Cut peppers and onions into medium strips
3. Season steak with half of the oil, salt, pepper, and spices to taste
4. In a hot skillet, grill steak. Remove meat
5. Add remaining oil to skillet and grill the peppers and onions
6. Divide the steak strips and the peppers and onions into 2 servings (11 oz portions or 1.5 cup each)
7. Layer on top of the tortillas or pita. Garnish with tomato, cheese and sour cream
8. 3-4 oz chicken strips, fish and lean pork can be used in place of beef
   Stats: 292 cal, 29g protein, 20g carb, 12g fat, 4g sat, 8g fiber, 492mg sodium, 40mg chol, 610mg potassium, 87mg calcium

**Seared Tuna With Fruit Salsa (Recipe 25)**

1 pound tuna steak, loin
1/8 tsp ground cumin
1 tsp ground cinnamon
½ tsp black pepper
¼ onion powder
¼ tsp garlic powder
½ tsp ground paprika

*Fruit Salsa:*

1 medium kiwi, diced
2 oz fresh papaya, diced
2 oz pineapple chunks, canned
2 oz mango, diced
1 oz strawberries, diced
1 tbsp fresh basil, chopped
1 tbsp fresh lemon juice
½ tsp sea salt

**Instructions:**

1. Combine all the spices and rub into the tuna, including 1 tsp sea salt if you want
2. Sear the tuna on a very hot griddle to rare, medium or done as you desire

3. Cool and slice on the bias into small portion
4. Gently combine the fruit salsa and serve with the tuna
5. Serving size is 4 oz tuna in 7 oz portion. Serves 4

   Stats: 158 cal, 26g protein, 10g carb, 1.4g fat, 0.4g sat, 2g fiber, 331mg sodium, 53mg chol, 620mg potassium, 60mg calcium

**Cheryl's Comfort Food (Recipe 26)**

3-4 oz or medium sweet potato with skin
1 tsp I can't believe it's not butter
1 tsp fresh ground cinnamon
½ tsp nutmeg
1 pkt Splenda or Stevia
Salt and pepper to taste

**Instructions:**

1. Baked sweet potato with skin
2. Slice open in the middle and scoop out the flesh into a bowl
3. Save the shell or skin
4. Combine to the potato fresh the butter, splenda, cinnamon and nutmeg
5. Mix well and restuff the flesh back into the shell

   Stats: 100 cal, 2g protein, 23g carb, 0.6g fat, 0.4g sat, 4g fiber, 12mg sodium, 0mg chol, 311mg potassium, 54mg calcium

*Cheryl*

**Fresh Mozzarella Pizza (Recipe 27)**

1 10-inch whole-wheat tortilla or oat bran/whole-wheat tortilla (*Joseph's*)
1 tbsp tomato or pizza sauce
2 oz low-fat mozzarella cheese, shredded
1 medium Roma tomato, sliced
1 oz Vegetarian pepperoni
1 tsp olive oil
Basil (fresh)

**Instruction:**

1. Preheat pan. Add olive oil to the pan
2. Place the tortilla in the pan and toast lightly on both sides
3. Spoon on sauce and top with sliced tomato, pepperoni and cheese
4. Top with fresh basil
5. Cook under broiler until the cheese is melted and slightly brown
6. Serving size is 7 oz. Serves 1.

   Stats: 264 cal, 25g protein, 17g carb, 12g fat, 4g sat, 7g fiber, 741mg sodium, 15mg chol, 163mg potassium, 210mg calcium

**Grilled Chicken Salad With Cheese (Recipe 28)**

3-4 oz grilled chicken breast, (recipe 18c)
2 tsp extra virgin olive oil

3 cups mixed green vegetables (spinach, romaine, arugula, etc), shredded
¼ cup cucumber, unpeeled, sliced
1 tsp Parmesan cheese, shredded
1 tbsp sliced almonds
6 cherry tomatoes
2 tbsp red wine vinegar
½ cup fresh medium strawberries cut in halves
1 oat bran/whole-wheat tortilla (*Joseph's*) or multigrain bread

**Instructions:**

1. In a medium bowl, combine chicken with salad dressing (olive oil and vinegar) and set aside
2. Place remaining ingredients in a large bowl, tossing to combine
3. Add cubed grilled chicken along with marinated liquid
4. Toss lightly to combine. Serve immediately
5. Serving size is 19 oz portion. Serves 1
   Stats: 267 cal, 31g protein, 11g carb, 11g fat, 2g sat, 5g fiber, 110mg sodium, 73mg chol, 860mg potassium, 114mg calcium

**Cucumber and Tomato Salad (Recipe 29)**

½ cup diced tomatoes
½ cup diced cucumbers
2 tsp red onion, chopped
1 tsp fresh parsley, chopped
¼ chopped cilantro
1 tbsp balsamic vinegar
1 tbsp fresh lemon juice
Salt, herbs and fresh ground pepper to taste

**Instructions:**

1. Combine chopped cucumber, tomatoes, onion, cilantro, and parsley in a bowl
2. Dress with the balsamic vinegar and lemon juice and season to taste
3. Serving size is 7 oz portion. Serves 1
   Stats: 49 cal, 2g protein, 12g carb, 0g fat, 0g sat, 3g fiber, 57mg sodium, 0mg chol, 269mg potassium, 11mg calcium

**Grilled Beef Tenderloin With Rosemary (Recipe 30)**

4 (4oz) beef fillets (½ inch thick or 16 oz beef tenderloin steaks)
¾ tsp steak seasoning
1 tsp olive oil
1 tsp rosemary, crushed
1 tsp parsley flakes
2 garlic cloves
Salt and freshly ground black pepper to taste

*Steak Sauce:*

2 cloves garlic
3 shallots, sliced
1 cup fresh parsley leaves
¼ cup chopped chives
¼ cup white wine vinegar
1 tbsp olive oil
Salt and ground black pepper

**Instructions for steak:**

1. Sprinkle steaks with the steak seasoning
2. Mix olive oil, rosemary, and parsley and blend until smooth
3. Brush on the steaks. Let marinate in refrigerator from 30-60 minutes
4. Grill steaks uncovered over high heat 4 to 6 minutes on each side or until done

**Instructions for sauce:**

1. Blend the garlic, shallots, vinegar and all the herbs until they are minced
2. Drizzle in the oil until the sauce becomes thick or to desired consistency
3. Season with salt and pepper to taste
4. Drizzle each steak with steak sauce
5. Serving size is 4 oz portion. Steaks serve 4
   Stats: 189 cal, 24g protein, 0.4g carb, 9.6g fat, 3.3g sat, 0g fiber, 83mg sodium, 70mg chol, 359mg potassium, 10mg calcium

**Crunchy Fennel Salad (Recipe 31)**

2 cups fresh string beans
2 cups fennel (anise), chopped
1 cup red pepper, chopped
1 can chickpeas, drained (can also use black or kidney beans)
1 cup red onion, chopped
4 oz (8 tbsp) Lite Balsamic Salad dressing

**Instructions:**

1. Combine vegetables and toss with dressing
2. Serving size is ½ cup. Serves 7
3. Prepare a big batch and refrigerate. Stays fresh for 5-7 days
   Stats: 113 cal, 3g protein, 15g carb, 5g fat, 0.6g sat, 4g fiber, 284mg sodium, 0mg chol, 210mg potassium, 37mg calcium

*Evelyn*

**Evelyn's Favorite Salad (Recipe 32)**

1 fresh Roma tomato, sliced
¼ cucumber, sliced
½-1 cup spinach
1 tsp chopped walnuts
1-2 tbsp red wine vinegar or lemon juice
Mrs. Dash seasoning or salt and ground black pepper

**Instructions:**

1. Assemble and toss with dressing
2. Serves 1

   Stats: 46 cal, 3g protein, 6g carb, 1.7g fat, 0g sat, 2g fiber, 28mg sodium, 0mg chol, 436mg potassium, 48 mg calcium

*Evelyn*

**Andreas Greek Salad (Recipe 33)**

1 large cucumber, sliced
4 fresh plum tomatoes
1 small whole red onion, julienne
12 black olives, canned
1 cup chopped fresh parsley
½ cup chopped fresh basil
1 tbs. extra virgin olive oil
2 tbs. vinegar, red wine
½ cup crumbled feta cheese
Salt and pepper to taste

**Instructions:**

1. Layer the ingredients following the listed order
2. Serving size is 1 cup. Serves 3

   Stats: 125 cal, 4g protein, 11g carb, 8g fat, 2g sat, 3.3g fiber, 212mg sodium, 6mg chol, 506mg potassium, 110mg calcium

*Andreas Restaurant*

**Andreas Lemon Chicken in a Pot With Potatoes (Recipe 34a)**

16 oz chicken breast, skinless, cut up into four large pieces and well seasoned (Mrs. Dash, herbs, spices)
2 tbsp olive oil
2 tbsp lemon juice
12 small-medium size new potatoes (about 3-5 oz per potato) or 4 medium sweet potatoes
¾ cup hot water
Salt, pepper and Oregano to taste

**Instructions:**

1. Heat pan over high heat in a large skillet containing oil
2. Add chicken and brown
3. Add the lemon juice, salt, and pepper
4. Add hot water and cover. Cook slowly over medium high heat
5. Clean and cut the potatoes into wedges, 15 minutes before the chicken is cooked add the potatoes and oregano

6. Serving size is 3-4 oz chicken in 13 oz portion. Serves 4. (Same recipe can be used with a lean cut of lamb, such as leg or blade chop)
   Stats: 264 cal, 28g protein, 20g carb, 6.5g fat, 1.3g sat, 3g fiber, 604mg sodium, 72mg chol, 227mg potassium, 44mg calcium

*Andreas Restaurant*

**Lentils (Recipe 34b)**

2 cups dried lentils (such as Chana dal)
1 small onion, chopped
2 tsp tomato paste
2 tbsp olive oil
1 tsp garlic, minced
1 tsp ginger, chopped
1 tsp whole cumin
¼ cup fresh cilantro, chopped
2 ½ cups water
Spices of your choice (salt, pepper, herbs, Mrs. Dash, etc.)

**Instructions:**

1. Sauté onions in olive oil. Add garlic, ginger, cumin, salt, and pepper to taste.
2. Stir for 2-3 minutes.
3. Add water and lentils. Cook until lentils are soft (no need to precook lentils).
4. Garnish with fresh cilantro.
5. Serving size is about 1 cup or 6oz. Serves 10.
   Stats: 148 cal, 9g protein, 22g carb, 3g fat, 0.5g sat, 8g fiber, 7mg sodium, 0mg chol, 383mg potassium, 24mg calcium

*Sonia*

**Pan-Roasted Lemon and Pepper Salmon (Recipe 34c)**

1 lb salmon filet
1 tbsp olive oil
1 tsp garlic powder
1 tbsp lemon pepper
Lemon wedges, 1 lemon
Black or crushed pepper to taste

**Instructions:**

1. Preheat oven to 400 degrees
2. Season salmon fillets with olive oil and seasonings
3. Roast in oven in a non-stick baking sheet 15-20 minutes or until fish is flaky and translucent
4. Serve with lemon wedges

5. Serving size is 4 oz salmon. Serves 4
   Stats: 199 cal, 23g protein, 2g carb, 10.7g fat, 1.6g sat, 0.3g fiber, 161mg sodium, 62mg chol, 587mg potassium, 20mg calcium
   *Cod, snapper or tuna steak can be substituted*

*Rosemary*

**Egg Salad Pocket (Recipe 35)**

2 medium cooked eggs, chopped
1 tbsp yogurt, plain
1 tbsp reduced fat mayonnaise
4 slices cucumber, peeled and chopped
½ cup fresh spinach, chopped
½ whole-wheat pita bread or 1 oat bran/whole-wheat pita or tortilla (*Joseph's*)
3 medium strawberries, sliced

**Instructions:**

1. In a bowl combine eggs, yogurt, mayonnaise and cucumber
2. Season with salt and black pepper to taste
3. Stuff into pita pocket with spinach and eat with strawberries
4. Serving size is 8 oz portion. Serves 1
   Stats: 255 cal, 15g protein, 21g carb, 12g fat, 3.9g sat, 4g fiber, 303mg sodium, 378mg chol, 484mg potassium, 115mg calcium

**Mushroom Soup (Recipe 36)**

1 lb. white button mushrooms, cleaned, and sliced
2 slices lean, low sodium bacon
3 cloves of garlic, finely minced
1 medium onion, chopped
¼ tsp Oregano
1 tsp vinegar
2-15 oz cans low sodium, fat free beef or chicken broth
1- 6 oz can low sodium V-8 juice or tomato juice
2 cups water

**Instructions:**

1. In pan, cook bacon until crisp. Remove from pan. Add onion and garlic. Sauté until translucent. Add bacon (chopped) back to the pan
2. Add mushrooms. Cook until water released from mushrooms evaporates
3. Add tomato juice, water, broth, and oregano. Season with salt and pepper. Let simmer
4. Add vinegar
5. Serving size is 1 cup. Serves 8
   Stats: 40 cal, 5g protein, 5g carb, 0.5g fat, 0g sat, 1g fiber, 70mg sodium, 2mg chol, 345mg potassium, 10mg calcium

**Grilled Salmon With Mixed Greens (Recipe 37)**

8 oz Salmon, grilled
4 cups mixed greens (baby spinach, arugula, romaine, etc), seasonal
6 artichoke hearts, canned (not marinade)
¼ cup red bell peppers, sliced
½ cucumber, sliced
2 medium tomato, chopped
2 tsp extra virgin olive oil
4 tbsp vinegar, Apple Cider
2 tbsp low-fat feta cheese, crumbled
Canola or olive oil cooking spray

**Instruction:**

1. Season salmon with salt and pepper to taste
2. Spray a hot grill pan lightly with cooking spray
3. Grill salmon until fish is flaky and translucent (3-5 minutes on each side)
4. Set aside to cool
5. Grill sliced red peppers
6. Add mixed greens to a bowl
7. Top with artichoke hearts, grilled red peppers, tomatoes, and cucumbers
8. Top with grilled salmon, broken into bite size pieces
9. Sprinkle on feta cheese and add vinegar and oil dressing
10. Serving size is 4 oz salmon. Serves 2

Stats: 290 cal, 28g protein, 13g carb, 14g fat, 3g sat, 5g fiber, 452mg sodium, 71mg chol, 1,102mg potassium, 132mg calcium

*You can also use snapper, cod or Tilapia*

*Karen*

**Tofu Omelet (Recipe 38)**

¼ cup silken soft tofu
1 whole egg + 2 egg white or ½ cup eggbeaters
2 button mushrooms, chopped
1 tbsp chopped green onion
1 tbsp chopped green bell pepper
1 medium tomato, sliced
¼ cup zucchini, thinly sliced
1 tsp olive oil
1 Oat bran/whole-wheat tortilla or pita bread (*Joseph's*)

**Instruction:**

1. Combine the eggs and tofu in a blender and whip to a smooth consistency
2. Heat a non-stick pan to medium high heat and add the oil
3. Sauté the vegetables for two minutes and add the egg-tofu

4. Stir occasionally until fully cooked
5. Place the scrambled egg into the tortilla and enjoy
6. Serving size is 15 oz portion. Serves 1
   Stats: 307 cal, 24g protein, 29g carb, 12g fat, 2g sat, 8g fiber, 549mg sodium, 187mg chol, 717mg potassium, 62mg calcium
   *You can accompany this meal with your choice of steamed vegetable (spinach, broccoli, chard, kale, etc.). Try it anytime - breakfast, lunch or dinner.*

**Lite Escarole Soup (Recipe 39a)**

1 lb escarole
7 turkey meatballs (see recipe 39b) or 4-6 oz chicken breast, chunks
2 bouillon cubes, low sodium
3-4 cups water
1 tbsp minced garlic
½ cup sliced mushroom
Black pepper and salt to taste

**Instructions:**

1. Cook until escarole is tender and meatballs are done about 20 minutes
2. Serving size is 1 cup. Serves 7
   Stats: 45 cal, 5g protein, 4g carb, 1g fat, 0.3g sat, 1g fiber, 169mg sodium, 14mg chol, 245mg potassium, 46mg calcium
   *You can also use chopped chicken, turkey breast, shrimps, etc.*

*Penny*

**Liz's Meat Balls (Recipe 39b)**

½ lb lean hamburger
¾ lb lean ground turkey
½ cup eggbeaters
¼ cup low sodium bread-crumbs (recipe 39d) or oat bran
1 tsp garlic powder or 1 tbsp fresh garlic, minced
1 tbsp parsley, dry
1 tbsp Italian seasoning or Mrs. Dash
¼ cup Parmesan cheese, low sodium

**Instructions:**

1. Mix all ingredients in a large bowl
2. Roll into ½ inch balls or meat loaf
3. Brown in 350-degree oven for 15 minutes
4. Remove from oven. Finish cooking in tomato sauce (recipe 39c)
   Stats: 112 cal, 13g protein, 4g carb, 4g fat, 1g sat, 1g fiber, 387mg sodium, 40mg chol, 104mg potassium, 29mg calcium

*Elizabeth*

**Liz's Tomato Sauce (Recipe 39c)**

4- 28 oz cans tomatoes
¼ cup olive oil

¼ cup onions, chopped
¼ cup celery, chopped
2 tbsp garlic, minced
2 tbsp Italian seasoning
1 tbsp basil, dry
4 bay leaves
2 tbsp Splenda sweetener
1 cup water

**Instructions:**

1. Sauté onion, celery, garlic, basil, bay leaves, and Italian seasonings in olive oil until transparent
2. Add tomatoes
3. Add water and sweetener
4. Cook on low for 1 hour
5. Add salt and pepper to taste
6. Serving size is 1 cup. Serves 15
   Stats: 85 cal, 2g protein, 9g carb, 3.6g fat, 0.5g sat, 2g fiber, 387mg sodium, 0mg chol, 364mg potassium, 38mg calcium

*Elizabeth*

**Bread Crumbs (Recipe 39d)**

4-6 slices multi grain bread or crackers with high fiber

Instructions:

1. Open bread to room temperature to harden over night, then toast
2. Put in food processor
3. Breadcrumbs can be seasoned with Italian Seasoning if desired
4. Place in a container for future use
5. Serving size is about 1 oz. Serves 5
   Stats: 37 cal, 2g protein, 8g carb, 0.4g fat, 0g sat, 2.2g fiber, 94mg sodium, 2mg chol, 32mg potassium, 15mg calcium

*Elizabeth*

**Three Bean Salad (Recipe 40a)**

½ cup kidney beans, canned, drained
½ cup black beans, canned, drained
½ navy beans, canned, drained
1 cup cilantro, fresh
2 cups fresh parsley
½ cup chopped scallions
2 tbsp chopped red onion
½ cup chopped sweet red pepper
½ cup chopped sweet green peppers
1 cup alfalfa seeds (sprouts)

2 tbsp Extra Virgin olive oil
2 tbsp flaxseed oil
4 tbsp Red wine vinegar
1 tsp black pepper

**Instructions:**

1. Canned beans are OK to use – look for low sodium canned beans and rinse before using to reduce sodium further
2. Combine all the solid ingredients
3. Wisk the dressing ingredients and drizzle into the salad
4. Toss thoroughly, chill and serve
5. Serving size is 1 cup. Serves 6
   Stats: 152 cal, 4g protein, 14g carb, 9.5g fat, 1g sat, 4g fiber, 6mg sodium, 0mg chol, 268mg potassium, 37mg calcium

**Seasoned Turkey Breast (Recipe 40b)**

8 oz turkey breast cutlets, pounded lightly to ½ inch thickness
2 tbsp season bread crumbs (recipe 39d) or oat bran
2 tsp Parmesan cheese, grated, low sodium
2 tsp olive oil
3 tbsp yellow onion, chopped
2 tsp garlic clove, minced
2 tsp poultry seasoning
Black pepper to taste
Other seasonings to taste (i.e. Ms. Dash)

**Instructions:**

1. Combine breadcrumbs or oat bran, cheese, and seasonings
2. Coat the turkey cutlets
3. In nonstick skillet, heat oil over medium high heat
4. Sauté breaded turkey cutlets about 3-5 minutes on each side until brown
5. In same pan, sauté garlic and onions until soft. Serve over turkey
6. Serving size is 4 oz portion. Serves 2
   Stats: 190 cal, 27g protein, 7g carb, 6.5g fat, 1g sat, 1g fiber, 51mg sodium, 63mg chol, 369mg potassium, 62mg calcium

*Elizabeth*

**Escarole Beans and Grilled Chicken Salad (Recipe 41)**

2 head escarole
19 oz Progresso Cannellini beans, canned
1 tbsp extra virgin oil
1 garlic clove
*Grilled chicken salad:*
9-12 oz chicken breast, grilled or roasted (recipe 18c)
2 Roma tomatoes

½ red bell pepper
½ green bell pepper
2 basil leaves
½ cup mushrooms
4 cups spinach
2 tsp extra virgin oil
2 tsp flaxseed oil
4 tbsp red wine vinegar

**Preparing Escarole:**

1. Wash escarole in cool water
2. Remove stem first to facilitate sand removal – save tender light green or white interior for salads
3. Boil or steam escarole until tender – drain and squeeze to remove bitterness
4. Sautee with olive oil, chopped garlic, and pepper flakes
5. Add Cannellini beans and cook until beans are heated through

**Preparing Grilled Chicken Salad:**

1. Arrange the sliced grilled or roasted chicken, tomato, peppers, and mushrooms over the salad greens
2. Combine the vinegar, oils, salt, and black pepper in a small bowl and dress the salad

**Preparing the escarole beans and grilled chicken salad:**

1. Combine the escarole beans and grilled chicken salad in a large bowl and mix well
2. Divide into 4 equal parts (about 22 oz) or about 2.5 cups per person. Serves 4
   Stats: 365 cal, 31g protein, 35g carb, 12g fat, 2g sat, 15g fiber, 488mg sodium, 55mg chol, 1,459mg potassium, 251mg calcium

**Tomato Basil Salad (Recipe 42a)**

6 fresh tomato slices
1 medium cucumber, slices
2 sprigs fresh thyme
3 fresh basil leaves
1 tbsp extra virgin olive oil
3 tbsp white rice vinegar
Salt, pepper and herbs to taste

**Instructions:**

1. Combine the tomatoes and cucumbers and season with salt, pepper, and herbs to taste
2. Layer the salad with the basil and thyme. Drizzle with the olive oil and vinegar mixture
3. Serving size is 9 oz portion or ½ of the salad. Serves 2

Stats: 104 cal, 3g protein, 12g carb, 5g fat, 1g sat, 2g fiber, 10mg sodium, 0mg chol, 471mg potassium, 213mg calcium

**Tomato Fennel Salad (Recipe 42b)**

1 fennel (bulb only, remove core) sliced thinly
3 orange tomatoes
3 cherry tomatoes
3 red radishes, sliced
1 tbsp olive oil
2 tbsp red wine vinegar
1 tbsp lemon juice
2 tbsp shredded carrots
Fennel prawns
Salt and pepper to taste

**Instructions:**

1. Add all the ingredients to a bowl and pour on dressing and toss
2. Top with fennel prawns
3. Divide into 3 portions or 1 cup serving. Serves 3
   Stats: 78 cal, 3g protein, 11g carb, 3.5g fat, 0.5 sat, 4g fiber, 92mg sodium, 0mg chol, 627mg potassium, 48mg calcium

**Grilled Shrimp Kabobs (Recipe 43)**

12 large shrimp or 8 oz, shelled and deveined
2 tsp fresh lemon juice
2 tsp canola oil
½ oz sun dried tomatoes
¼ tsp crushed red pepper flakes
¼ cup boiling water
Salt and black pepper to taste

**Instructions:**

1. Soak sun-dried tomatoes in ¼ cup boiling water for few minutes
2. Then add lemon juice, canola oil, and pepper flakes
4. Blend the mixture until smooth
5. Season with salt and black pepper
6. Pour the mixture over the shrimps and then thread on skewers
7. Grill over medium heat
8. Turn occasionally. Brush with remaining mixture as needed
9. Serving size is 5 oz portion. Serves 2
   Stats: 185 cal, 24g protein, 6g carb, 7g fat, 1g sat, 1g fiber, 176mg sodium, 172mg chol, 225mg potassium, 74mg calcium

**Lemon Salmon in Foil (Recipe 44)**

8 oz salmon fillet
1 cup celery, chopped

¼ cup red onion, thinly sliced
4 cups spinach, chopped
¼ cup fresh lemon juice
2 tsp olive oil
Salt and black pepper to taste

**Instructions:**

1. Cut a sheet of foil to one square foot
2. Combine the celery, onions, spinach, and olive oil
3. Place the salmon over the vegetables and season as desired
4. Pour the lemon juice over the salmon
5. Fold the foil unto itself and seal into a package
6. Bake in a preheated oven (toaster oven ok) at 350°F for about 25 minutes
7. Serving size is 4 oz fish in 11 oz portion. Serves 2
   Stats: 272: cal, 31.5g protein, 10g carb, 11.8g fat, 1.8g sat, 3.5g fiber, 165mg sodium, 81mg chol, 1,319mg potassium, 111mg calcium
   *Substitutes: red snapper fillet, Tuna fillet, swordfish fillet and tilapia fillet*

**Omega Flax Butter (Recipe 45a)**

4 oz soft margarine or butter, unsalted
4 oz flaxseed oil/linseed oil

**Instructions:**

1. Let butter stand at room temperature until soft
2. Place butter in a mixing bowl and whip with an electric mixer until butter starts to turn lighter in color
3. With the mixer still running, slowly add in the flaxseed oil allowing it to incorporate into the butter
4. When all of the flaxseed oil has been incorporated into the butter continue mixing for one minute
5. Place mixture in a covered container and refrigerate
6. Serving size is 1 tsp. Serves 42
   Stats: 33 cal, 0g protein, 0g carb, 3.8g fat, 1g sat, 0g fiber, 0mg sodium, 4mg chol, 0mg potassium, 0mg calcium

**Ginger Chicken With Garlic (Recipe 45b)**

16 oz (1lb.) chicken breast (boneless/skinless)
4 tsp extra virgin olive oil or canola oil
1 tbsp fresh minced ginger or ½ tbsp ground ginger
1 clove garlic, crushed, or 2 tsp minced garlic
2 tbsp fresh lime juice
Salt and black pepper to taste

**Instruction:**

1. Marinade chicken with all ingredients for about 30 minutes
2. Grill or broil chicken, baste with marinade until cooked

3. Serving size is 4 oz. Serves 4
Stats: 176 cal, 26g protein, 2g carb, 6g fat, 1g sat, 0.2g fiber, 74mg sodium, 66mg chol, 321mg potassium, 17mg calcium

**Mixed Veggies (Recipe 46a)**

4 cups broccoli pieces
½ red onion, chopped
⅛-¼ chicken broth bouillon pkt., dry, or Mrs. Dash seasoning
1.5 cup water
¼ cup carrots, frozen slices
¼ cup green peas, frozen

**Instructions:**

1. Bring water to a boil and add boullion and vegetables
2. Cook for about 5-6 minutes
3. Serving size is 1 cup. Serves 4
Stats: 59 cal, 5g protein, 11g carb, 0.6g fat, 0.1g sat, 6g fiber, 95mg sodium, 0mg chol, 555mg potassium, 84mg calcium

*Penny*

**Sautéed Spinach and Roasted Red Peppers (Recipe 46b)**

1 (16 oz.) bag Baby Spinach or 6 cups fresh or frozen
2-3 cloves garlic, sliced
2 oz roasted red pepper (pimento), cut in slices
2 tsp olive oil
1/8 tsp nutmeg
Salt and ground black pepper to taste

**Instructions:**

1. Add olive oil to skillet. Add garlic. Sauté until brown
2. Add spinach. Toss lightly
3. Add roasted red pepper (pimento) and nutmeg
4. Serving size is about 1 cup.. Serves 3
Stats: 70 cal, 4g protein, 7g carb, 3.7g fat, 0.5g sat, 1g fiber, 227mg sodium, 0mg chol, 637mg potassium, 121mg calcium

**Baked Tuna Fillet With Potatoes (Recipe 47)**

16 oz tuna fillet, seasoned and coated with oat bran
2 tbsp canola oil
2 garlic cloves, chopped
1 red onion, chopped into big chunks
1 cup fresh mushroom, chopped
¼ cup fresh chopped parsley
8 new potatoes, cut into 4 slices each and seasoned
¼ cup oat bran

**Instructions:**

1. Preheat oven to 350 degrees
2. Coat fish fillets with seasoning salt, black pepper, and oat bran
3. Brown fillet in oil and put aside
4. Cut new potatoes into four slices and rub salt and black pepper all over and brown them also
5. Layer fish fillets on the side of the potatoes and add the remaining ingredients
6. Cook in the oven at 350 degrees until done
7. Garnish with parsley
8. Serving size is 4 oz tuna in 12 oz portion. (2 potatoes per person). Serves 4
   Stats: 272 cal, 28 protein, 21g carb, 8.5g fat, 0.9g sat, 4g fiber, 406mg sodium, 53mg chol, 654mg potassium, 71mg calcium

**Grilled Chicken Salad With Almonds (Recipe 48)**

4 oz grilled or roasted chicken breast, diced into bite-size pieces
2 cups romaine lettuce, chopped
2 cups red leaf lettuce, chopped
3 thin slices red bell peppers
3 thin slices green bell pepper
¼ cup orange wedges
½ apple, slices
1 tsp roasted almonds or walnuts, sliced
2 tbsp red wine vinegar
1 tsp olive oil
1 tsp canola oil or flax oil
Salt and black pepper to taste

**Instructions:**

1. Combine and mix the canola oil, black pepper, and salt
2. Season the chicken breast with the canola oil, salt, and pepper mixture
3. Heat grill pan until hot. Spray with cooking spray
4. Add seasoned chicken over a medium – high heat and grill until done
5. Dice the chicken and chill
6. In a medium bowl, layer the lettuces, peppers, diced chicken breast, orange wedges, apples slices, and sliced almonds
7. Add the vinegar and the olive oil dressing and serve
8. Serving size is 15 oz portion. Serves 1
   Stats: 325 cal, 27g protein, 25g carb, 14g fat, 1.9g sat, 8g fiber, 77mg sodium, 63mg chol, 1,008mg potassium, 141mg calcium

**Fresh Cucumber and Tomato Salad (Recipe 49)**

½ cup diced tomatoes
½ cup diced cucumbers

2 tsp red onion, chopped
1 tsp fresh parsley
1-2 tbsp red wine vinegar
Mrs. Dash or salt and black pepper to taste

**Instructions:**

1. Assemble the ingredients and drizzle with dressing and seasoning
   Stats: 68 cal, 3g protein, 15g carb, 0.7g fat, 0g sat, 3g fiber, 35mg sodium, 0mg chol, 544mg potassium, 71mg calcium

**Sautéed Scallops (Recipe 50)**

12 frozen Atlantic scallops, large
1 tbsp olive oil
1 tbsp soft margarine
2 tbsp balsamic vinegar
1 tsp low sodium chicken bouillon, dry
¼ tsp garlic powder
¼ tsp onion powder

**Instructions:**

1. Melt margarine in a sauté pan with olive oil
2. Add scallops. Cook for 2 or 3 min
3. Add balsamic vinegar, bouillon and garlic powder. Turn frequently until caramelized
4. Serving size is 4 oz portions with 6 scallops. Serves 2
   Stats: 216 cal, 23g protein, 5g carb, 10g fat, 2g sat, 0g fiber, 310mg sodium, 60mg chol, 309mg potassium, 32mg calcium

*Elizabeth*

**Southwestern Scrambled Eggs (Recipe 51)**

½ cup eggbeaters or 1 whole egg + 2 egg whites
1 tbsp red pepper, chopped
1 tbsp roasted bell peppers
2 button mushrooms, sliced
1 tbsp chopped tomato
1 tbsp onion, chopped
1 slice, 1oz, extra lean ham, cut in small pieces
½ tsp extra virgin olive oil
3 medium strawberries
1 oat bran/whole-wheat pita bread (*Joseph's*) or ½ whole-wheat pita
3 medium strawberries, ½ cup berries or ½ cup melons (cantaloupe, honeydew, etc.)

**Instructions:**

1. Scramble eggbeaters or eggs in a nonstick skillet with red peppers, mushrooms, ham, and onion
2. Serve with small whole-wheat pita bread and berries
3. Serving size is 16 oz portion. Serves 1

Stats: 317 cal, 30g protein, 31g carb, 10g fat, 2g sat, 9g fiber, 903mg sodium, 200mg chol, 518mg potassium, 45mg calcium

**Bleu Cheese Stuffed Cherry Tomatoes (Recipe 52a)**

5 cherry tomatoes
1 tbsp crumbled bleu cheese
1 tbsp chopped parsley
½ tsp extra virgin olive oil
¼ tsp fresh ground black pepper

**Instructions:**

1. Cut a small, round piece off the tomatoes to expose the inside
2. Gently squeeze out the seeds and liquid. Set aside
3. Combine remaining ingredients
4. Use a small spoon or the tip of a butter knife to fill each tomato. Enjoy chilled
5. Serving size is 3 oz. Serves 1
   Stats: 67 cal, 2.4g protein, 5g carb, 4.6g fat, 1.6g sat, 1g fiber, 107mg sodium, 5mg chol, 209mg potassium, 49mg calcium

**Turkey Wrap (Recipe 52b)**

4 thin slices cooked turkey breast, low sodium (such as *Louis Rich* thin smoked turkey breast or 97% fat free oven roasted turkey breast)
1 tbsp low sodium lite mayonnaise
¼ tsp garlic powder
½ tsp oregano leaves, chopped
2 tsp extra virgin olive oil
¼ red bell pepper cut into strips
4 cucumber slices cut into strips
1 oat bran/whole-wheat tortilla or pita bread (*Joseph's*)
Salt and pepper to taste

**Instructions:**

1. Mix the mayonnaise, garlic powder, oregano leaves, and olive oil
2. Spread the dressing mix on top of the tortilla or pita
3. Add the turkey slices on the tortilla or pita
4. Top with the bell peppers and cucumber strips
5. Roll up and enjoy or wrap in plastic wrap and refrigerate until ready to serve
6. The turkey wrap can be served as a whole sandwich wrap or bite size slices
7. Serving size is 6 oz portion. Serves 1
   Stats: 224 cal, 17g protein, 15g carb, 13g fat, 2g sat, 7g fiber, 884mg sodium, 22mg chol, 59mg potassium, 10mg calcium

**Mixed Berry Sorbet (Recipe 53)**

4 large fresh strawberries (freeze before use) or use frozen fruits

6 fresh raspberries (freeze before use) or use frozen fruits
½ cup whole milk
2-pct splenda, stevia, or 2 tsp sugar

**Instructions:**

1. Blend until smooth
2. Serve immediately or freeze
3. Serving size is 4 oz portion. Serves 2
   Stats: 48 cal, 2g protein, 9g carb, 0.7g fat, 0.4g sat, 1.4g fiber, 31mg sodium, 2mg chol, 172mg potassium, 144mg calcium

**Mixed Fruit Salad (Recipe 54)**

½ cup berries (strawberries, blueberries, etc.)
¼ cup grapes, seedless
1 cup melon chunks (cantaloupe, honeydew, watermelon etc.)
½ tbsp chopped almonds
½ tbsp chopped walnuts
½ tbsp sunflower seeds
1 cup low-fat cottage cheese

**Instructions:**

1. Combine fruit and nuts
2. Serve along with cottage cheese
3. Serving size is 1.5 cup or 12 oz portions. Serves 2
4. Snack: ½ cup portion
   Stats: 282 cal, 21g protein, 26g carb, 11g fat, 2.5g sat, 6g fiber, 604mg sodium, 17mg chol, 862mg potassium, 237mg calcium (for 1.5 cup)

**Roasted Chicken (Recipe 55)**

3 lb roasting chicken, skinless (farm raised or free range)
2 sprigs tarragon, fresh
10 fresh garlic cloves
1 Spanish or yellow onion, chopped
1 lemon
2 tbsp extra virgin olive oil or unsalted omega flax butter (see recipe 45a)

**Instructions:**

1. Preheat oven to 425° F
2. Wash chicken inside and out with salt and water. Rinse well and pat very dry
3. Cut garlic in half width wise and cut lemon in fourths
4. Rub chicken inside and out with black pepper and salt
5. Stuff garlic heads, lemon, and about 2 sprigs tarragon (may substitute with other herbs like Rosemary) into cavity of chicken
6. Rub outside of chicken with olive oil or omega butter and add one Spanish onion, chopped to roasting pan

7. Roast at 425 degree preheated oven for about 1 ½ hours or until the internal thigh temperature reads 180 degrees with a probe thermometer
8. Remove from the oven and allow resting for 15 minutes before carving
9. Serving size is 6 oz portion containing 4 oz chicken. Serves 11
   Stats: 157 cal, 25.5g protein, 2g carb, 4.6g fat, 1g sat, 0.3g fiber, 94mg sodium, 80mg chol, 326mg potassium, 21mg calcium

*Rosemary*

**Zucchini Soup (Recipe 56)**

2 (10 oz.) cans whole tomatoes
1 small onion
3 zucchini chopped into pieces
1 (15 oz.) can lentils (rinsed)
1 (14 oz.) can chicken broth (low sodium)
3.5 cups water

**Instructions:**

1. Add vegetables and broth to a saucepan
2. Add additional water just to cover
3. Boil for approximately 20 minutes or until vegetables are tender
4. Serving size is 1 cup. Serves 3
   Stats: 51 cal, 4g protein, 8g carb, 0.4g fat, 0g sat, 2.4g fiber, 123mg sodium, 1mg chol, 292mg potassium, 35mg calcium

**Flax Caesar Salad (Recipe 57)**

¼ tsp crushed garlic
1 tbsp flaxseed oil, *Barlean's Organic Flax Oil*
½ tsp Dijon mustard
1 tbsp lemon juice
1 tbsp white wine vinegar
6 Greek olives, pitted
24 oz Romaine lettuce, torn into bite-size pieces (2 bundles)

**Instructions:**

1. Combine the first 5 ingredients in a jar with a lid. Shake until emulsified
2. Place the lettuce in a large bowl and toss with dressing
3. Serving size is 1 cup. Serves 3
   Stats: 95.5 cal, 4g protein, 7g carb, 6g fat, 0.5g sat, 4g fiber, 330mg sodium, 0mg chol, 666mg potassium, 84mg calcium

*Barlean's Organic Oils (modified)*

**Granny Smith Apple With Cheddar (Recipe 58)**

1 Granny Smith apple
½ cup diced low-sodium, low-fat cheddar cheese
4 medium fresh strawberries

**Instructions:**

1. Wash and dice the apple, omitting the core
2. Remove the green tops from the strawberries
3. Quarter the strawberries
4. Combine all the ingredients
5. Divide into two portions and bag
6. Enjoy chilled
7. Serving size is 10 oz. Serves 1
   Stats: 197 cal, 17g protein, 24g carb, 4.6g fat, 2.9g sat, 5g fiber, 15mg sodium, 14mg chol, 361mg potassium, 481mg calcium

**Spinach Ham Quiche (Recipe 59)**

3 whole eggs, beaten
2-cups egg white or eggbeaters
¼ cup heavy whipping cream
4 sheets phyllo dough
2 cups spinach, cooked and drained (frozen ok)
2 cups small-diced lean ham
1 cup chopped mushrooms
1 cup onion, julienne
2 cloves minced garlic
1 tsp salt
½ tsp black pepper
½ tsp nutmeg
4 tbsp shredded Parmesan cheese
6 tbsp olive oil

**Instructions:**

1. Measure out the olive oil into a 4 tbsp portions (for the phyllo sheets) and a 2 tbsp portion for sautéing
2. Brush the bottom and sides of a 10” cake pan with olive oil
3. Brush one phyllo sheet with olive oil and place into the pan. Follow this procedure with the other phyllo sheets
4. Cut off the excess phyllo, leaving some above the side of the pan. Set aside
5. Heat a pan to medium heat and add 2 tbsp of olive oil
6. Cook the ham, mushrooms, onion, garlic, and seasoning until wilted. Remove from the pan, set aside
7. Combine the beaten eggs with the egg whites and heavy cream
8. Partially cook the egg product to curd-like consistency and remove from the heat
9. Fold the vegetables into the egg product
10. Place the batter into the phyllo sheet layered mold and bake in a pre-heated oven at the 350 degrees F for 15 minutes
11. Remove from the oven and allow the quiche to rest a few minutes before cutting into 16 pieces
12. Serving size is 4 oz portion using a 10-inch mold. Serves 16

Stats: 132 cal, 9g protein, 5g carb, 8.4g fat, 2.3g sat, 1 fiber, 631mg sodium, 14mg chol, 225mg potassium, 46mg calcium

**Easy Quiche (Recipe 60)**

16 oz Egg Beaters or egg substitute
16 oz chopped frozen broccoli or spinach (thawed and well drained)
¼ cup Parmesan cheese, low sodium
Garlic powder, salt and pepper to taste

**Instructions:**

1. Combine all ingredients
2. Pour into a 10" inch glass dish (pie pan)
3. Bake 1 hour in a 350 degree oven
4. Serving size is ¼ pie. Serves 4
   Stats: 109 cal, 17g protein, 7g carb, 2g fat, 1g sat, 2.4g fiber, 337mg sodium, 5mg chol, 410mg potassium, 164mg calcium

*Elizabeth*

**Baked Salmon With Beets and Goat Cheese (Recipe 61)**

6-8 oz Atlantic salmon fillet
2 garlic cloves, minced
1 cup fennel bulb, slices
1 cup beets, canned, diced, drained
½ green onions, chopped
2 tbsp goat cheese, soft type
4 tsp red wine vinegar
Salt and black pepper or Mrs. Dash to taste

**Instructions:**

1. Finely mince the garlic
2. Combine the garlic, beets, fennel, green onions, and vinegar
3. Place the vegetables in oven ware plate
4. Season the salmon with salt and pepper and place over the vegetables
5. Bake in a preheated oven at 350°F for 20 minutes. If well-done fish is preferred, cook for an additional 15 minutes
6. Remove from oven and crumble the soft goat cheese over the fish
7. Serving size is 3-4 oz salmon in 9 oz portion. Serves 2
   Stats: 249 cal, 26g protein, 12g carb, 10g fat, 3g sat, 4g fiber, 286mg sodium, 67mg chol, 916mg potassium, 73mg calcium

*Goat cheese is lactose-free.*

**Baked Spaghetti Squash With Meatballs (Recipe 62)**

1 spaghetti squash (about 2 lbs.), raw
¾ lb lean hamburger
1 lb lean ground turkey
½ cup eggbeaters

¼ cup low sodium breadcrumbs (recipe 39d) or oat bran
1 tsp garlic powder
1 tbsp dry parsley
1 tbsp Italian seasoning or Mrs. Dash
¼ cup Parmesan cheese
1- 15 oz can Contadina tomato sauce or your favorite brand

**Instruction:**

1. Slice squash in half, remove seeds and bake at 350 degrees for 45 minutes to 1 hour or until tender
2. Using fork, remove squash from shell (it will come out in spaghetti-like strands)
3. Mix hamburger, turkey, eggbeaters, oat bran or breadcrumbs, seasonings, and cheese in a large bowl. Mix well
4. Roll into ½ inch balls
5. Brown in 350-degree oven for 15 minutes
6. Remove from oven and finish cooking in tomato sauce
7. Serve over spaghetti squash
8. Sprinkle with Parmesan cheese
9. Serving size 1.5 cup or 12 oz portions. Serves 6
   Stats: 284 cal, 30g protein, 19g carb, 10.5g fat, 3g sat, 4g fiber, 579mg sodium, 91mg chol, 414mg potassium, 78mg calcium

**Grilled Eggplant With Mozzarella (Recipe 63)**

1 large eggplant, cut into ½ inch slices
1 large Roma tomato, cut into thin slices
Cooking spray, canola, or olive oil
1 tsp minced garlic
4 tsp mozzarella cheese, shredded
Salt and pepper to taste

**Instructions:**

1. Place sliced eggplant on a large bakery sheet
2. Spray lightly with cooking spray
3. Season with salt, pepper and garlic and a sprinkle of mozzarella cheese
4. Flip eggplant over and repeat the procedure – spray and seasoning
5. Place eggplant in oven for 15 minutes
6. Remove from oven and top with tomato slices
7. Put eggplant and tomato under broiler about 3-4 minutes
8. Serving size is 5 oz or 1 eggplant slice. Serves 4
   Stats: 48 cal, 2g protein, 10g carb, 0.7g fat, 0.3g sat, 4g fiber, 20mg sodium, 1mg chol, 341mg potassium, 28mg calcium

*Penny*

**Veggie Marinara (Recipe 64)**

15 oz can tomatoes, crushed
1 garlic clove

2 tbsp extra virgin olive oil
1 large zucchini, sliced (about 12 oz)
1 large yellow squash, sliced
1 medium onion, chopped
10 button mushrooms, sliced
¼ tsp basil, dry
¼ cup parsley, fresh, chopped
½ cup water
Salt and black pepper to taste

**Instructions:**

1. In a pan, heat the oil
2. Sauté onion and garlic until tender
3. Add sliced squash and zucchini
4. Sauté about 5 minutes
5. Add remaining ingredients
6. Simmer for 10-15 minutes
7. Serving size is 10 oz portion. Serves 4
   Stats: 136 cal, 4g protein, 14g carb, 7g fat, 1g sat, 4g fiber, 171mg sodium, 0mg chol, 289mg potassium, 64mg calcium

**Oriental Blend Vegetables (Recipe 65)**

16 oz bag of frozen vegetables (green beans, broccoli, onions, and mushrooms) (*Stop and Shop* Brand or other brands or 1 cup of each vegetables).

**Instructions (See directions for preparation on package )**

1. 1 Measure 8 oz (½ bag) of Oriental Blend Vegetables
2. Bring ¼ cup water to a boil
3. Add vegetables and ¼ bullion cube or Mrs. Dash and bring to a second boil
4. Reduce heat and cover
5. Simmer 6-8 minutes, just until tender
6. Drain and season to taste
7. Serving size is 1 cup (95grams). Serves 5
   Stats: 35 cal, 1g protein, 5g carb, 0g fat, 0g sat, 2g fiber, 10 mg sodium, 0 mg chol

**Instructions (Stir-fry):**

1. Heat 1 tsp oil in a skillet over high heat or use cooking spray
2. Add the vegetables and stir fry, turning frequently
3. Pour in ½ cup of low sodium chicken broth
4. Add 1 tsp low sodium soy sauce
5. Stir for about 2 minutes
6. Season salt and pepper to taste
7. Serving size is 1 cup. Serves 5
   Stats: 80 cal, 3g protein, 6g carb, 5g fat, 1g sat, 2g fiber, 254 sodium, 2mg chol, 10mg potassium, 11mg calcium

**Grilled Tuna Pita Pocket (Recipe 66)**

2 tsp light low sodium mayonnaise
3 oz or ½ can regular tuna, drained and flaked
¼ tsp lemon juice
¼ tsp Dijon mustard or yellow mustard
2 tsp celery, finely chopped
½ tbsp red onions, finely chopped
½ tsp fresh cilantro, chopped
1 tsp extra virgin olive oil
1 slice (1oz) low-fat Provolone cheese
3 slices Dill pickle, low sodium
½ whole-wheat pita pocket or 1 oat bran/ whole-wheat pita or tortilla *(Joseph's)*

**Instructions:**

1. Combine all ingredients and stuff into pita pocket bread
2. Add cheese and broil until cheese melts
3. Serving size is 7 oz portion. Serves 1
   Stats: 332 cal, 32g protein, 20g carb, 13g fat, 4g sat, 3g fiber, 679mg sodium, 59mg chol, 314mg potassium, 276mg calcium

**Tofu Vegetable Soup (Recipe 67a)**

1 cup frozen snow peas, thawed, trimmed, and cut in half
2 tbsp sliced scallions
2 cups spinach, frozen
½ cup sliced Bok choy (Chinese cabbage)
8 oz firm tofu, well blotted, cut into small cubes
15-oz can cut baby corn, liquid drained
½ medium red bell pepper, cut into short strips
1 ½ cups chicken or vegetable broth, low sodium
1 cup water
2 eggs white
Salt and pepper to taste

**Instructions:**

1. Add the water with the vegetable broth, bell pepper, corn, tofu, and snow peas in a soup pot. Bring to a simmer
2. Cook covered for about 5 minutes
3. Rinse spinach, remove stems and chop coarsely
4. Add the egg white and spinach to the soup and cook until spinach is done
5. Season with pepper and salt to taste
6. Serving size is 1 cup. Serves 5
   Stats: 67 cal, 6g protein, 7g carb, 2g fat, 0.4g sat, 1g fiber, 83mg sodium, 1mg chol, 311mg potassium, 61mg calcium

**Greek Style Lemon Soup (Recipe 67b)**

4 cups low sodium chicken broth

2 tbsp raw egg white or eggbeaters
1 whole egg
1.5 tbsp fresh parsley
2.5 tbsp lemon juice
1 tbsp fresh oregano
2 tbsp long grain white rice, dry
Mrs. Dash lemon pepper seasoning

**Instructions:**

1. In a pot, bring chicken broth to a boil. Add the rice, cover. Lower the heat. Let rice cook until tender (about 15 minutes)
2. In a small bowl mix lemon juice and eggs
3. Slowly pour the lemon mixture into the broth. Stir gently
4. Let simmer for 2-3 minutes
5. Add the parsley, oregano, and seasoning
6. Serving size is 1 cup. Serves 4
   Stats: 78 cal, 6g protein, 8g carb, 2.8g fat, 1g sat, 0g fiber, 137mg sodium, 58mg chol, 57mg potassium, 33mg calcium

*Aronis*

**UDP Tofurkey Meatloaf (Recipe 68)**

10 oz Tofu (firm) or lean ground beef
1 pound 8% fat lean ground turkey
½ cup portabella mushrooms, chopped
¼ cup onion, chopped
1 cube vegetable bouillon, low sodium
1 cup cooked white rice
2 tbsp soy sauce, low sodium
2 tbsp whole-wheat bread crumbs or whole-wheat flour
2 tbsp carrots, grated
1 teaspoon ground black pepper
¼ cup water, hot
1 tsp black ground pepper
8 tsp canola oil

**Instructions:**

1. Combine all ingredients by kneading the mixture into a uniform consistency and shape into 8 patties
2. Fry in a non-stick pan with 1 teaspoon of canola oil per patty
3. The oil should be very hot to prevent the patties from breaking apart
4. Cook a few at time; do not crowd your pan. Drain well and serve
5. Serving size is 5 oz portion. Serves 8
   Stats: 187 cal, 14g protein, 11g carb, 9.6g fat, 1.6g sat, 0.5g fiber, 322mg sodium, 45mg chol, 220mg potassium, 27mg calcium

**Mashed Cauliflower (Recipe 69a)**

3 cups raw cauliflower
1/3 cup skim milk
3 tbs. soft margarine, Benecol, or Smart Balance with omega plus

**Instructions:**

1. Boil cauliflower until soft. Put in food processor or blender.
2. Add skim milk and soft margarine or Benecol.
3. Whip on high until smooth. Season to taste.
4. Serving size is 1 cup. Serves 3.
   Stats: 53.5 cal, 3g protein, 6.5g carb, 2g fat, 0.3g sat, 3.3g fiber, 55mg sodium, 0mg chol, 207mg potassium, 53mg calcium

*Donna*

**Citrus Marinated Skinless Chicken Breast Skewers (Recipe 69b)**

(*For the Marinade*)
1 lemon
1 tsp Dijon mustard
1 tsp salt
½ tsp dried coriander leaf
½ tsp black pepper
2 fresh garlic cloves
½ cup dry white wine
2 tbsp extra virgin olive oil
(*For the Skewer*)
1 skinless, boneless chicken breast (about1 lb. – divide into 4 parts and cut each into bite-size chunks)
1 yellow onion
4 cherry tomatoes
4 portabella mushrooms (about 4 oz)
½ cup shredded Parmesan cheese
4 10-inch bamboo skewers
1 lemon
Olive or canola oil spray

**Instructions:**

*For the marinade:*

1. Cut one lemon into smaller, easy to blend pieces and place in a blender along with rest of the marinade ingredients
2. Blend on high until mixture is smooth
3. Marinade the chicken for at least 15 minutes or preferably overnight

*For the skewers:*

1. Soak the bamboo skewers in water until ready for use
2. Cut the onion in half, then into quarters, and set aside
3. Skewer the chicken and vegetables in any order you desire

*To cook*:

1. You may cook over a charcoal flame, oven broiler, or a non-stick sauté pan on your stovetop. For best results, cook over a charcoal or wood flame
2. Cook the skewer for a total of 7-10 minutes, spraying occasionally with olive oil spray to enhance favor and to prevent drying out
3. At the end of the cooking process, squeeze the juice of the remaining lemon unto the skewers
4. Your chicken is done when it has become "springy" to the touch. Also the vegetables should acquire a charred, caramelized look
5. Shortly before removing the chicken, sprinkle with the parmesan cheese
6. Serving size is 4 oz chicken breast plus vegetables. Serves 4
   Stats: 324 cal, 26g protein, 9g carb, 17.9g fat, 3.7g sat, 2g fiber, 736mg sodium, 68mg chol, 496mg potassium, 102mg calcium

**Basic Cucumber Tomato Salad (Recipe 70)**

2 Roma tomatoes, sliced
½ whole cucumber, sliced
2 red radishes, sliced
1 tsp fresh parsley, chopped
1 tbsp fresh cilantro
1-2 tbsp red wine vinegar
Mrs. Dash or salt and black pepper to taste

**Instructions:**

1. Assemble the ingredients and add dressing and seasonings
2. Serving size is 10 oz. Serves 1
   Stats: 48 cal, 2g protein, 10g carb, 0.6g fat, 0g sat, 3g fiber, 19mg sodium, 0mg chol, 525mg potassium, 33mg calcium

**Tuna Pasta Salad (Recipe 71)**

¼ cup whole-wheat pasta (macaroni, cooked) or Barilla Plus (see recipe 44)
3 oz (½ can) water packed regular tuna
4 tbsp red onion, chopped
4 tbsp red bell pepper, chopped
4 tbsp green bell pepper, chopped
2 tbsp light mayonnaise
1 tbsp lemon juice
Combine pasta with remaining ingredients. Salad can be served warm or cold

Stats: 282 cal, 26g protein, 27g carb, 9g fat, 1.5g sat, 4g fiber, 587mg sodium, 41mg chol, 519mg potassium, 80mg calcium

**Vegetable Pot Soup (Recipe 72)**

1 big or 2 small broccoli heads or cauliflower
½ cauliflower head
10 baby carrots, chopped

½ medium onion, chopped
½ big or 1 small whole zucchini, chopped into pieces
1 medium summer squash, chopped into pieces
1 cup mushrooms, cut into halves
2 cans or 4 cups low sodium chicken broth or water
Salt and black pepper to taste or Mrs. Dash seasoning

**Instructions:**

1. Cook in a Dutch oven or cooking pan
2. Add all the vegetables and broth into a pot and simmer 12-15 minutes or until vegetables are cooked – tender but firm and crispy
3. Serving size is 1 cup. Serves 8
   Stats: 47 cal, 4g protein, 7g carb, 1g fat, 0.4g sat, 3g fiber, 74 mg sodium, 2mg chol, 557mg potassium, 38mg calcium

*Anne*

**UDP Signature Vegetable Soup (Recipe 73)**

6 cups water
2 low sodium chicken cubes
1 medium yellow onion, chopped
1-cup low sodium V-8
1 large green bell pepper, sliced in strips
1 large red bell pepper, sliced in strips
1 cup sliced mushrooms
10 cups Bok Choy (1-inch pieces)
1 Whole Eggplant
3 garlic cloves, finely chopped
1 cup frozen mixed vegetables
½ cup green soybeans (edamame)
2 lbs. chicken breast cut in 1-inch pieces
2 eggs
1 tbs. cornstarch
1 tbs. toasted sesame oil or canola oil
1 tsp. paprika
2 tbs. soy sauce (low sodium)
1 tbs. black peppercorns
1 small jalapeno, chopped

**Instructions:**

Add water and V-Juice to a large pot. Bring to a boil. Add chicken breast, chicken bouillon, onions, peppercorns, chopped jalapeno, green and red bell peppers, edamame, paprika, sesame oil, chopped garlic and chicken. Bring back to a boil. Add frozen mixed vegetables. Cook until chicken is done. Add chopped Bok Choy, mushrooms and soy sauce. Reduce heat. Simmer 4-6 minutes. Mix cornstarch with 1 cup of cold water. Stir well to eliminate lumps. Add to the pot,

stirring constantly. Beat eggs with 1 tbsp. cold water. Slowly stir egg mixture into the pot, stirring constantly. Shut off heat.
Serving size is 2 cups. Serves 12.

Stats: 196 cal, 25g protein, 13g carb, 5g fat, 0.9g sat, 4g fiber, 438mg sodium, 75mg chol, 638mg potassium, 118mg calcium

* Other protein sources such as turkey breast; tofu chunks, fish or lean meat can be substituted (about 2 lbs).

* Chinese Cabbage, Spinach, Watercress, Escarole, Broccoli, Romaine Lettuce or any other leafy greens can be used as a substitute for the Bok Choy.

** Vegetarian Alternative. Substitute chicken bouillon and water with low sodium vegetable broth. Substitute meat with firm Tofu. (Cut tofu into 1-inch cubes. Season with 1 1/2 tbs. low sodium soy sauce. Brown in a non-stick pan with a small amount of cooking spray or canola oil. Add to cooked soup.

Barley, pearled: You can also add 4 cups cooked parley to soup and serve as a complete meal.

*Therese*

**Chicken Picata Platter (Recipe 74)**

4- (4) oz boneless/skinless chicken breast (1lb)
1 cup oat bran
1 tbsp extra virgin olive oil
1 tbsp margarine or I can't Believe It's Not Butter
8 oz low sodium chicken broth
1 tbsp capers, washed
1 tsp garlic powder
3 tbsp fresh lemon juice
Seasoning salt-pinch or Mrs. Dash
Salt and black pepper to taste
Chopped basal or cilantro for garnish

**Instructions:**

1. Heat oil and butter in a large skillet
2. Coat each chicken breast in oat bran., seasoning salt, and garlic powder
3. Place in a pan and cook 5-7 minutes on each side over medium heat
4. Remove from pan
5. Add broth and capers and bring to a boil
6. Reduce heat and add chicken with liquid
7. Cook 1-2 minutes over medium heat
8. Remove chicken and place on platter
9. Pour liquid over chicken and garnish with chopped fresh basil or cilantro and lemon juice, including salt and black pepper to taste
10. Serving size is 4 oz chicken in a 6 oz portion. Serves 4

Stats: 245 cal, 28g protein, 18 g carb, 10.6g fat, 2g sat, 4g fiber, 170mg sodium, 64mg chol, 344mg potassium, 31mg calcium

*Cheryl*

**Zesty Gazpacho With Seafood (Recipe 75a)**

2 cups low sodium V-8 juice
2 cups low sodium tomato juice
1 cucumber, cut into small chunks
2 tbsp celery, finely chopped
1 garlic clove, crushed
2 tbsp extra virgin oil
2 tbsp fresh lemon juice
3 tbsp fresh cilantro, chopped
1 cup crushed canned tomatoes
1 sweet yellow onion, chopped
4 oz clams, canned, drained
6 oz shrimp, cooked
Salt, ground black pepper, tobacco sauce to taste

**Instructions:**

1. Cut the cucumber into small chunks and chop coarsely in food processor. Transfer to a mixing bowl
2. Cut the following vegetables (pepper, onion, garlic) in chunks and process until finely chopped. Add to the cucumber bowl
3. Cut celery into small chunks and add to cucumber mixture
4. Add to the cucumber mixture the crushed tomatoes, tomato juice, V-8 juice, lemon juice, olive oil, cilantro, salt, black pepper, and Tabasco sauce to taste
5. Refrigerate to chill for about 2 hours
6. Serving size is about 2 cups. Serves 3
   Stats: 273 cal, 25g protein, 18g carb, 11g fat, 1.4g sat, 3.3g fiber, 316mg sodium, 137mg chol, 637mg potassium, 110mg calcium

**Grilled Tuna Steaks (Recipe 75b)**

4- (4 ounce steaks) of tuna or salmon
1tsp lemon juice
¼ tsp dill weed (dry or fresh)
Salt and black pepper to taste

**Instructions:**

1. Season steaks with lemon juice, salt, and black pepper
2. Spray inside a grill pan with canola oil cooking spray
3. Layer steaks and cook until done
4. Turn the steaks every few minutes
5. Garnish with dill and lemon wedges

6. Serving size is 4 oz Serves 4
   Stats: 163 cal, 26g protein, 0g carb, 5.5g fat, 1.4g sat, 0g fiber, 44mg sodium, 43mg chol, 286mg potassium, 9mg calcium

**Couscous Salad (Recipe 76)**

¾ cup water (boiled)
½ cup couscous, dry
2 tbsp chopped, scallions
½ cup chickpeas (canned, drained)
1 English cucumber, chopped
2 tbsp lemon juice
1 tbsp olive oil
Salt and pepper to taste.

**Instructions:**

1. In a pot bring water to a boil. Add couscous and scallions. Shut off heat. Cover and let stand for 5 to 10 minutes. Liquid should be absorbed
2. In a bowl, combine lemon juice and olive oil. Season with salt and pepper
3. Pour over chickpeas and chopped cucumber
4. Stir in couscous. Serve warm or cold
5. Serving size is 1 cup. Serves 5
   Stats: 135 cal, 5g protein, 21g carb, 3.7g fat, 0.5g sat, 2g fiber, 79mg sodium, 1mg chol, 144mg potassium, 23mg calcium

*Sonia*

**String Beans Casserole (Recipe 77)**

2.5 pkg (10oz each) green snap/string beans, frozen
2 medium onions, chopped
2 tbsp fresh parsley, chopped
4 garlic cloves, chopped
2 tbsp extra virgin olive oil
6 oz *Progresso* tomato paste, canned
Salt and pepper to taste

**Instructions:**

1. Sauté onion and garlic in olive oil, add tomato paste
2. Simmer adding a little water, salt, and pepper
3. Add string beans and enough water to cover the beans
4. Cook for 1.5 hours until beans are tender
5. Serving size is 1 cup. Serves 6
   Stats: 130 cal, 5g protein, 20g carb, 5g fat, 0.7g sat, 5.3g fiber, 23mg sodium, 0mg chol, 315mg potassium, 68mg calcium

*Aronis*

**Chickpea and Tuna Salad (Recipe 78)**

2 cans chickpeas w/fluid (low sodium)
2 cans Italian tuna (Torino or Genova)
½ cup fresh parsley
1 small red onion, thinly sliced
4 tsp olive oil
1 tbsp Vinegar
2 red wine vinegar or fresh lemon juice
Salt and pepper to taste
1 tsp *Good Seasons* salad dressing (dry)

**Instructions:**

1. Pour chickpeas w/fluid into a small pan
2. Simmer gently for 2 hours, adding water as needed
3. Drain peas and transfer into a bowl. While the chickpeas are still hot, add tuna (but break apart before adding to chickpeas)
4. Add chopped parsley, sliced red onion and olive vinegar dressing
5. Salt and pepper to taste along with 1 tsp *Good Seasons* salad dressing, dry
6. If made one day ahead, it tastes even better
7. Serving size is 1.5 cup or 12 oz portion. Recipe serves 4
   Stats: 285 cal, 26g protein, 15g carb, 13g fat, 2g sat, 4g fiber, 525mg sodium, 26mg chol, 340mg potassium, 42mg calcium

*Joan*

**Baked Chicken With Stuffed Sun Dried Tomatoes and Feta Cheese (Recipe 79)**

2 boneless chicken breasts, skinless (about 32 oz)
2 tbsp feta cheese, crumbled
2 cups chopped fresh spinach
1 cup chopped cilantro
1 oz sun dried tomatoes, cut in strips
1 tsp minced garlic
2 tbsp olive oil
Salt and ground black pepper to taste

**Instructions:**

1. Preheat oven to 350 degrees F
2. In a skillet, wilt spinach in a small amount of oil
3. Add tomatoes and garlic and cook an additional 1 minute
4. Season with salt and pepper. Let cool
5. Cut a pocket lengthwise on each chicken breast
6. Stuff each breast with half of the filling
7. Top filling with feta cheese
8. Secure with a toothpick
9. Season chicken with salt and black ground pepper to taste

10. In the cleaned skillet heat the remaining 1-tablespoon oil over moderately high heat until hot but not smoking
11. Brown the chicken on both sides
12. Transfer skillet to oven and bake until cooked through
13. Serving size is 5-6 oz portion. Serves 6
    Stats: 242 cal, 33g protein, 6g carb, 9g fat, 2g sat, 1.4g fiber, 312mg sodium, 86mg chol, 687mg potassium, 62mg calcium

**Roasted Asparagus and Zucchini (Recipe 80)**

1 red bell pepper, cut in lengthwise strips
1 green bell pepper, cut in strips
1 ½ red onion, sliced
1 large tomato, cut in chunks
1 zucchini, sliced
1 bunch asparagus
1 small-medium sized eggplant, cut in chunks
½ tbsp extra virgin olive oil
½ tsp garlic, minced
Salt and pepper to taste

**Instructions:**

1. Chop veggies into large cubes or slices, add to bowl - toss with ½ tbsp olive oil and add garlic, salt, and pepper to taste. You may add herbs (thyme, rosemary, basil, etc.) to taste
2. Spread veggies on baking sheet or heavy-duty aluminum foil. Double fold top and ends to seal, leaving some room for steam
3. Roast at 450° F for 20-25 minutes or 10-15 minutes in covered grill
4. Serving size is about 1 cup or 7 oz portion. Serves 4
   Stats: 67 cal, 2g protein, 12g carb, 2g fat, 0.3g sat, 4g fiber, 6mg sodium, 0mg chol, 379mg potassium, 22mg calcium

*Rosemary*

**Pan –Roasted Lemon and Pepper Salmon With Spinach (Recipe 81)**

4- (4 ounce) portions salmon fillet, skin on
1 tbsp extra virgin olive oil
4 tbsp chopped celery
2 cloves minced garlic
1 tsp cracked black pepper
1 each bay leaf
1 tsp lemon pepper or Mrs. Lemon Pepper Seasoning
1 medium lemon juice
4 cups fresh spinach
¼ cup water
½ tsp salt
Garlic powder, black or crushed pepper to taste

**Instructions:**

1. Heat a non-stick skillet to medium-high heat
2. Place the oil in the pan and swirl to coat the bottom
3. Add the celery, garlic, and bay leaf and cook for 1 minute
4. Rub the salmon with salt, pepper, and garlic
5. Place the fish skin-side down on the skillet and cook for 5 minutes and turn
6. Move the fish to the sides of the pan
7. Add the spinach in the middle
8. Add the lemon juice and water
9. Reduce heat to medium-low and cook for 5 minutes
10. Serving size is 4 oz salmon in 8 oz portion. Serves 4
    Stats: 225 cal, 25g protein, 7g carb, 11g fat, 1.7g sat, 1g fiber, 394mg sodium, 62mg chol, 937mg potassium, 112mg calcium
    *Cod, snapper or tuna can be substituted.*

**Baked Chicken Thighs With Fennel (Recipe 82)**

6 chicken thighs or 24 oz boneless chicken breast, cut into 4 oz portions
2 tbsp extra virgin olive oil
1 fennel bulb
1 red onion, chopped
3 garlic cloves, chopped
½ tsp oregano, dried
½ cup sun dried tomatoes
Salt and black pepper to taste

**Instructions:**

1. Preheat oven to 450 degrees
2. Season the chicken thighs with salt and pepper
3. In a skillet heat oil until hot or shimmering, but not smoking
4. Cook chicken thighs (skin down) over medium heat until golden and crispy, 8-10 minutes
5. Turn the chicken thighs and brown for about 2-3 minutes more
6. Transfer chicken to a plate
7. Add the onions, garlic, oregano, red pepper flakes, and fennel and cook for about 3 minutes or until the vegetables begin to wilt
8. Add the tomatoes and the chicken (skin side up) on top of the vegetables
9. Transfer skillet to oven and bake uncovered until the chicken is cooked through (about 20-30minutes)
10. Serving size is 1 thigh. Serves 6
    Stats: 222 cal, 23g protein, 8g carb, 11g fat, 0.7g sat, 2g fiber, 115mg sodium, 0mg chol, 353mg potassium, 32mg calcium

**Chicken Noodle Soup (Recipe 83)**

4 cups low sodium chicken broth
½ tsp ground basil

1 tsp minced garlic
½ whole onion
3 oz chicken breast, cut into small chunks
1 cup water
½ cup vermicelli pasta noodles
Salt and black pepper to taste

**Instructions:**

1. Add all the ingredients, except vermicelli, and bring to a boil
2. Add noodles and cook over medium heat for about 3-5 minutes
3. Serve one or cold
4. Serving size is 1 cup. Serves 6
   Stats: 82 cal, 6g protein, 9g carb, 2.5g fat, 0.9g sat, 0.5g fiber, 82mg sodium, 12mg chol, 53mg potassium, 19mg calcium

*Anne*

**Turkey Meatloaf (Recipe 84)**

1 lb lean ground turkey
¼ cup salsa (see recipe 18b or 39c)
2 whole eggs
¼ cup oatmeal
1 tbsp wheat germ
¼ cup oat bran
1 tsp minced garlic
Salt and pepper to taste

**Instructions:**

1. Combine all ingredients
2. Shape into a loaf
3. Bake in preheated oven at 350
4. Serving size is 5 oz portion. Serves 5
5. Serving suggestions: 1) Serve meat loaf wrapped in two lettuce leaves and top with salsa. 2) Wrap in a pita or tortilla with shredded lettuce and salsa. 3) Make a sandwich with lettuce, salsa, and a slice of low-fat cheese
   Stats: 290 cal, 29g protein, 11g carb, 13.5g fat, 4.6g sat, 3g fiber, 520mg sodium, 166mg chol, 359mg potassium, 308mg calcium

*Karen*

**Romaine Radish Salad (Recipe 85)**

2 cups romaine, arugula or escarole
2 red radishes, sliced
1 fresh Roma tomato, sliced
1 large red onion slice

***Dressing:***

1 tsp extra virgin olive oil
1 tbsp apple cider vinegar
1 tbsp fresh lime juice

½ tsp yellow mustard or Dijon mustard
¼ tsp mined garlic
Salt and black pepper to taste

**Instructions:**

1. Combine all the ingredients and dress with mustard dressing
   Stats: 94 cal, 3g protein, 11g carb, 5g fat, 0.7g sat, 4g fiber, 50 mg sodium, 0mg chol, 566mg potassium, 58mg calcium

**Steamed Cabbage/Chinese Cabbage (Recipe 86)**

4 cups cabbage, shredded (kale, Napa cabbage or mustard greens)
1 tsp minced garlic
½ cup water
Salt and pepper to taste

**Instructions:**

1. Steam seasoned cabbage until tender
2. Serving size is slightly over 1 cup. Serves 2
   Stats: 26 cal, 2g protein, 5g carb, 0g fat, 0g sat, 0g fiber, 26 mg sodium, 0mg chol, 189mg potassium, 64mg calcium

**Italian Style Peas and Mushroom Sauté (Recipe 87)**

2 cups green peas, frozen
1 small red onion, chopped
1-cup mushroom, slices/pieces, canned
1 tbsp canola oil

**Instructions:**

1. Sauté chopped onions in olive oil
2. Add 2 cups frozen green peas or 10oz pkg frozen, thawed/drained
3. Add 1 cup chopped button canned mushroom
4. Sauté mixing frequently to prevent burning
5. Add salt and black pepper to taste
6. Transfer to oven and bake in 350 degree until tender
7. Serving size is ¾ cup. Serves 4
   Stats: 102 cal, 5g protein, 13g carb, 3.8g fat, 0.3g sat, 4.5g fiber, 247mg sodium, 0mg chol, 182mg potassium, 23mg calcium

*You can substitute the peas with soybeans or edamame*

*Karen*

**Spinach and Feta Wrap (Recipe 88)**

2 cups fresh whole leaf spinach (escarole, arugula or romaine)
1 tbsp olive oil
½ tsp chopped garlic or onions
½ cup jumbo pitted black olives, sliced
¼ cup low-fat Feta cheese
8 oz chicken breast, without skin

1 tbsp fresh lemon juice
3 tbsp apple cider vinegar
½ cup strawberries, whole
2 small oat bran/whole-wheat tortillas or pita bread (*Joseph's*) or ½ whole-wheat pita per person
Salt, peppers and seasonings to taste

**Instructions:**

1. Wash spinach and set aside
2. Finely mince the garlic and combine with olive oil and lemon juice
3. Marinade chicken breast in balsamic marinade (balsamic vinegar, pepper, salt, and seasonings)
4. Broil chicken breast until done (about 30 minutes)
5. Fill the wrap with spinach and remaining ingredients
6. Cut chicken into strips
7. Season with the lemon juice mixture and roll closed
8. Serving size is 6 oz portion. Serves 2
   Stats: 285 cal, 29g protein, 18g carb, 12.7g fat, 1.5g sat, 7g fiber, 641mg sodium, 51mg chol, 641mg potassium, 79mg calcium

*Doreen.*

**Roast Beef Pocket Sandwich (Recipe 89)**

1 tbsp low sodium lite mayonnaise or ½ tsp Dijon mustard
½ tsp horseradish
2 tbsp fat free sour cream
1 oz lite provolone cheese or 1 tbsp feta cheese, crumbled
1 cup shredded lettuce leaves (romaine, spinach, or arugula)
3 oz thinly sliced roasted lean roast beef
1 oat bran/whole-wheat tortilla or pita (*Joseph's*), or sourdough bread

**Instructions:**

1. Combine the mayonnaise, horseradish, and sour cream in a small bowl
2. Cut the tortilla or ½ whole-wheat pita pocket in half crosswise
3. Spread the mayonnaise or mustard mixture on the inside of the bread
4. Top with cheese, roast beef slices, and shredded lettuce leaves
5. Season with salt and pepper to taste
6. Close the sandwich and enjoy
7. Serving size is 8 oz portion. Serves 1
   Stats: 282 cal, 35g protein, 17g carb, 9.5g fat, 3.6g sat, 7g fiber, 626mg sodium, 81mg chol, 709mg potassium, 136mg calcium

**Seafood Picata Platter (Recipe 90)**

8 oz medium-large shrimps, cut
8 oz scallops, cut
1 tsp garlic powder
¼ cup fresh chopped parsley or cilantro
1 tbsp capers

1 tbsp *I Can't Believe It's Not Butter* or tub margarine
1 tbsp canola oil
3/4-cup oat bran
1-cup low sodium chicken broth
Salt and black pepper or red pepper flakes to taste

**Instructions:**

1. Heat oil and butter in a large skillet
2. Coat shrimp and scallops with oat bran, garlic powder, seasoning salt or salt, and pepper to taste
3. Place in pan. Lightly brown seafood/cook until done
4. Remove seafood from pan
5. Add broth and capers to pan. Bring to a boil
6. Reduce heat and add seafood with liquid
7. Cook 1-5 minutes over medium heat
8. Remove seafood and place on platter
9. Pour liquid over seafood
10. Garnish with chopped fresh parsley, lemon juice, salt, and pepper to taste
11. Serving size is 4 oz seafood in 7 oz portion. Serves 4
    Stats: 218 cal, 25g protein, 15g carb, 9g fat, 1.4g sat, 3g fiber, 293mg sodium, 106mg chol, 417mg potassium, 64mg calcium
    *You can use white fish, such as cod, swordfish, scrod or halibut--cut into chunks.*

**Sugar Snap Peas With Lemon Basil (Recipe 91)**

1 cup sugar snap peas
1 tbsp canola oil
2 cups chopped fresh basil
½ tsp grated lemon zest
Salt and black pepper to taste

**Instructions:**

1. Heat oil in nonstick skillet
2. Add peas and stir-fry until tender (but still crisp)
3. Sprinkle in basil, lemon zest, salt, and black pepper to taste
4. Serving size is 2 oz or ¼ cup. Serves 4
   Stats: 68 cal, 3g protein, 9g carb, 2g fat, 0.9g sat, 2g fiber, 28mg sodium, 0mg chol, 51mg potassium, 112mg calcium

**Sharon's Lunch: Fresh Seasonal Vegetables (Recipe 92)**

¼ summer squash or zucchini, raw, slices
3 asparagus spears
1-cup spinach
½ red tomato, slices
½ cup romaine or arugula lettuce
½ orange, slices
¼ cup eggplant, boiled/drained

3-4 oz chicken breast, roasted, baked, or grilled
1 tsp extra virgin olive oil
2 tbsp red wine vinegar
½ cup skim or 1% milk
3 fat free whole-wheat crackers or 1 slice toasted multigrain bread
Salt and black pepper to taste

**Instructions:**

1. Combine all the vegetables and fruit and toss well
2. Add the oil and season with Mrs. Dash or salt and black pepper to taste
3. Break baked or broiled fish in bite size pieces and add to the salad
4. Serve with crackers or toasted bread
5. Serving size is 3-4 oz chicken in 19 oz portion. Serves 1
   Stats: 330.5 cal, 35.6g protein, 30g carb, 8.6g fat, 2g sat, 8g fiber, 208mg sodium, 69mg chol, 1,313mg potassium, 396mg calcium

*Sharon*

**Beef and Mushroom Stir-Fry (Recipe 93)**

3/4 lb (12 oz) beef top round steaks (cut into thin slices)
3 cups fresh shiitake or button mushrooms, chopped, stems removed
3 tbsp chopped green onion, including tops, sliced
3 tsp minced garlic
3 cups chopped bok choy or Chinese cabbage
3 tbsp chopped sweet red bell peppers
½ cup chicken broth (low sodium)
3 tbsp lite soy sauce (low sodium)
3 tsp olive oil
1 ½ tsp sesame oil or canola oil
2 tbsp sherry wine
1.5 cup vermicelli noodles, cooked (recipe 22)
Salt and pepper to taste

**Instructions:**

1. Very thinly slice the flank steak and add the soy, sherry, and oils
2. Marinate for 5 minutes
3. Heat a non-stick skillet to high heat and add the beef. Sauté for 5 minutes and set aside
4. Using the same skillet, add the garlic, onions, and vegetables and cook for 5 minutes stirring constantly
5. Turn off heat, return the beef and combine
6. Place the cooked, warm noodles (about ½-1 cup) on a plate and serve the stir-fry over the noodles. The noodles will soak up the sauce
7. Serving size is 4 oz meat in 12 oz portion. Serves 3
   Stats: 368 cal, 28g protein, 27g carb, 16g fat, 4.7g sat, 3g fiber, 220mg sodium, 95mg chol, 987mg potassium, 48mg calcium

*You may substitute the beef with chicken or turkey meat. You may also substitute the noodles for ½-1 cup cooked Brown rice or stuffed into 1 oat bran/whole-wheat pita bread (Joseph's).*

**Garlic and Herb Crusted Salmon (Recipe 94)**

4 (4 ounces) salmon fillets
2 tbsp Dijon mustard
¼ cup white rice vinegar
2 garlic cloves, thinly sliced or 1 tsp minced garlic
½ red onion, thinly sliced
2 tbsp chopped fresh basil
2 tbsp chopped fresh thyme
2 tbsp chopped fresh sage
2 tbsp chopped fresh thyme
2 tbsp chopped fresh rosemary
2 tbsp chopped fresh oregano
Salt and pepper to taste

**Instructions:**

1. Preheat broiler
2. Spay a baking pan with cooking spray
3. Season the fish fillets with salt and pepper and marinade in vinegar for about 30-60 minutes
4. When ready arrange the salmon skin side down in the baking pan lined with baking sheet
5. Spread mustard on salmon fillets and then top with the herbs
6. Finish with minced garlic and onion slices on top salmon fillets
7. Season with salt and fresh ground black pepper to taste
8. Broil evenly: for about 6-10 minutes in one direction and turn pan 180 degrees and broil another 6-10 minutes or until done
9. Fish is done when easily flaky with a fork or garlic is crusted (brown)
10. Serves with lemon wedges
11. Serving size is 4 oz salmon. Serves 4
    Stats: 184 cal, 23.5g protein, 4g carb, 8g fat, 1g sat, 1g fiber, 240mg sodium, 62mg chol, 634mg potassium, 53mg calcium

*Karen*

**Escarole and Beans (Recipe 95)**

2 heads escarole
1- 19 oz can Cannellini beans
1 tbsp extra virgin olive oil
1 clove garlic, chopped
Salt and crushed red pepper flakes to taste

**Instructions:**

1. Wash escarole in cool water

2. Remove stem first to facilitate sand removal - save tender light green or white interior for salads
3. Boil or steam escarole until tender - drain and squeeze to remove bitterness
4. Sautee with olive oil, chopped garlic and pepper flakes
5. Add Cannellini beans and cook until beans are heated through
6. Serving size is 1 cup. Serves 7
   Stats: 103 cal, 5g protein, 16g carb, 2.5g fat, 0.3g sat, 8g fiber, 192mg sodium, 0mg chol, 462mg potassium, 101mg calcium

*Rosemary*

**Haddock Fillets (Recipe 96)**

1 lb haddock fillet (4 x 4 oz fillets)
1 can plum whole tomatoes
1 small onion, chopped
2 cloves garlic, chopped
¾ cup white wine
1 head fennel, thinly sliced
2 tbsp extra virgin olive oil
1 tbsp capers
12 green olives, silted

**Instructions:**

1. Cook onion and garlic in olive oil until translucent
2. Drain tomatoes and save liquid for another use if desired, coarsely chop or break up tomatoes
3. Add tomatoes and wine to onions and garlic
4. Add fish, some leaves from the fennel and thin slices of fennel
5. Cover and poach for 20 minutes. May be garnished with capers and green olives
6. Serving size is 4 oz fish in 13 oz portion. Serves 4
   Stats: 261 cal, 23g protein, 13g carb, 10g fat, 1g sat, 3g fiber, 559mg sodium, 65mg chol, 887mg potassium, 107mg calcium

*Rosemary*

**Mashed Celeriac (Recipe 97)**

1 lb celeriac, peeled and cut into small pieces
2 tbsp non-fat yogurt or plain
1 tsp ground cinnamon

**Instruction:**

1. Peel off the outer skin. Cut into small pieces and boil in water until soft
2. Put soft, hot celeriac pieces in food processor and puree
3. Add yogurt and cinnamon. Mix well
4. Serving size is ½ cup. Serves 3
   Stats: 99 cal, 3g protein, 18g carb, 3g fat, 0.5g sat, 5g fiber, 186mg sodium, 0mg chol, 563mg potassium, 86mg calcium

*Sharon*

**Cucumber Tomato Salad (Recipe 98)**

½ cup red tomatoes, chopped
½ cup cucumber slices
2 tsp red onion slices
1 tsp fresh parsley, chopped
2 tbsp red wine vinegar
Salt and black pepper or Mrs. Dash to taste

**Instructions:**

1. Assemble vegetables and dress with dressing
2. Garnish with parsley
   Stats: 29 cal, 1g protein, 6g carb, 0.4g fat, 0g sat, 1.5g fiber, 13mg sodium, 0mg chol, 289mg potassium, 16 mg calcium

**Grilled Eggplant (Recipe 99a)**

½ whole eggplant, raw, unpeeled
¼ yellow summer squash, sliced
¼ red bell pepper, sliced
1 tsp garlic powder
1 tsp onion powder
1 tsp canola oil

**Instruction:**

1. Make a paste of the garlic powder, onion powder, and canola oil
2. Brush the paste on sliced vegetables and grill until brown on both sides
3. Serving size is 5 oz portion. Serves 2
   Stats: 59 cal, 2g protein, 9g carb, 2g fat, 0g sat, 3g fiber, 4mg sodium, 0mg chol, 307mg potassium, 14mg calcium

*Sharon*

**Eggplant and Cheese Wrap (Recipe 99b)**

1 large eggplant or 8-10 ounce
2 garlic cloves, finely chopped
1 cup Contadina tomato sauce
1 tsp canola oil
1 package frozen spinach, thawed and strained
4 tbsp grated Parmesan cheese
3 tbsp shredded mozzarella
4 large romaine leaves
Salt and ground black pepper to taste

**Instructions:**

1. Preheat the oven to 350 degrees F
2. Wash the eggplant, cut off the tips and slice lengthwise into thick slices and spread in a baking sheet that has been sprayed with cooking spray
3. Coat eggplants with salt and ground black pepper

4. Combine the spinach, garlic, oil, Parmesan, and mozzarella cheese in a bowl and mix well. Season to taste with salt and pepper
5. Cover the eggplants with the spinach, garlic, oil, and cheese preparation.
6. Top with tomato sauce
7. Cover with aluminum foil and bake for 35-45 minutes or until done.
8. Put aside to cool
9. Place 2 large romaine leaves on a plate (serves 2)
10. Top with half the baked eggplant. Roll and enjoy
11. Serving size is 1 cup or 10 oz portion. Serves 2
    Stats: 256 cal, 28g protein, 25g carb, 7g fat, 3g sat, 9.4g fiber, 520mg sodium, 15mg chol, 990mg potassium, 505mg calcium

**Garlic Tilapia (Recipe 100)**

2- (4 oz) tilapia fillet
6 garlic cloves
4 tsp olive oil
2 eggs white
4 tbsp whole-wheat flour or unprocessed bran
½ cup dry white wine
½ tsp ground white pepper
4 tsp capers
¼ tsp Tabasco pepper sauce (optional)
Salt and pepper to taste

**Instructions:**

1. Combine the flour, salt, and white pepper
2. Dust the fish with the seasoned flour
3. Beat the egg white until frothy and cover the dusted fillet with the beaten egg white
4. Heat a non-stick skillet to medium-high heat
5. Add the oil and garlic. Cook until garlic turns brown. Turn frequently
6. Add the fillet
7. Cook for about 3 minutes on each side to golden brown
8. Add the remaining ingredients (white wine, capers, and Tabasco sauce)
9. Bring to a simmer to burn off alcohol completely
10. Serve hot
11. Serving size is 4 oz fish in a 8 oz portion. Serves 2
    Stats: 255 cal, 26g protein, 14g carb, 10g fat, 1g sat, 1g fiber, 332mg sodium, 49mg chol, 553mg potassium, 41mg calcium

    *Salmon, halibut, catfish, cod are all good substitutes*

**Rosemary Apple Baked Pork Tenderloin (Recipe 101)**

12-16 oz pork tenderloin, lean
1.5 tsp canola oil

2 tbsp rosemary, crushed
1 tbsp parsley, flakes
½ medium red onion, slices
1.5 tbsp minced garlic
2 Granny Smith apples
2 cup low sodium chicken broth
Salt and black pepper or Mrs. Dash to taste

**Instructions:**

1. Preheat oven to 400 degrees
2. Line a baking pan with foil, spray with cooking spray and place in oven
3. Trim fat from pork tenderloins and butterfly the meat – cutting nearly half lengthwise
4. Open the pork tenderloins and lay out and then pound to flatten with the bottom of a heavy skillet
5. Mix the minced garlic, salt, black pepper, or Mrs. Dash seasoning and oil into a paste
6. Rub pork tenderloins all over with the paste, then sprinkle chopped rosemary and chopped parsley on both sides and let marinate in refrigerator 30-60 min
7. Two Granny Smith apples: peel, core and slice
8. Spoon the apple mixture around the pork tenderloins
9. Add chicken broth and onion slices
10. Cover with foil and bake 30-40 minutes
11. Remove the lid or foil and spoon the apple mixture and juice over the tenderloin
12. Return to the oven and bake for another 10-15 minutes without the foil or lid or until pork tenderloins are browned at the top and cook through; apples shrink down and onions are nice and soft
13. Take out of oven and cover again with foil for 5 minutes
14. Take out the pork tenderloins and cut on a board, then place on a platter
15. Arrange apple slices and onion around pork slices
16. Pour broth over dish
17. Serving size is 3-4 oz portion pork in 9 oz meal portion. Serves 4
    Stats: 216 cal, 26g protein, 13g carb, 7g fat, 2g sat, 2g fiber, 104mg sodium, 69mg chol, 523mg potassium, 27mg calcium

*Cheryl*

**Lemon Chicken With Avocado Salad (Recipe 102)**

¼ small ripe avocado, cubed
¼ small red onion, chopped
¼ tsp garlic, minced
¼ cup fresh cilantro, chopped
½ medium tomato, chopped
¼ medium cucumber, seeded and cubed

1 tsp olive oil
1-2 tbsp fresh lime juice
4 oz grilled or baked chicken breast, chopped
Salt and ground black pepper to taste

**Instructions**:

1. Mix all together in a small bowl
2. Chill before serving
3. Serving size 10 oz portion. Serves 1
   Stats: 267 cal, 26g protein, 12g carb, 13.7g fat, 2.6g sat, 5.5g fiber, 60mg sodium, 63mg chol, 683mg potassium, 40mg calcium

**Sushi Tuna Tortilla (Recipe 103)**

1- 6 oz can tuna, drained
½ cup celery, chopped
2 tbsp light mayonnaise, low sodium
1 cup chopped romaine lettuce
½ cup chopped red bell pepper
2 tsp chopped red onion
1 tsp fresh lemon juice
½ tsp black pepper
2 oat bran/whole-wheat tortillas or 1 whole-wheat pita bread

**Instructions:**

1. Break up large chunks of tuna into smaller pieces
2. Mix tuna, mayonnaise, peppers, onion, and celery
3. Place half the tuna salad and lettuce on each tortilla
4. Roll tortillas or whole-wheat pita bread and trim the ends off
5. Cut each roll into 4 pieces and close with toothpick
6. Serving size is 3 oz tuna in 8 oz portion. Serves 2
   Stats: 226 cal, 28g protein, 17g carb, 6g fat, 1.7g sat, 8g fiber, 769mg sodium, 41mg chol, 451mg potassium, 41mg calcium

**Vegetable Stir-Fry (Recipe 104)**

2 cups medium diced tofu or 2 cups diced chicken or white fish
1 cup snow peas (stems removed)
1 cup chopped mushrooms
½ cup chopped onion
½ cup chopped red peppers
2 tbsp canola oil
½ tsp sesame oil
3 tbsp low sodium soy sauce (*Kikkoman* lite soy sauce)

**Introductions:**

1. Heat a pan to high heat and add the oil
2. Add the vegetables and pan fry for 4 minutes, turning constantly

3. Add the tofu and cook for 4 additional minutes
4. Finish with the soy sauce, mix well and serve
5. Serving size is 1 cup. Serves 4
   Stats: 136 cal, 11g protein, 9g carb, 7.5g fat, 1g sat, 2g fiber, 199mg sodium, 0mg chol, 472mg potassium, 61mg calcium

**Sauteed Garlic Shrimp (Recipe 105)**

12 medium-large shrimp, cleaned, shelled deveined
1 tsp minced garlic
¼ small onion slices
1 tsp soft margarine
¼ tsp red pepper flakes
1 tbsp old bay
1 tsp olive oil or canola oil
Salt and black pepper to taste
Lemon wedges

**Instructions:**

1. Season shrimp with old bay, pepper flakes and garlic
2. Saute shrimp with onions in margarine and oil until done
3. Serve with lemon wedges. Serving size is 4 shrimps. Serves 3
   Stats: 46 cal, 5g protein, 3g carb, 1.5g fat, 0.2g sat, 0.5g fiber, 65mg sodium, 47mg chol, 87mg potassium, 16mg calcium

**Tofu Steak Saute (Recipe 106)**

8 oz extra firm tofu or 4 oz lean steak
2 tbsp chopped yellow onion
1 garlic clove, chopped
¼ chicken bouillon, dry, low sodium or Mrs. Dash
1 tbsp fresh parsley, chopped
¼ cup water
1 cup green peas, canned, drained
1 cup mushrooms, sliced
½ cup strawberries
Cooking spray, olive, or canola

**Instructions:**

1. Use 8 ounces of tofu at 4 ounces per piece
2. Season the tofu with the bouillon powder or Mrs. Dash
3. Heat a non-stick pan to medium-high heat and spay lightly with cooking spray
4. Sauté the tofu on both sides to a crispy texture
5. Add the onions, garlic mushrooms and parsley and cook until translucent. Add the water and peas and cook for 2 minutes
6. Place the cooked tofu on plate and accompany with strawberries
7. Serving size is 4 oz tofu in 18 oz portion. Serves 2

Stats: 196 cal, 17g protein, 18g carb, 8g fat, 1g sat, 5g fiber, 369mg sodium, 0mg chol, 522mg potassium, 150mg calcium

**Blueberry and Yogurt Sorbet (Recipe 107)**

½ cup frozen blueberries, unsweetened
¼ cup frozen strawberries, unsweetened
½ cup 2% milk, cold
2 pct Splenda or 2 tsp sugar
3 kiwi slices, for garnish
6 oz yogurt-plain or non-fat, low sugar
2 tsp canola, sesame, or olive oil

**Instructions:**

1. Combine all the ingredients and blend until smooth
2. Garnish with kiwi slices
3. Serving size is 4 oz (snack size) portion. Serves 4
   Stats: 89 cal, 4g protein, 10.6g carb, 5g sugar, 3.7g fat, 1g sat, 1g fiber, 49mg sodium, 7mg chol, 196mg potassium, 124mg calcium

**Sweet Fruits Sorbet (Recipe 108)**

1 cup ripe cantaloupe, slices
1 cup watermelon, diced
½ cup pineapple, chunks, canned
1 tsp sugar
2-pct Splenda/Stevia
1 tsp fresh peppermint

**Instructions:**

1. Remove the seeds from the cantaloupe and watermelon
2. Place the melon flesh in a blender
3. Add the rest of the ingredients and blend until smooth
4. Pour into plastic containers and freeze until firm
5. Serve chilled
6. Serving size is 4 oz portion or snack size. Serves 4
   Stats: 45 cal, 0.8g protein, 10.5g carb, 8g sugar, 0.2g fat, 0g sat, 1g fiber, 4mg sodium, 0mg chol, 198mg potassium, 13mg calcium

**Chocolate Pineapple Sorbet (Recipe 109)**

½ cup 2% cold milk
4 oz non-fat, low sugar yogurt or plain yogurt
1 ½ tbsp Hershey's unsweetened cocoa powder
2 tsp sesame seed oil or vegetable oil
½ cup pineapple chunks in water
3 pct Splenda/Stevia
½ tsp vanilla extract
5 ice cubes

**Instructions:**

1. Combine all ingredients and blend to a smooth consistency
2. Serve immediately or freeze
3. Serving size is 6 oz portion. Serves 3

   Stats: 86 cal, 4g protein, 10g carb, 4g sugar, 3.8g fat, 1g sat, 0.7g fiber, 49mg sodium, 7mg chol, 49mg potassium, 125mg calcium

**Baked Sirloin Steak (Recipe 110)**

2-(4 oz), ½ inch thick, select sirloin steak
4 cloves garlic
2 sprigs fresh rosemary
2 tbsp fresh chopped parsley
2 sprigs fresh thyme
1/8 tsp crushed dry pepper
1 tsp extra virgin olive oil
Salt and black pepper to taste

**Instructions:**

1. In food processor, combine, garlic, fresh herbs, pepper, and olive oil
2. Blend until smooth. Rub the paste on the steak. Let marinade in the refrigerator from 30 minutes to 1 hour
3. Grill steak, uncovered over high heat 4 to 6 minutes on each side in
4. Place in a 350-degree preheated oven
5. Cook for an additional 15 to 20 minutes or until desired doneness
6. Serving serve is 4 oz portion. Serves 2

   Stats: 177 cal, 25g protein, 3g carb, 7g fat, 2g sat, 1g fiber, 69mg sodium, 67mg chol, 484mg potassium, 39mg calcium

**Lemon String Beans (Recipe 111)**

1 frozen 10 oz pkt string beans
½ medium onion, chopped
¼ tsp sweet basil, dried
1.5 tbsp lemon juice or ½ lemon
2 cans or 4 cups low sodium chicken broth
1 tsp garlic powder
2 tsp olive oil
¼ tsp dried dill weed

**Instructions:**

1. Add all the ingredients and simmer 20-25 over low heat
2. Cool and add 1-2 tbsp Mrs. Dash salad dressing, *Walden Farms* dressing, or Diet Italian Salad Dressing, no salt added
3. Serving size is 1 cup. Serves 5

Stats: 66 cal, 4g protein, 7g carb, 3g fat, 0.9g sat, 2g fiber, 88mg sodium, 3mg chol, 132mg potassium, 41mg calcium

*Anne*

## Extra Recipes

**Signature Barley**

1 cup Pearled Barley (dry)
2-½ cups low sodium chicken or vegetable broth
1 cup sliced mushrooms
3 tbsp. Chopped scallions
¼ cup fresh Cilantro, chopped
2 tsp canola or toasted sesame oil

Bring broth to a boil. Add oil. Rinse the barley in cold water. Add barley to the pot along with the sliced mushrooms. Cook for 45 minutes over low heat until barley is tender but chewy. Add chopped scallions and chopped cilantro. Season to taste with black pepper and salt.

Serving size is 4 oz (½ cup). Serves 8.

Stats: 110 cal, 4g protein, 20g carb, 2g fat, 0g sat, 4g fiber, 37mg sodium, 1mg chol, 101mg potassium, 15mg calcium

** For women: Serve with 3-4 oz grilled or baked (skinless) chicken, turkey or other lean cut of meat. For men: Serve with 4-6 oz. grilled or baked (skinless) chicken, turkey or other lean cut of meat.

**Maria's Soup**

1 yellow onion, chopped
1 small green pepper, chopped
5 stalks celery, chopped
2 cups cauliflower
2 cups broccoli flowerets
1 cup summer squash, sliced
1 small eggplant, peeled and chopped
1 chicken cube
4 cups water
8 oz chicken breast, chopped in ½ inch pieces

Bring water to a boil. Add chicken broth, onions and chopped chicken (cook until chicken is well done). Add chopped vegetables and simmer for additional 3-5. Vegetables should be cooked al dente to preserve nutrients. Serving size is 1 cup. Serves 9.

Stats: 66 cal, 4g protein, 7g carb, 3g fat, 0.9g sat, 2g fiber, 184mg sodium, 15mg chol, 462mg potassium, 39mg calcium

## Chapter 18

# Testimonials

### In Their Own Words

In this chapter, diverse selections of patients are presented – giving us their own experience, in their own words. Their story and struggle should be an inspiration to you as you use their experience as a guide for your own adjustments. The names of the contributors in this book have been changed to protect their privacy:

### Sophia, Medical Student At Brown University

**Diagnosis:** Syndrome X, high cholesterol, fatigue, and carbohydrate cravings
**Motivation:** Searching for a permanent solution to her lifelong weight problems

Sophia, a medical student at Brown Medical School, Providence, Rhode Island, has struggled with her weight as long as she could remember. She was also troubled by her family history and didn't want to share the same fate as some of her very close relatives.

"I was tired of the cycles of losing and gaining weight. My most recent attempt left me desperately frustrated, as my weight remained the same for six months. And, frankly, I didn't know what else to do. I had joined a gym and was trying to be faithful to my exercise program but it didn't seem to make a difference. I was at the point of giving up when I came across an article in *The Woman's Page* written by Dr. Billy Johnson, founder of the UDP program. The article immediately caught my interest and I decided to check them out.

"I was impressed by the fact that there were no pre-packaged foods or foods that I had to purchase at a specialty store. There were no diet pills or stimulants. I ate regular grocery foods that I considered healthy for my body. The program was well-structured and held me accountable for my actions. I have better self control than I ever had. That only came after months of hard work.

"I'm still not perfect. But this program does not demand that you be perfect and that's a good thing. I still make bad choices – especially when I'm stressed – but the tendency for me to do so is far less. The good thing is that I'm in control and that has made a big difference.

"Making proper food choices has really made a difference in my energy level. Eating the right kinds of food helps me maintain my energy and concentration.

"Since I've been on the program, I have lost a total of 30 pounds and have lost 5 percent of body fat. I achieved all this in only three months and have been able to maintain it. My concentration and focus are better; I feel great and I am in the best and healthiest physical condition I have ever been in my life. I have made believers of my family and friends and my mother is now in the program as well. It surprises me how simple and easy it was to change my lifestyle. It is not all based on will power, but on giving the body the right nutrients it needs to function properly.

"The main point that UDP has taught me is not to go on a low-carb or low-fat diet because the success of these methods is short lived. Instead, I learned how to eat carbohydrates, proteins and fats according to my body's ability to burn these energy sources. This has made all the difference because I can really do this for the rest of my life without missing out on anything. This is the principle that sets UDP apart from any other program that I have known.

"I am studying to be a physician and I am hoping that what I'm learning here will make me a better and more prepared doctor who will deliver a better quality of care to my patients."

| Stats | Start | Now |
|---|---|---|
| Weight | 160 | 130 |
| Waist | 34½ | 30 |
| Fat | 44 | 34 |
| Total Fat | 74 | 45 |
| Muscle | 86 | 85 |

Update: It has been three years since Sophia reached her weight goal and she has maintained it with ease. I recently saw her, she looked radiant and beautiful and it's amazing how well she is handling her clinical rotations at Brown Medical School.

"What I learned with UDP has definitely helped me to handle the stress of medical school. For one thing, I eat consciously and I do my best to tailor my food intake to my level of physical activity. I'm also handling stress in a positive way giving the pressures of clinical rotation in a major hospital center," she said.

**Melinda, a Nurse**

**Diagnosis:** Inflammatory Bowel Syndrome, Multiple Sclerosis
**Motivation:** To improve the quality of her life

Melinda was 35 when she was diagnosed with inflammatory bowel syndrome and Multiple Sclerosis seven years ago, and had to deal with the psychological trauma that there is no real cure for her diseases.

"Prior to my diagnosis in 2001, I kept going to doctors complaining of severe abdominal bloating, pain and diarrhea, but I was never taken seriously. They gave me pills to take and said that it would be fine. It appeared to me that they were taking my condition lightly. I was angry and frustrated and I wanted somebody to do something about my situation, which was getting worse. Everything I ate rushed out of me in few hours, and I was losing weight. They thought I was suffering from anxiety and stress (my favorite sister-in-law had suddenly died of cerebral hemorrhage at age forty and three days later I had my first symptom). So, it was easy to assume that her death triggered my condition.

"After many months of going to the doctor's office, I was so seriously sick that my husband had to rush me to the emergency room. I was admitted and I stayed in the hospital for an entire month. I was so weak that I was receiving TPN (intravenous nutrition) through a PICC (intravenous line) line for nutrition. After I was sent home I came right back to the hospital with an infection from the PICC line. Following my discharge, I would be right back in the hospital for readmission for abdominal pain and diarrhea. It took me seven months to get back to feeling better after the ordeal, but it didn't last long. I had several flare ups and struggled with my disease for three years until I finally found a doctor that truly understands Chron's disease.

"On top of it all, I was also diagnosed with Multiple Sclerosis (MS) that was characterized by severe and crippling aches and pain throughout my body that made even walking difficult. My legs were so painful it felt like sharp needle pricks. High doses of steroids relieved some of the symptoms, but caused me to gain weight. This was very distressing to me, because I only became overweight as an adult, and being a nurse, I was well aware that the steroids and the other anti-inflammatory medications were the likely culprits. But, I couldn't dare stop them. In addition, I was having other minor health problems that included frequents headache, fatigue, insomnia and anxiety."

"Attacks or flare ups with Multiple Sclerosis was usually in the summer as a result of heat intolerance related to the MS, which some people are prone to for unknown reasons. I knew that I would have to exercise in order to lose the weight that I put on taking steroids, but the MS made it very difficult.

"I did my best to eat a reasonably healthy diet and kept a slightly active lifestyle (yard work and walking outdoors). I also tried to lose weight, and had no success. I was at the point of giving up when my daughter met a friend who told her about the UDP program. I decided to check them out after my daughter encouraged me to join the program.

"Looking back now I can truly say that joining UDP is the best thing that ever happened to me. It only took a few weeks to start feeling better. My energy was up and the pain and aches were not as intense, and I could exercise without difficulty. After a couple of months, I hardly needed medication for pain, which was quite surprising to me and to my doctor too.

"My Crohn's disease is now very well controlled through diet and exercise and using limited amounts of medications. In addition, I have had no need for steroids since starting the UDP program about a year ago, and I continue to eat and enjoy vegetables and fruits that were responsible for triggering Crohn's flare up—causing me so much pain that I avoided them completely.

"My doctor was surprised to find out that I was still eating these foods, especially in the winter with no problems. Usually, I would get a Crohn's flareup in the fall and winter, and my last attack was in late fall of last year before joining UDP. I remembered being in the hospital getting medications and feedings through my veins, and wondering if this is what I would have to put up with for the rest of my life. After I was discharged from the hospital, my daughter suggested trying the UDP program.

"Since joining the UDP program, I have changed my eating and physical activity habits and at the present time I have had no flare up or hospital stay for Crohn's for about a year, which surprised both me and my doctor. I remember that prior to UDP, I had flare up frequently and was never in remission from diagnosis. In order to be in remission you have to be symptom free continuously for six months. I can truly say that there is hope that I can truly enjoy life again, and not worry about crippling abdominal pain and diarrhea when I eat salads and fruits."

Looking back, Melinda recalled the first month with UDP, " I am amazed at how well I feel and look. After just few months into the program, I lost 26 pounds and more importantly, 21 pounds of fat. When I first started, my legs were very painful, and I was on high dose of medication for MS. But, with exercise, almost daily, I felt great improvement with my legs and body pain. My energy was up. "

Melinda lost about forty-five pounds of total weight and 37 pounds body fat in a couple of months, and continues to do substantially well. Even though, the weight loss is quite impressive in itself, but what is truly remarkable, are the improvements in most of her symptoms. As a result, her physicians have reduced the dosage of her medications, thereby, minimizing unwanted side effects, and she has not been on steroids for a long time (which is unusual for MS and Crohn's).

The UDP approach has been to increase the levels of antioxidants and anti-inflammatory foods sources (Omega-3 fatty acids, vitamins and minerals, including vitamin D) in combination with a tolerable level of physical activity that is in line with her food consumption. However, the extent to which she responded is quite unexpected, and may suggest that people with MS and Crohn's could benefit using minimal medical therapy if it is also accompanied with appropriate anti-inflammatory dietary and exercise intervention. Both MS and Crohn's are believed to be due to autoimmune diseases, which are mediated by inflammatory cells (such as T cells). In both cases, the deficiency of activated vitamin D (which is actually a steroid hormone that can turn or inhibit specific gene expression) has been implicated. This would suggest that dietary and physical therapy in these diseases could be highly beneficial.

Melinda still has some distance to go, but she is well aware that this whole process involves a life long commitment, and not a temporal superficial fix. The future for Melinda is brighter today, and holds more promise for health and longevity than she could have ever imagined.

| Stats | Start | Now |
|---|---|---|
| Weight | 249 | 200 |
| Waist | 47 | 37 |
| %Fat | 50 | 43 |
| Total Fat | 126 | 89 |
| Muscle | 124 | 116 |

Note: TPN stands for Total Parenteral Nutrition. This is a complete form of nutrition. It is a technique in which nutrients are given to a person through an intravenous infusion line. TPN is a lifesaver for people who are unable to absorb adequate nutrients from the gut. A PICC line is a special IV line used to provide fluids into a large vein. In general, a PICC line is very stable and lasts longer than a typical intravenous line.

**Michael, Retired Law Officer:**

**Diagnosis:** High cholesterol, chronic pain and low energy
**Motivation:** To lower his cholesterol without medication

Michael retired from law enforcement at age 55, and started a second career in the private sector. A routine visit to his private physician office left him stoned cold and upset. He was told that his total cholesterol and LDL (bad) cholesterol were dangerously high and he needed medication. Concerned about the side effects of cholesterol reducing drugs, he decided to try alternative therapy for a couple of months, and then return for reevaluation. Though his doctor reluctantly agreed, he sent him off with a strong warning and the danger of procrastinating.

Michael came to UDP with mixed emotions, not sure whether he had really made the right decision. It would take at least six weeks for him to find out. He was 6' 2" and weighed 260 pounds with 38% body fat. His BMI was 34---placing him at a higher risk for cardiovascular disease and diabetes, especially with the abnormal lipid profile he had gotten from his doctor (total cholesterol was 257 and LDL (bad) cholesterol was 164).

After the initial complete evaluation and analysis, he was started on an anti-inflammatory diet that was tailored to his level of physical activity and he could not have been happier. Within two weeks, he was feeling good, his energy improved greatly, and he was eating more food than before. By the fifth week, he had enough energy to increase his physical activity level. He had started off concentrating on muscle growth, instead of burning body fat (most men make this mistake). Focusing on aerobics during this early stage worked very well for him.

"I was kind of surprised how quickly I felt more vibrant, healthier and full of energy. It took only 12 weeks to lower my cholesterol from 257 to 176 and my bad cholesterol from 164 to 94. I have no problem staying on the program for the long haul. It is simple and easy to follow and you can make it your own. No calorie counting and definitely no dieting."

Michael's doctor agreed that he had made the right decision, but nevertheless, was skeptical about him staying in the program on a long-term. Michael had no hesitation in assuring him that this was a lifestyle change to which he was totally committed.

"I have forgotten what it feels like to have this amount of energy. This was a big surprise to me. I had no idea that it was possible to still feel the caliber of energy and stamina that I now have."

Michael's progress is steady and will continue to evolve because it's based on the ideal concept of acquisition of new sets of eating and physical activity habits, in combination with stress reduction –such changes can be learned and become a permanent part of one's life.

In three months, Michael lost 37 pounds of body fat and increased his muscle mass by 14 pounds; see the rest of his stats below:

| Stats | Start | Now |
|---|---|---|
| Weight | 260 | 237 |
| Waist | 43 | 41 |
| %Fat | 38 | 26 |
| Total Fat | 99 | 62 |
| Muscle | 161 | 175 |

**Tony, Gentleman and Businessman**

**Diagnosis:** High cholesterol and high blood pressure
**Motivation:** To have a good quality of life

Tony is one of the most gentle and polite persons I have ever known. As a successful businessman, Tony was able to have his own personal trainer to help with his blood pressure and cholesterol. But two years of intensive exercise did very little to change his situation and he was getting frustrated. He realized that medications alone with exercise were inadequate and he wanted to learn how to eat right without giving up on the foods that he liked. His trainer realized that things were not going well and recommended UDP. Tony was surprised that he didn't have to diet or eat pre-packaged foods and drinks. He had choices and he learned to pick ones that were right most of the time. He was never deprived or starved.

Tony lost approximately 37 pounds of body fat while maintaining a healthy muscle mass for over two years running. Though his total weight changed only slightly (judging by the bathroom scale) his progress was extremely good: He lost 18 percent of his body fat and increased his muscle mass by 4-5 percent. This is a classic textbook case that demonstrates the concept that healthy weight loss maintains or promotes muscle growth while melting body fat. As a result, it's easy to maintain the weight loss over a long period of time. In addition, he showed all the benefits of a healthy metabolism – his blood pressure and cholesterol are much better controlled and his energy is up.

"I soon realized that I was learning habits and methods that would result in permanent weight loss. I needed a structured environment and someone who could explain everything so clearly that I truly understand what I need to do to be successful. There is nothing like being perfect in this program and that's what I like about it. I still eat some foods that I know are not good for my cholesterol or blood pressure, but the difference is that I'm more aware and can make up for it or balance the bad foods with lots of good and healthy foods. In fact, sometimes when I eat badly, my body reacts in such a way that I can tell. It is like someone sucked the energy and stamina out of me. The funny thing is that this is the way I used to feel most of the time and thought it was normal. I never want to feel like that anymore. And this motivates me to make better choices most of the time. It is an education and experience that, once you get the knowledge, you can do it forever. This is what sets UDP apart from any other program that I know."

| Stats | Start | Now |
|---|---|---|
| Weight | 197 | 190 |
| Waist | 42 | 36 |
| %Fat | 45 | 27 |
| Total Fat | 89 | 52 |
| Muscle | 133 | 138 |

Update: Tony continues to maintain a healthy body weight and percent body fat. His blood pressure and cholesterol have steadily improved and his energy remains strong.

**Salvatore, Workout Fanatic**

**Diagnosis:** High blood pressure, low HDL (good) cholesterol, high triglycerides, fatigue, and carbohydrate cravings
**Motivation:** To get off medications and build a better quality of life

"Prior to UDP, I was never able to keep the weight off even though I exercised regularly at the gym. I have lost and gained weight on different diets, even on a high-protein diet. My problem was I did not know what and how to eat. Before, I was trying to cut down on a lot of things. With UDP I learned to make better food choices. There are foods that help your body burn calories and fat and there are foods that will do exactly the opposite. These are foods that are right in the regular grocery store and the funny thing is that most of these foods I was already eating. I'm still eating the same foods, but I am more consistent. I could not have made this transformation without understanding the effect of the food I eat on my body and my mood.

"Diets fail because they are not natural. What I'm doing now has helped to keep my mind at ease and body in the shape of fitness that I always wanted it to be. The most important thing is that I'm doing it for myself. Sometimes, when I eat certain foods, it affects my body in a negative way. This makes me believe that it is important to keep my body healthy and fit; otherwise I won't feel right.

"UDP taught me the skills and knowledge that are needed to make the right food choices. I reached my goal in three months and I've kept the weight off since. I'm not worried about gaining weight anymore because I know exactly what to do now, even on holidays. I'm eating real food that I like, my energy is good, my blood pressure is much better controlled, my good cholesterol (HDL) is up by several points and my triglycerides are down to normal."

| Stats | Start | Now |
|---|---|---|
| Weight | 195 | 182 |
| Waist | 42 | 35 |
| %Fat | 36 | 16 |
| Total Fat | 70 | 30 |
| Muscle | 125 | 152 |

Update: Salvatore has maintained a healthy weight and body fat percentage for close to three years now. His blood pressure, cholesterol, and triglycerides are all perfectly normal and his physician has since lowered his medications. He occasionally comes to the office for briefs casual visits. "There is no turning back after you have tasted how it feels to be healthy and full of energy and life," he said.

**Dorothy, Retired School Teacher**

**Diagnosis:** High blood pressure, diabetes, high cholesterol, tarchycardia, depression, carbohydrate cravings, and fatigue
**Motivation:** Tired of being sick and wanted a better quality of life

Dorothy, 68, was eager to find a healthier lifestyle but she didn't know how to go about it. She was frustrated with her life and worried to death that the medications that she was taking were like a bandage that only provided superficial relief. She wanted something more definitive – a cure that worked at the cellular level. A childhood friend that she trusted recommended UDP.

"I was never overly concerned about my weight. I would have loved to be thinner but I enjoyed food too much to switch to low-fat foods. I felt I would rather enjoy what I ate than eat food that did not taste good. I have type 2 diabetes and, when my sugar started to rise out of control, I decided it was time to make my health my first concern. I decided to get help from UDP. I found that, with careful thought, I could eat the right foods for my sugar and still enjoy the food I ate. I did not have to starve myself and I did not have to eat food that did not taste good. I also learned that when I made bad food choices it showed in my sugar level and in my weight or muscle. I know what I can eat if I want to keep my weight and sugar level down. I now enjoy what I eat and it is nothing that is so far away from what I ate before. Because of the loss in weight and the lowering of my sugar level, I have more energy. I now exercise five mornings a week and I also bowl once a week. Feeling better is a great incentive for me to be conscious about my eating habits.

"Another thing that bothered me very much was my heart rate. My heart rate goes over a hundred beats per minute and no body has been able to tell me why."

Most normal hearts beat between 60-80 times per minute – so you can understand why this would keep Dorothy up at night wondering if she was slowly dying. To make matters worse, tests after tests and advanced studies turned out nothing. Finally, she was told that she would have to live with it.

Feeling hopeless and heartbroken, Dorothy sank deeper into depression and even entertained the thought that it was probably in her head. Nonetheless, within a couple of months after she began the UDP program, her heart rate returned to normal. The reason for this is not really clear, but it surely gave Dorothy peace of mind that she had long sought. A possible explanation is that Dorothy's new anti-inflammatory diet was rich in antioxidants and Omega-3 fatty acids, which are protective to the heart and blood vessels---- help to normalize the beating of the heart. Omega-3 fatty acids have anti-inflammatory properties that could have also helped to lower her blood pressure, blood sugar, and cholesterol after only few months. It didn't stop there – she had a dramatic increase in energy, which allowed her to incorporate a tolerable level of regular physical activity into her lifestyle. Her mood and sleep improved too, all due to the Omega-3 fatty acids and, of course, the rich supply of antioxidants and phytonutrients.

Dorothy's hemoglobin A1C prior to UDP was 8.4 and a few months later it was down to 5.8, suggesting excellent blood-sugar control, which made her physician so pleased that he discontinued one of her medications and reduced the second oral medication to a very low dose with less side effects. She successfully reached her goal weight, losing a total of 34 pounds and lowered her body fat to 34 percent (normal for her age is 23-36%).

"I feel liberated that I have taken charge of my own health and really know how to keep my blood sugar and cholesterol under control."

| Stats | Start | Now |
|---|---|---|
| Weight | 196 | 161 |
| Waist | 39 | 34 |
| %Fat | 45 | 34 |
| Total Fat | 93 | 56 |
| Muscle | 103 | 105 |

Update: Dorothy has successfully kept the weight off for over three years and enjoys the best of physical and mental health in her seventies than she had at any other age. She is now involved in helping to nourish other relatives that have chronic health problems. Last year, her older brother had a massive heart attack and stroke that left him partially paralyzed. He also has diabetes but, unlike his sister, it has never been well controlled. It's very likely that his diabetes brought about the heart attack. Dorothy quickly went to work applying the knowledge that she has learned from the UDP program to nurse her brother back to health.

Dorothy also shared with us other good news that she is very proud of (even though she does not want to take the credit for it). Her oldest daughter (a nurse in a prestigous hospital in Boston) decided to follow in her mother's footsteps and sought professional help to become healthy. That will make any mother happy and, these days, Dorothy has so many things to be happy about – she is enjoying health and vitality regardless of her age.

**Irene, Executive Secretary**

**Diagnosis:** High cholesterol, fatigue, carbohydrate cravings, anxiety, and mood swing
**Motivation:** Tired of dieting and wanted to learn how to do it right

Irene, 48 years old, came to UDP because she wanted to learn how to lose weight and improve the quality of her life without dieting.

"I have struggled with my weight for as long as I can remember. Like so many others, I tried Weight Watchers, fasting, cabbage soup diet, grapefruit diet, vegetarianism, and even macrobiotics – along with countless other 'get skinny fast' fads – in my attempt to get thin and stay thin. They all worked for a while but, inevitably, I would slowly but surely see the scale (my dreaded enemy) creep up.

"I was on a daily roller coaster ride of energy highs and lows. No breakfast, little if any lunch, my main meal for dinner, and unhealthy snacking before bed contributed to this steady weight gain. A sedentary job and an exercise routine consisting of sporadic walking and yoga did little to burn off the excessive calories I consumed.

"Not until I made the conscious decision to get healthy and become more energetic (with losing weight as a secondary goal) did my journey find me at the doorstep of UDP. Dr. Billy Johnson's intelligent, scientific, no-nonsense approach is a recipe for success. This is not a fad or a quick fix, but a real lifestyle change. It is a process, not an event.

"With the UDP Program, I am now eating whole foods, lots of green leafy vegetables, salads, and fruits in sensible quantities. With Dr. Billy's guidance I have watched my weight decline at a steady pace. I am down two dress sizes and have lost about 30 pounds, which I know I will not find again. The scale is no longer my enemy. Regular exercise has become part of my daily life."

| Stats | Start | Now |
|---|---|---|
| Weight | 190 | 162 |
| Waist | 33 | 29 |
| %Fat | 44 | 35 |
| Total Fat | 83 | 57 |
| Muscle | 107 | 105 |

Update: Irene continues to follow the healthy practice of a proper meal, physical activity and stress reduction. She graduated from the UDP program three years ago and has never looked back.

## Natasha, Child With a Heavy Load

**Diagnosis:** Fatigue and carbohydrate cravings
**Motivation:** To improve her self-esteem, increase her energy, and decrease her risk of diabetes

Natasha, 8 years old, stood 4'9½" and weighed 133 pounds. She also led a sedentary lifestyle. Her parents, who were concerned that schoolmates were making fun of their daughter, enrolled her in UDP. Natasha told Barbara Morse Silva of NBC 10 that people made fun of her because of her weight.

"They said, 'You're overweight, you can't ride the pony rides' and I said 'I want to,'" she shyly reported.

According to Natasha's mother, "She would come home to me with tears in her eyes and say 'Mommy I couldn't ride on it.' I'd say 'Why?' 'Because it's only 80 pounds and I'm overweight.' That's when I started to think I have to do something for her because her self-esteem was too low."

Natasha wanted to lose weight so she could fit in, but she wasn't sure whether she could do what was necessary to reach her goal. But, just five weeks into the program, Natasha had a change of heart.

"Now I feel that I have more energy than before and I think that a lot of overweight children can do it, too. I do feel proud of myself."

Natasha learned at this crucial age how to make better choices and eat food in line with her level of physical activity. Whereas previously she ate fast foods, sodas, and snacks, she resolved to incorporate healthier choices into her diet and she felt good about herself. "

Both parents were encouraged by their young daughter's transformation that they became UDP members. It didn't take long before they too saw the quality of their health and lives improve dramatically within a short period of time. The father was overweight and had trouble controlling his diabetes and that quickly changed. The mother, who had no known health problems, reached her weight goal and had good energy.

Natasha was on television and, considering this new-found fame, some of the classmates who had once teased her wanted to be her friend. Gaining confidence and a positive self-image, Natasha became more sociable and her grades also improved significantly. Her parents were so impressed with her progress that they enrolled her in a dance school. When she was asked what she would like to be when she grows up, she replied, "When I grow up, I want to be a pediatrician in order to help other young people like myself."

Natasha lost 20 pounds and 13 percent body fat and was considered to be at the normal weight for her age and height by her pediatrician.

| Stats | Start | Now |
|---|---|---|
| Weight | 133 | 113 |
| Waist | 39 | 28½ |
| %Fat | 37 | 24 |
| Total Fat | 52 | 27 |
| Muscle | 81 | 86 |

Update: Natasha graduated from the UDP program almost four years ago and has been doing quite well since then. She is growing beautifully and continues to strive for a healthy mind and body.

Intervention or preventive measures at a very early age, like in the case of Natasha, offers the best opportunity to slow or reverse the trend of obesity and its associated health risks. Most of the chronic health problems (heart disease and diabetes) that we encounter as adults originate as a result of cellular changes during childhood, continue to progress silently through the adolescent period, and may become full-blown in mid life. That's why appropriate intervention during childhood is highly effective and beneficial and must be a primary goal in the fight against obesity.

**Rebecca, Retired Office Manager**

**Diagnosis:** High cholesterol, high triglycerides, high LDL (bad) cholesterol, and high blood pressure

**Motivation:** To decrease or come off medications

Rebecca, 64, was concerned about the several medications she was taking and wanted to reduce or come off some of them. She also wanted to increase her energy level as well as prevent bone and muscle loss. She was encouraged to join UDP by a close friend who was concerned about her blood pressure and cholesterol.

At one point, Rebecca's cholesterol was close to 300, her triglyceride level was over 600 and LDL (bad) cholesterol was over 400. But with the help of UDP, Rebecca's blood work became normal in just a few months.

"By eating the right foods, I was able to lower my cholesterol without too much exercise. I like what I am eating and what I am doing. I am very happy and I feel so good. I did want to lose weight, but that wasn't my primary reason."

Rebecca lost 14 lbs and reached her ideal weight. Her body fat is down to 34%, which is normal for her age. She surprised herself when she went through the Thanksgiving and Christmas holidays and was still able to lose body fat and maintain muscle mass.

"It is a lifestyle change and a very positive experience for me and my family. I am not dieting and this is something I can do for the rest of my life. My blood pressure is down, my primary physician reduced my medication to the lowest dose – and I am very pleased about that."

| Stats | Start | Now |
|---|---|---|
| Weight | 149 | 135 |
| Waist | 37¼ | 33 |
| %Fat | 39 | 34 |
| Total Fat | 58 | 45 |
| Muscle | 90 | 89 |

Update: Rebecca continues to do well, graduating from the UDP program over three years ago. She is on a very low dose of medication for her blood pressure and cholesterol. She is determined to keep it that way.

**Ellen, Retired School Teacher**

**Diagnosis:** Headache, heartburn/indigestion, carbohydrate craving, menopausal symptoms, and back pain
**Motivation:** Worried about getting diabetes (it runs in her family)

After having tried Weight Watchers and several other weight loss programs, Ellen, 68 said, "I'm finally learning how to incorporate healthy food choices and eliminate bad ones. Frankly, I don't miss the bad foods that I used to eat. For me, it was more of a social thing. I remember after church service, we'd drive by the bay and have coffee and doughnuts. I don't do that anymore.

"There is no such thing as dieting in the program. They even took my own recipes and made them over. I'm not missing anything because the flavor is still there.

"I lost the weight that I've been trying to lose for a long time and I feel very good. I have more energy now and, when I walk three miles first thing in the morning, I feel great afterwards. I believe a lot of it is mental and it makes me feel good that I can actually change my life for good."

| Stats | Start | Now |
|---|---|---|
| Weight | 178 | 157 |
| Waist | 37½ | 33½ |
| %Fat | 44 | 35 |
| Total Fat | 78 | 60 |
| Muscle | 100 | 97 |

Update: Ellen is doing extremely well after graduating from the UDP program over three years ago. She continues to eat healthy and maintain a regular level of physical activity. For her, this is a way of life and there is no need to change it for anything else.

**Sharon, Corporate Executive With a Heart**

**Diagnosis:** High cholesterol, high LDL (bad) cholesterol, Syndrome X, fatigue, headaches, and carbohydrate cravings
**Motivation:** To take control of her fate and take the guesswork out of what she was eating and doing

"I am a 61-year-old female who has been struggling with my weight since I was 14 years old – when I gained 30 pounds after being bedridden with encephalitis. Throughout my life, I have tried every diet imaginable with varying degrees of success.

"Approximately 15 years ago, I began to notice that I had certain drastic reactions to food. Whenever I ate high-carbohydrate foods I got reactions. First, a rash appeared on my hips and legs; then my eyes would swell. One day, I ate some roast beef with cooked carrots at a company cafeteria. Within 15 minutes of completion my eyes were swelled shut.

"I began experimenting with the foods I ate and started reading popular press on foods, food combinations, theories on eating, etc. After a lot of experimentation I settled on eating no more than 10 grams of carbohydrates per meal. For many meals, I ate low-fat proteins only. I never ate processed foods, only fresh vegetables, fruit, and fresh fish, chicken, and beef. For years, this kept my weight in check but every so often I would have tremendous binges, cravings for sugar, chocolate, etc.

"My physical examination also showed that I had high total cholesterol plus high LDL and low HDL. I continued reading and found that newer studies show that too few carbohydrates in the diet produced some of the same symptoms as too many carbohydrates. I found that, after five years, I had gained about 25 pounds and, no matter how little I ate or how much I exercised, I could not lose any weight.

"I read about Dr. Johnson's program in a local newspaper and decided that I had had enough guesswork. I began the UDP program primarily to get regular laboratory tests of my blood and insulin/cortisol levels. What I found was much more than that. Dr. Johnson helped me understand that proper balance is most important. I still have sensitivity to carbohydrates but I can now accommodate approximately 60-130 grams of carbohydrates a day (real carbs through vegetables and beans) but no sugar, processed or junk food.

"I read the nutrition labels on everything I buy in the grocery store and am thoughtful about everything I eat. Dr. Johnson's idea of eating meals in courses and beginning every meal with nutrients and antioxidants rich dark green leafy vegetables (including breakfast) and having the right balance of low-fat proteins, carbs, and good fats has changed how I feel. I also take multivitamins and minerals, including Omega-3. I feel better than I ever have more consistently. I also lost 22 pounds and decreased my body fat percentage by 4%. I have retained my muscle but, more importantly, I feel happy, healthy and in control of my fate."

| Stats | Start | Now |
|---|---|---|
| Weight | 175 | 153 |
| Waist | 40 | 32 |
| %Fat | 44 | 39 |
| Total Fat | 75 | 61 |
| Muscle | 94 | 92 |

Update: Sharon's cholesterol decreased from 284 mg/dl to 193 in nine weeks. LDL (bad) cholesterol normalized within six weeks without prescribed medications and has remained in the healthy range since. She has also maintained a steady healthy weight and body fat for the last three years. She travels overseas quite often on business trips, and continues to make healthier choices when ever possible.

**Adlene, College Student With Plans on Hold**

**Diagnosis:** Syndrome X, fatigue, carbohydrate, and fat cravings
**Motivation:** To improve her chance of getting pregnant

Adlene, 29, was married and frustrated that she was unable to get pregnant after almost six years of trying. Meanwhile, she put that on hold and went back to finish her education. She ate very poorly and, though she exercised occasionally, it was not enough. As a result, her weight soared and she had no energy. She noticed that she was not alone in this struggle. Some of her best friends were having even bigger problems.

"I see my best friend going through so much. She goes to the gym to lose weight and eats so little, yet she doesn't lose any weight. She was so frustrated that she went to her doctor to check her thyroid and have lots of other tests. They all came back normal and she doesn't understand why she is not losing weight.

"I used to be just like my friend. I ate less, exercised a lot, and thought I was doing the right thing. Now, it is different; I really know what to do. In fact, I eat more and I'm losing body fat. What a big difference! I'm losing weight and enjoying it. People are asking me to tell them my secret because they think it is not normal to eat like a regular person and not take drugs or eat pre-packaged food or omit carbs and still lose weight consistently."

She learned how to plan her meals, such that she was able to eat healthy even at school. She also started a tolerable level of physical activity and it paid off. She lost a total of 23 pounds, 20 pounds fat, and 5 percent body fat in a short eight weeks. But there was a bigger surprise that was totally unexpected. She became pregnant without even trying.

| Stats | Start | Now |
|---|---|---|
| Weight | 229 | 206 |
| Waist | 45 | 41½ |
| %Fat | 53 | 48 |
| Total Fat | 121 | 101 |
| Muscle | 108 | 105 |

**Theresa, Retired School Principle**

**Diagnosis:** Dehydration, carbohydrate cravings, joint pain, heartburn, and hair loss
**Motivation:** To improve the quality of her life.

Theresa, 63, came to UDP because her eating habits were erratic and she wanted a healthier and more structured lifestyle.

"I seldom ate breakfast or lunch. I would, however, eat a medium portion for dinner and usually after 7 p.m. I was also an emotional eater and would eat ice cream and other snacks at night. All this changed when I joined UDP after I was inspired by the success of a friend of mine who was on the program. She had transformed herself so nicely and didn't look her age at all.

"With UDP, I learned that you have to eat in order to lose weight. I am eating three meals daily, plus healthy snacks, but I make sure I eat appropriate portions by paying attention to food labels. Breakfast is now my biggest meal and it has helped me deal with my addiction to sugary foods. I eat less at lunch and dinner and never after 7 p.m.

"UDP has taught me to eat foods (whether it is carbohydrates, proteins, or fats) according the level of my physical activity. I also learned to listen to my body and this has helped me to make better food choices and also to know when to stop eating. I don't count calories. I simply eat to fullness and I found out that I am not getting hungry between meals. I am so amazed that I am even able to control my cravings.

"I can't believe my energy level. I have even incorporated simple regular physical activity (such as brisk walking) daily in my life. Now I really appreciate and enjoy being healthy and I am in better physical condition."

| Stats | Start | Now |
|---|---|---|
| Weight | 176 | 150 |
| Waist | 38 | 32 |
| %Fat | 41 | 22 |
| Total Fat | 72 | 32 |
| Muscle | 104 | 118 |

Update: Theresa lost 26 pounds and 17 percent of her body fat three years ago and had since maintained it. She continues to eat healthy and tailors her food intake to her level of physical activity.

**Martina, Homemaker**

**Diagnosis:** Craving carbohydrates and heartburn/indigestion
**Motivation:** Losing her pregnancy weight

After having given birth to her third child, Martina wanted to shed pounds and regain her pre-pregnancy weight. She had tried many diets and exercise programs and failed. Her husband, who knew about the UDP program through a friend, encouraged her to enroll.

"I learned the proper food choices and ate real grocery foods with my entire family. I was never dieting and, with what I learned, I was still able to eat out without sabotaging my weight-loss goal. I feel energetic, lively and my self-esteem is high. My relationship with my husband is at its best. I have recommended several of my friends to UDP because the program is real and it works."

Martina lost 38 lbs and reduced her percentage body fat from 44% to 31% – which is normal for her age. She has reduced her dress size from a 14 to 6.

| Stats | Start | Now |
|---|---|---|
| Weight | 174 | 136 |
| Waist | 38 | 30 |
| %Fat | 44 | 31 |
| Total Fat | 77 | 42 |
| Muscle | 97 | 94 |

Update: Martina graduated from the UDP program about two years ago and comes in for maintenance occasionally. She is doing very well and continues to apply the knowledge and resources that she acquired from the UDP program.

**Carmen, Homemaker**

**Diagnosis:** Fatigue, anxiety, headaches, depression, heartburn/indigestion, dehydration, and carbohydrate cravings

**Motivation:** To reduce depression and anxiety and improve her ability to get along with others

Carmen, 4'11½", weighed 163 pounds. She was constantly hungry even though she ate frequently. Little did she know that her symptoms and the way she felt were due to the poor food choices that she was making on a daily basis.

"I felt like I was drowning; I didn't know what to do. I was so depressed that it was hard for me to get along with anyone, including my immediate family. I was angry all the time and hated to see myself in the mirror. Things that I cared about in my life were falling apart – until a friend recommended UDP. That changed my life for the better. The first day I went there, I knew that they would help me. They gave me sincere support and attention on a one-on-one basis and my confidence grew. I became more aware of food and the choices I was making and I was amazed by how much power food had over me.

"I am in my mid-forties and I feel like I am in my twenties. People are asking me what I'm taking to look so young and energetic. When I tell them that it is just making the proper food choices in combination with my multivitamins, they don't believe me. I feel so proud of my accomplishment and myself. I believe I really learned how to eat all over again.

"What UDP has taught me is not to be afraid of food, but to enjoy it. The other thing that is most important to me is my relationship with my father, family, and kids, which is much better than it's ever been. When I was feeling bad, I did not always get along with others. My advice to others is to enjoy the program because it really works and it can work for you, too."

| Stats | Start | Now |
|---|---|---|
| Weight | 164 | 140 |
| Waist | 36 | 29 |
| %Fat | 40 | 34 |
| Total Fat | 66 | 47 |
| Muscle | 98 | 93 |

Update: Carmen reached her goal weight within seven weeks. She has not gained back the weight over the course of two years.

**Rosalyn, Homemaker**

**Diagnosis:** Diabetes, high blood pressure, spinal stenosis, and sleep apnea
**Motivation:** To improve the quality of her life

Rosalyn, at the age of 68, found herself having to think seriously about her mortality. She was diabetic and was taking about 130 units of insulin every day. She was over a hundred pounds overweight and sedentary. To make matters worse, she was gaining weight rapidly and was totally miserable.

"Moving was difficult and painful. My diabetes was out of control," she explained, almost in tears, "Having had many unsuccessful attempts at improvement, I had given up hope. I had a negative attitude."

In addition to diabetes, Rosalyn had high blood pressure, spinal stenosis, acid reflux, sleep apnea, severe shortness of breath, and pain in the spine and joints. Her ankles, lower extremities, and legs were badly swollen, making it very painful if not impossible to walk even short distances. High doses of water pill did not resolve the water retention. As expected, she was on several medications and recently had cataract surgery caused by the uncontrolled blood sugar. Blood sugar readings were in the 300's in spite of the very high doses of insulin she was injecting daily (20 units regular and 45 units NPH in the morning; 20 units regular and 45 units NPH in the evening).

It wasn't easy at first. In the beginning, she could only manage to work on improving her diet (anti-inflammatory). Then, in the third week, she tried to exercise on a stationary bike for few minutes without running out of breath. She also needed assistance to get on and off the bike. But she persisted, exercising a few minutes several times per day. Her resolve began to pay off. Not long, she was exercising up to thirty minutes at a time. She also added variety to her workouts – swimming, walking, and weights.

She acquired the skill to eat to fullness without counting calories and also became familiar with the glycemic index of food and its impact on the blood sugar. She acquired new information about the relationship between food (especially carbohydrates) and activity level. She became more aware of portion sizes and learned how to use food labels to estimate the amount of any given food that is appropriate for her level of activity. She also made sure to measure out her food portions until she reached a level of certainty. She followed the UDP model very closely to make sure that every meal had enough nutrients, antioxidants, and soluble fiber. She was not restricted to eating only at home. She and her husband went out to eat once or twice a week.

The pay off was beyond her wildest imagination. After only four weeks of following the UDP program, Rosalyn, with her doctor's permission, was able to reduce her insulin dosage by one third. Her blood sugar levels were within the normal healthy range most of the time and she also lost forty pounds in three months. Her leg and ankle edema resolved, and she was able to move more freely. She could now exercise on the stationary bike without help. There is remarkable improvement in her blood pressure, spinal stenosis, acid reflux, and sleep apnea, and shortness of breath, including back pain.

She is turning her life around and enjoys tremendous energy and vitality.

"The UDP program has enabled me to lose weight, vastly improved my health and helped me to understand how to keep on the right track. This program and Dr. Johnson have given me a new lease on life."

Rosalyn continues to make steady progress, has made healthy eating, and exercises a part of her life. The entire family is supporting and motivating her and she is committed for life because she knows very well that her old lifestyle of making very poor food choices and inactivity only made her miserable and hopeless.

**Dominique, Construction Worker**

**Diagnosis:** Diabetes and low energy
**Motivation:** To improve image and health

Dominique, 40 years old, is diabetic and on oral medication to control his blood sugar. He was sixty pounds overweight and moderately active. He paid attention to exercise but his diet was very unhealthy. His diabetes was getting out of control and he was afraid of having to take insulin injections. Dominique had other concerns too. His daughter, Kate, was eleven years old and weighed 161 pounds. So, he decided it was time to seek help for the both of them.

Dominique was used to a regular exercise regimen so, when he began to eat a proper meal, he quickly had remarkable results. He saw his energy improve and he did not need medication to control his blood sugar after only two weeks. Following the UDP program, he lost twenty-one pounds (about three pounds per week) and lowered his body fat percentage from 42% to 36% in two months. His progress is expected to continue because he is truly committed to living healthy and making it a way of life. In spite of his limited English (which sometimes makes communication difficult) he is absorbing the information that he is given and applying it to his life.

| Stats | Start | Now |
|---|---|---|
| Weight | 243 | 222 |
| Waist | 49½ | 44 |
| %Fat | 42 | 36 |
| Total Fat | 103 | 81 |
| Muscle | 140 | 141 |

**Kate, Child Struggling With Weight**

**Diagnosis:** Attention Deficit Disorder (ADD)
**Motivation:** To improve image and health

Kate is only eleven years old and weighs 161 pounds (more than 50% of her body weight is fat). Like most children her age, she eats very poorly and exercise is out of the question. When her father, Dominique, decided to join the UDP structured program, he brought his daughter along. At first, the easily distracted little girl thought it was a joke and paid no attention to what she was being taught. But, after few weeks in the program, she surprised everybody by showing keen interest. It paid off – as she began eating balanced meals and cutting down junk foods. She went as far as bringing the school cafeteria menu to the office so that the healthy choices could be pointed out. When there were no healthy selections, her mother would prepare her lunch from home.

After only two months of following the UDP program, there were already noticeable improvements in her concentration and focus as a result of the anti-inflammatory diet. According to her parents, she was much calmer and more attentive than she had ever been. She also began to pay attention to things that she hardly cared for in the past, including healthy food choices. This new attitude paid off high dividends when Halloween came and she lost body fat in a situation were most children her age gain fat.

Kate also took part in recreational activities at least 3-5 times per week both at school and at home. She and her mother enrolled in a state-funded program at the YMCA recently. The future looks brighter for this youngster, who is keenly aware at this age that the quality of her adult life depends solely on what she does at this early age. To this end, the entire family, including her younger brother, Joshua, are all helping and supporting her all the way. It's a worthy course and investment that every parent should make for their child. Attacking the obesity crisis at the very root should be a goal that we should all strive for, as this can assure health and vitality no matter the age. It's indeed the only security to health.

| Stats | Start | Now |
|---|---|---|
| Weight | 161 | 146 |
| Waist | 42½ | 38 |
| %Fat | 65 | 55 |
| Total Fat | 105 | 81 |
| Muscle | 56 | 66 |

# SELECTED REFERENCES

Agatston, Arthur. The South Beach Diet: The Delicious, Doctor-Designed, Foolproof Plan for a Fast and Healthy Weight Loss. New York: Random House, 2003.

Anderson, RA, Chen N, et al. Elevated intakes of supplemental chromium improves glucose and insulin variables in individuals with type 2 diabetes. Diabetes, 1997; 46:1786-1791.

AICR/WCRF Expert Report, Food, Nutrition and the Prevention of Cancer: a global perspective – background on the leading scientific report on diet and cancer, including the Report's *Summary* and information on the second Expert Report. www.aicr.org.

Al, MDM. Essential fatty acids, pregnancy and pregnancy outcome. Relationship between mother and child. CIP-Gregevens Kuninklijke Bibliotheck, Den Haag, The Netherlands, 1994.

Alden, Lori: The Cook's Thesaurus: www.foodsubs.com; 2001.

Allred, JB. Too much of a good thing? An overemphasis on eating low-fat foods may be contributing to the alarming increase in overweight among US adults. J Amer Dietetic Assoc, 1995; 95(4) 417-18.

American Diabetes Association Complete Guide To Diabetes. New York. Bantam Books. 1997.

American Diabetes Association, Nutritional recommendation and Principles for people with diabetes mellitus, Diabetes Care 1994; 17:519-22

American Diabetes Association. Gestational diabetes mellitus. Diabetes Care, volume 22, Supplement 1, 1999.

Anderson, JW, Story L, Zettwoch N et al. Diabetes care 1989; 12:337-44

Anderson, RL, Kaiser DL. Effects of calorie restriction and weight loss on glucose and insulin levels in obese humans. J Am Coll Nutr. 1985; 4: 411-9

Anderson, JW. Hypocholesterolemic effects of oat and bean products. Am. J. Clin. Natr., 1988, 48,749-753.

Artal, R.: Exercise: An Alternative Therapy for Gestational Diabetes. The Physician and Sportsmedicine. March 1996. 24 (3): 54-6.

Ascherio, A, et al. Health Effects of Trans fatty acids. Am J. Clin Nutr (1997) Oct. 66 (4 Suppl): 1006S-1010S

Astrup, A. "Healthy lifestyles in Europe: Prevention of obesity and Type II diabetes by diet and physical activity" Public Health Nutrition (2001) 4: 499-515.

Atkins, Robert C., MD. Dr. Atkins' new diet revolution. New York: Avon Books 1999.

Augustin, LS, et al. Dietary glycemic index and glycemic load and breast cancer risk: a case-control study. Ann Oncol. 2001; 12(11): 1533-1538.

Axelrod, L. Omega-3 fatty acids in diabetes mellitus. Gift from the sea. Diabetes 1989 May; 38(5): 539-43

Bantle, JP, Raatz SK, Thomas W, Georgopoulos A. (2000). Effects of dietary fructose on plasma lipids in healthy subjects. American Journal of Clinical Nutrition, 72, 1128-1134.

Barilla, J. et al. The Nutrition Superbook: The Antioxidants. New Canaan, Conn. Keats Publishing, Inc. 1995.

Bassuk, SS, et al. High-sensitivity C-reactive protein: clinical importance. Curr Probl Cardiol 2004 Aug; 29(8): 439-93.

Battezzati, A, et al. Drugs and Foods for Chronic Subclinical Inflammation in Humans. Current Medical Chemistry- Immunoly, Endocrine and Metabolic Agents, April 2005, vol. 5. no.2, pp. 149-155(7).

Bell, SJ, Sears B. Low-glycemic load diets: impact on obesity and chronic diseases. Crit. Rev. Food Sci Nutr 2003; 43(4): 357-77

Bellerson, Karen J. The Complete and Up-to-date fat book: A Guide to the fat calories and fat percentages in your food, NY: Avery 1991

Bloch, A., Thomson CA.: Position of the American Dietetics Association: Phytochemicals and functional foods. J Am Diet Assoc 1995; 95:493-96

Block, JB, Evans S. Clincal evidence supporting cancer risk reduction with antioxidants and implications for diets and supplements. JANA. 2000; 3(3); 6-16

Braaten, JT, Scott FW, et al. "High beta-glucan oat bran and oat gum reduce postprandial blood glucose and insulin in subjects with and without type 2 diabetes. Diabetes Med 1994 Apr; 11(3); 312-8

Brand, JC, Nicholson PL et al. Food processing and the glycemic index. Am J Clin Nutr 1985; 42: 1192-6.

Brand-Miller, J, et al. The Glucose Revolution: the authoritative guide to the glycemic index. New York: Marlowe and Co. 1999.

Brand-Miller, J, Hayne S. et al. Low- Glycemic Index Diets in the Management of Diabetes: A meta-analysis of randomized controlled trials. Diabetes Care. 2003;26 (8):2261-2267.

Bouche, C, Rizkalla SW, et al. Five-week, low-glycemic index diet decreases total fat mass and improves plasma lipid profile in moderately overweight nondiabetic men. Diabetes Care. 2002; 25 (5):822-828.

Campbell, CW. The truth about fitness. Organic Style. May/June 2003. Also see Gina Kolata below.

Carroll, KK. Review of Clinical studies on cholesterol lowering response to soy protein. J Am Diet Assoc 1991; 91:820-7

Casey, BM, et al. Pregnancy outcomes in women with gestational diabetes compare with the general population. Obstetrics and Gynecology, volume 9, number 6, December 1997, pages 869-873

Challem, J. "The anti-inflammation diet" Letsliveonline.com – March 2003.

Challem, J. The inflammation Syndrome. Hoboken, NJ: John Wiley and Sons. 2003.

Challem, J. " Is Fructose Dangerous". The Nutrition Reporter, 1995.

Chen, YD, Coulston AM, et al. "Why do low-fat, high carbohydrate diets accentuate post prandial lipemia in patients with NIDDM. Diabetes care 1995 Jan; 18(1): 10-6.

Chow, CK, Fatty acids in foods and their health implications. 1992, New York: Marcek Dekker, Inc. 889.

Coulston, AM, Hollenbeck CB, Swislocki AL, Chen YD, Reaven GM. Deleterious metabolic effects of high-carbohydrate, sucrose-containing diets in patients with non-insulin-dependent diabetes mellitus. Am J Med 1987 Feb; 82 (2): 213-220

Crawford, MA. Fatty-acid ratios in free-living and domestic animals. The Lancet, 1968; 1: 1329-33.

Crowley, MA, Matt KS. Hormonal regulation of skeletal muscle hypertrophy in rats: The testosterone to cortisol ratio. Eur J Appl Physiol Occup Physiol. (1996) 73(1-2):66-72.

Cummings, JH et al. Diet and the prevention of cancer. BMJ. 1998; 317: 1636-40.

Davis, J. (2000) "Weight-loss tip: Add extra calcium to a low-fat diet. Low-fat dairy products may help weight loss control." My.webmd.com/content/article/1728.56703

Del Toma, E, Lintas C. et al. Soluble and insoluble dietary fibre in diabetic diets. Eur J Clin Nutr 1988 Apr; 42 (4): 313-9.

De Lorgeril, M, Reraud S, Delaye J. Mediterranean alpha-linolenic acid-rich diet in secondary prevention of coronary heart disease. The Lancet, 1994; 343-1454-145.

DeLorgeril, M, Salen P, Delaye J: "Effect of Mediterranean type of diet on the rate of Cardiovascular complications in patients with coronary heart disease," J. Amer. Cell Cardiology. 1996;28 (5):1103-8

Demark-Wahnefried, Wendy, M.D. Weight gain after chemotherapy tied to inactivity. OB/GYN NEWS, May 2000.

Denkins, Y. et al. Fish Oil Helps Prevent Diabetes. This study was presented at the Experimental Biology 2002 Conference in New Orleans, April 21, 2002.

Devaraj, S. Jiaial I. Alpha tocopherol supplementation decreases serum C-reactive protein and monocyte interleukin-6 levels in normal volunteers and type 2 diabetic patients. Free Rad Biol Med 2000:29:790-792.

Diet and Cancer: Food additives, coffee and alcohol," Nutrition and Cancer, 1983

Dietary Guidelines for Americans (2005) U. S. Department of Agriculture. www.ars.usda.gov/dgac/dgacguidexp.htm

Doll, R et al: The Causes of Cancer. J Nat; Cancer Insti. 1981;66:1191

Dosch, HM. "The Possible Link Between Insulin Dependent (Juvenile) Diabetes Mellitus and Dietary Cow Milk," Clinical Biochemistry 26 (4), 307-8,1993

Dreon, DM, Krauss RM. "A very low-fat diet is not associated with improved lipoprotein profiles in men with a predominance of large low-density Lipoproteins," American Journal of Clinical Nutrition 69(3), 411, 1999

Duyff, RL. The American Dietetic Association's Complete Food and Nutrition Guide. Minneapolis: Chronimed; 1998

Dye, TD et al. Exercise Cuts Rate of diabetes in Pregnancy in Obese Women. American Journal of Epidemiology. December 1997. Also www.psgroup.com/dg/4a5cc.htm.

Eades, Michael R, Mary Dan Eades, Protein Power. NY: Bantam Books 1998.

Epel, ES, McEwen B, Seeman T et al, "Stress and body shape: Stressed-induced cortisol secretion is consistently greater among women with central fat". Psychosomatic Medicine (2000) 62:623-634.

Exchange lists for meal planning. The American Diabetic Association, 1995.

Fabricant, Florence. Why do Americans weigh more? We eat more: *Self Magazine* August 2001.

Fahey, J, Zhang Y, Talalay P. Broccoli sprouts: an exceptionally rich source of inducers of enzymes that protect against chemical carcinogens. Proc Natl Acad Sci USA. 1997;94:10367-10372

Fannain, M, Szilasi J, Storlein L, Calvert GD. The effect of modified fat diet in insulin resistance and metabolic parameters in type II diabetes. Diabetologia, 1996; 39(1): A7.

Finley, J. et al: Selenium content of foods purchased in North Dakota. Nutr. Res. 1996; 16:726-28, 1991.

Flegal, KM, Carroll MD, Kuczmarski RJ, Johnson CL. Overweight and Obesity in the United States: prevalence and trends, 1960-1994. Int J Obes Relat Metab Disord. 1998; 22: 39-47

Ford, ES et al. Increasing Prevalence of the Metabolic Syndrome Among U.S. Adults. Diabetes Care, October 1, 2004; 27(10): 2444-2449.

Ford, ES, Giles WH, Dietz WH. Prevalence of the metabolic syndrome among US adults: findings from the third National Health and Nutrition Examination Survey. JAMA. 2002; 287: 356-359.

Ford, ES, Liu S. Glycemic index and serum high-density lipoprotein cholesterol concentration among US adults. Arch Intern Med. 2001;161(4):572-576.

Foster, GD, Wyatt HR, Hill Jo, McGuckin BG, Brill C, Mohammed BS, et al. A randomized trial of a low-carbohydrate diet for obesity. N Eng J Med. 2003; 348: 2082-90.

Foster-Powell, K, Holt SH, Brand- Miller JC. "International Table of Glycemic Index and Glycemic Load Values: 2002." AJCN 76:1, p 5-56.

Giacco, R, Parillo M, et al. Long-term dietary treatment with increased amounts of fiber-rich low-glycemic index natural foods improves blood glucose control and reduces the number of hypoglycemic events in type 1 diabetic patients. Diabetes Care. 2000;23 (10):1461-1466.

Gibson, RA, Neaumann MA, Makrides M. Effect of dietary docosahexaenoic acid on brain composition and neural function in term infants. Lipids, 1996; 31 (supplement):S-177-181.

Gitlin, MJ, Pasnau RO. Psychiatric syndrome linked to reproductive function in women: A review of current knowledge. Am. J. Psychiatry. 1989; 146(11) 1413-1422.

Golay, A. et al. Weight loss with a low or high carbohydrate diet? Int J Obesity, 1996; 20: 1062-72.

Goldbeck, N, Goldbeck D. The Healthiest Diet in the World, Penguin-Putnam: NY, 2001.

Grimble, RF. Modification of inflammatory aspects of immune function by nutrients. Nutrition Research 1998; 18:1297-1317.

Grimble, RF. Nutritional modulation of cytokine biology. Nutrition, 1998; 14:634-640.

Gulliford, MC, Bicknell EJ, Scarpello JH. Differential effect of protein and fat ingestion on blood glucose responses to high-and low- glycemic- index carbohydrates in noninsulin-dependent diabetic subjects. Am J Clin Nutr 1989 Oct; 50 (4):773-7.

Hainault, I, Carlotti M, Lavau M. Fish oil in a high lard diet prevents obesity, hyperlipemia and adipocyte insulin resistance in rats. Annals of New York Academy of Sciences 1993 683: 98-101.

Harper, CR, Jacobson TA. The fats of life: the role of Omega-3 fatty acids in the prevention of coronary heart disease. Arch Intern Med. 2001; 161: 2185-92.

Harris, S, PhD. Moderate Physical Activity Prevents Breast Cancer Recurrence. Active Living. Summer 2004 Vol. 5 no. 3.

Herber, D. What Color Is Your Diet? Regan, 2002.
Also see: The California Cuisine Pyramid. UCLA Center for Human Nutrition or http://www.cellinteractive.com/ucla/center_overview/pyramid.html.

High calcium intake can lead to weight loss in women. Reuters Health. (2001). www.heartinfo.com/reuters2001/010125elin011.htm

Hirano, T, Fukuoka K., Oka K et al. Antiproliferative activity of mammalian lignan derivatives against the human breast carcinoma cell line, ZR-75-1. Cancer Invest 1990; 8:595-601.

Holmes, Michelle, et al. Exercise after breast cancer treatment may improve survival and reduce recurrence. J Am Med Assoc 2005; 293: 2479-2486. Also see www. Breastcancer.org

Holman, RT, Johnson SB, Ogburn PL. Deficiency of essential fatty acids and membrane fluidity during pregnancy and lactation. Proc Natl Acad Sci, USA, 1991; 88: 4835-9

Houston, MD, Strupp JS. Prevention and treatment of cancer: Is the cure in the produce aisle? JANA 2000; 3(3); 27-30.

Hu FB, et al. "Dietary Intake of Alpha-Linolenic Acid and Risk of Fatal Ischemic Heart Disease among Women," American Journal of Clinical Nutrition 69(5), 890-97, 1999.

Hudgins, LC, Hellerstein M. Seidman C, Hirsch J. Human fatty acid synthesis is stimulated by a eucaloric low-fat, high carbohydrate diet. Amer. J Clin Nutr, 1994; 60: 470-5.

Institute of Medicine: Committee on nutritional status during pregnancy and lactation. Nutrition during pregnancy: Part 1, Weight Gain: Part 2, Nutritional Supplement, Washington, DC: National Academy Press, 1990.

James, MJ, et al. Dietary polyunsaturated fatty acids and inflammatory mediator production. Am J CLIN Nutr 2000; 71(Suppl): 3435-3485.

Jankun, J. et al (1997). "Why drinking green tea could prevent cancer." Nature; 387 (6633): 561.

Jayagopal, V, Albertazzi P, Kilpatrick ES et al. Beneficial effects of soy phytoestrogen intake in postmenopausal women with type 2 diabetes. Diabetes Care. 2002 Oct; 25(10): 1709-14.

Also see: Laird Harrison (MSNBC staff writer): Soy Comparable to some Diabetes drugs. http://content.health.msn.com/content/article/48/39149.htm? Printing-true, 2002.

Jenkins, DJ, Axelsen M, et al. Dietary Fibre, lente carbohydrates and the insulin-resistant diseases. Br J Nutr 2000 Mar; 83 Suppl 1: S157-63.

Jenkins, DJ, et al. "Glycemic Index of Foods: A Physiological Basis for Carbohydrate Exchange." The American Journal of Clinical Nutrition, Vol. 34, March 1981, pp. 362-366

Johnson, SR, Kolberg BH, Varner MW, Railsback LD. Maternal obesity and pregnancy. Surg Gynecol Obstet. 1987; 164: 431-437.

Johnston, CS, Day CS, Swan PD. Postprandial thermogenesis is increased 100% on a high-protein, low-fat diet versus a high-carbohydrate, low-fat diet in healthy young women. J AM Coll Nutr. 2002; 21:55-61.

Kaizer, L, Boyd N, Tritchier D. Fish Consumption and Breast Cancer Risk: An Ecological Study. 1989. 12(1): pp. 61-68.

Kanter, M "Lower Cholesterol Naturally." Health Smart Today. Winter 2002-03. p 97

Kasim, SE. Dietary marine fish oils and insulin in type 2 diabetes. Annals of the New York Academy of Sciences, Vol 683, June 14, 1993. pp 250-57.

Keys, Ancel: Ancel B. Keys, Eat Well, Stay Well the Mediterranean Way. Garden City, New York: Doubleday, 1975.

Khan, A, Hermansen K, Rasmussen O, et al. Influence of ripeness of banana on the blood glucose and insulin response in type 2 diabetic subjects. Diabetes Med 1992 Oct; 9(8): 739-43.

Khan, A, Safdar M, Ali Khan MM, Khattak KN, Anderson RA. Cinnamon improves glucose and lipids of people with type 2 diabetes. Diabetes Care. 2003 Dec; 26 (12):3215-8

Kirschmann, G, Kirschmann JD. Nutrition Almanac, New York: McGraw Hill Book Co., 1996.

Kitzmiller, JL, Garin LA, Gin GD, et al. Preconception care of diabetes. Glycemic control prevents congenital anomalies. JAMA 1991, 265:731-736.

Kolata, G. Ultimate Fitness: The Quest for Truth about Exercise and Health. New York. Farrar, Straus and Giroux, 2003.

Krezowski, PA et al. The effect of protein ingestion on the metabolic response to oral glucose in normal individuals. Am J Clin Nutr 1996; 44: 847-56.

Krumhout, D, Bosschieter EB, Lezenne-Coulander C. "The inverse relation between fish consumption and 20 year mortality from coronary heart disease. New Engl. J. Med. 1985, 312, 1205-1209.

Kushi, LH, Folsom AR, Prineas RJ, Bostick RM. Dietary antioxidant vitamins and health from coronary heart disease in postmenopausal women. N Eng J Med, 1996; 334: 1156-62.

La Chance, PA. How should the food guide pyramid be updated? Food Tech. 2003; 57(7): 128.
Also see: Eller D. (Staff writer) "The absolute healthiest way to eat" (featuring Dr. David Heber and Professor Paul LaChance). New Women, August 1999.

Larosa, JC, Fry AG, Muesing R, Rosing. DR. Effects of high-protein, low-carbohydrate dieting on plasma lipoproteins and body weight. J Am Diet Assoc. 1980; 77: 264-70

Lasslo-Meeks, Millicent, MS, RD. Weight gain liabilities of psychotropic and seizure disorder medications: SCAN'S PULSE, WINTER 2001.

LaValle, James B. RPh. Belly Fat- when stress is the culprit: HearthSmart today, Winter 2002-03.

Layman, DK, Boileau RA, Erickson DJ et al "A reduced ratio of ratio of dietary carbohydrate to protein improves body composition and blood lipid profiles during weight loss in adult women." Journal of Nutrition (2003) 133: 411-417.

Leeds, AR. " Glycemic Index and heart disease." AJCN 76:1, p 286s-298s, July 2002.

Lin, HJ. et al. Glutathione transferase null genotype, broccoli and lower prevalence of colorectal adenomas. Cancer Epidemiol Boimarkers Prev. 1998 Aug; 7(8): 647-52.
Lin, HJ. et al. Glutathione transferase GSTT1, broccoli and prevalence of colorectal adenomas. Pharmacogenetics. 12(2): 175-179, March 2002.

Lin, YC. et al. (2000). "Dairy calcium is related to change in body composition during a two-year exercise intervention in young women." Journal of the American College of Nutrition; 19(6): 754-60.

Litin, L, Sacks F. Trans-fatty acid content of common foods. N Engl J Med, 1996; 329(26).

Liu, S, Manson JE, Buring, HE et al. Relation between a diet with a high glycemic load and plasma concentrations of high sensitivity C-reactive protein in middle-aged woman. Am J Clin Nutr (2002) 75(3): 492-498.

Liu, S, Stampfer MJ, Manson JE, Hu FB, Franz M, Hennekens CH, Willet WC. A prospective study of dietary glycemic load and risk of myocardial infarction in women. FASEB 1998; 124: A260 (abstract #1517).

Liu, S, Willet WC. Dietary glycemic load and atherothrombotic risk. Curr Atheroscler Rep. 2002;4(6):454-461.

Liu, S. Willet WC, Stampfer M, et al. A prospective study of dietary glycemic load, carbohydrate intake and risk of coronary heart disease in US women. Am J Clin Nutr 2000; 71(6):1455-61.
Also see: Liu, S. Diet, The Glycemic index and Coronary Heart Disease in the Nurses' Health Study. http//www.lipid.org/clinical/artcles/100004.php.

Ludwig, DS. The glycemic index: physiological mechanisms relating to obesity, diabetes and cardiovascular disease. JAMA. 2002;287(18):2414-2423.

Ludwig, DS. Dietary glycemic index and the regulation of body weight. Lipids. 2003;(2):117-121.

Lutz, CA, Przytulski KR. Nutrition and Diet Therapy, Philadelphia: FA Davis, 1994.

McArdle, WD, Katch FI, Katch VL. Essential of Exercise Physiology. Philadelphia: Lea and Febinger, 1994.

McCullough, ML., Feskanich D, Stampfer MJ, et al. Diet quality and major chronic disease risk in men and women: moving toward improved dietary guidance. Am J Clin Nutr 2002; 76:1261-71.

McDonalds Nutrition Facts. www.mcdonalds.com

McGee, D.L., et al. "Ten year incidence of Coronary Heart Disease in Honolulu Heart Program: Relationship to Nutrient Intake," American Journal of Epidemiology 119(5), 667-76, 1984.

Mckeown, NM et al. Carbohydrate Nutrition, Insulin Resistance and the Prevalence of the Metabolic Syndrome in the Framingham Offspring Cohort. Diabetes Care 2004 Feb; (2): 538-546.

Mendosa, R. Revised International Table of Glycemic Index (GI) and Glycemic Load (GL) values – 2002.
www.mendosa.com/gillists.htm.

Mensink, RP and Katan MB: effect of dietary trans fatty acids on high-density and low-density lipoprotein cholesterol levels in healthy subjects. New Engl J Med 323:439-45, 1990.

Messina, M, Messina V. The Simple Soybean and Your Health. Avery Publ. Comp; NY, 1994.

Messina, MJ, "Soy intake and cancer risk: a review of the in vitro and in vivo data," Nutrition and Cancer 21(2), 113-28, 1994.

Metzger, BE, Freinkel N: Amniotic fluid insulin as a predictor of obesity. Arch Dis Child 65: 1050-1052, 1990

Middleton, E. "Biological Properties of Plant Flavoniods: An overview" International Journal of Pharmacognosy (1996) 34: 344-348

Mimura, et al., "Nutritional factors for Longevity in Okinawa- Present and Future," Nutrition and Health 8(2-3), 159-63,1992.

Mokdad, AH. et al. (2001). The continuing epidemics of obesity and diabetes in the United States." JAMA; 286(10): 1195-1200.

Mokdad, AH. et al. "The spread and the obesity epidemic in the Untied States, 1991-1998," Journal of American Medical Association 282(16), 1519-22, 1999.

Montignac, Michael. Eat Yourself Slim. Baltimore: Erica House 1999.

Mori, TA, Bao DQ, et al. Dietary fish as a major component of weight-loss diet: effect on serum lipids, glucose and insulin metabolism in overweight hypertensive subjects. Am. J. Clinical Nutrition, November 1, 1999: 70(5): 817-825.

Moyad, MA. "Soy, Disease prevention and Prostate Cancer," Seminars in Urologic Oncology 17 (2), 97-102, 1999

Nestle, M. Broccoli sprouts in cancer prevention. Nutr Rev. 1998; 56:127-130.

Nettleton, J. Comparing nutrients in Wild and Farmed Fish. Aquaculture Magazine. Jan/Feb. 1999.

Netzer, Corinne T. The Complete Book of Food Counts. New York: Dell Publishing 2000

Nomura, AMY, Le Marchard L, Hankin JH. The effect of dietary fat on breast cancer survival among Caucasian and Japanese women in Hawaii. Breast Cancer Research and Treatment, 1991. 18: pp. S135-S141.

Nutritional Recommendation and Principles for Individuals with Diabetes Mellitus. American Diabetes Association Position Statement.
Diabetes Care, vol. 13, supp. 1, 1990.

Obesity Research, vol. 6 Suppl. 2 1998 Clinical Guidance on the Identification, Evaluation and Treatment of Overweight and Obesity in Adults – The Evidence Report.

Okuyama, H., et al. Dietary fatty acids- the N-6/N-3 balance and chronic elderly diseases. Excess linoleic acid and relative N-3 deficiency syndrome seen in Japan. Prog. Lipid Res, 1997; 3 (4): 409-457.

Olszewski, AJ. Fish oil decreases homocysteine in hyperlipemic men. Coron Arter Dis, 1993; 4:53-60.

Ornish, Dean. Eat More, Weigh Less. New York: Harper Perennial Library, 1994.

Patel, A et al. Exercise may lower breast cancer risk. Cancer, November 15, 2003. Also see: Exercise Helps Breast Cancer Fight (Medical Editor Q. Haney is a special correspondent for The Associated Press). Health. May 23, 2005.
http://www.aacr.org/2004AM/2004AMasp.
http://www.breastcancer.org/research_exercise_111503_pf.html.

Pavlov, K. et al. Exercise as an adjunct to weight loss and maintenance in moderately obese subjects. Am J Clin Nutr 1989; 49: 1115-23.

Peeke, Pamela, MD. Fight Fat after Forty: The Revolutionary Three-Pronged Approach that will Break your Stress-Fat Cycle and Make you Healthy, Fit and Trim for Life. New York: Viking Penguin, 2000.

Perricone, Nicholas, MD. The Perricone Prescription: A Physician's 28-Day Program For Total Body and Face Rejuvenation. New York: Harper Resource, 2002.

Pick, ME, Hawrysh ZJ, et al. Oat bran concentrate bread products improve long-term control of diabetes: A Pilot Study. J Am Diet Assoc 1996 Dec; 96(12):1254-61.

Pi-Sunyer, FX. "Glycemic Index and Disease." AJCN 76:1, p 290s-298s, July 2002.

Plumb GE. et al. Antioxidant properties of the major polyphrnolic compounds in broccoli. Free Radic Res, 1997 Oct, 27:4, 429-35.

Prakash, C, et al. Decreased systematic thromboxane A2 biosynthesis in normal human subjects fed a salmon-rich diet. *Am J Clin Nutr* 1994; 60:369-73.

Pucher, J, Dijkstra L. Making walking and cycling safer: Lessons from Europe. *Transpotation Quarterly* 2000; 54(3):25-50.

Pucher, J, Dijkstra L. Promoting Safe Walking and Cycling to Improve Public Health: Lessons from The Netherlands and Germany. American Journal of Public Health, Vol. 93, No. 9, September 2003.

Radack, K, Deck C, Huster G. Dietary Supplementation with low-dose fish oils lower fibrinogen levels: A Randomized, Double-Blind Controlled Study. Ann Int Med,1989; 11(9): 757-58

Rasmussen, O, Gregersen S. Influence of the amount of starch on the glycemic index to rice in non-insulin dependent diabetic subjects. Br J Nutr 1992; 67:371-7.

Ravussin, E, Bogardus C. Relationship of genetics, age and physical fitness to daily energy expenditure and fuel utilization. Am J Clin Nutr 1989; 49: 968-75.

Reaven, GM. "Pathophysiology of insulin resistance in human disease, " Physiological Reviews 75(3), 473-87, 1995

Reichman, Judith, MD. Slow Your Clock Down: The Complete Guide to a Healthy Younger You," William Morrow/HarperCollins, 2004. Also see " Is a glass of wine (or two) good for you? http://www.msnbc.msn.com/id/4779784/.

Ridker, PM et al. Inflammation, aspirin and the risk of cardiovascular disease in apparently healthy men. N Engl J Med, 1997; 336(14): 973-9
Rodale Press, 1981.

Ridker, PM, et al. C-reactive protein and other markers of inflammation in the prediction of cardiovascular disease in women. N Engl J Med 2000 Mar 23; 342 (12): 836-43.

Rolls, Barbara J, Barnett, R. Volumetric Weight-Control. HarperCollins Publisher, 2002.

Romieu, I. et al. Carbohydrates and the Risk of Breast Cancer among Mexican Women. Cancer Epidemiology Biomarkers and Prevention. Vol 13, 1283-1289, August 2004.

Salmeron, J, Manson JE, et al. Dietary fiber, glycemic load and risk of non-insulin dependent diabetes mellitus in women. JAMA 1997 Feb 12; 277 (6): 472-7

Salmeron, J, Manson JE, Willett WC. Dietary fiber, glycemic load and risk of non-insulin dependent diabetes mellitus in women. JAMA, 1997; 277(6): 472-477.

Samaha, FF, Iqbal N, Seshadri P, Chicano KL, Daily DA, McGroy J, et al. A low-carbohydrate as compared with a low-fat diet in severe obesity. N Engl J Med. 2003; 348: 2074-81.

Satter, E. Child of Mine: Feeding with love and good sense. Bull Publishing CO., 2000.

Schardt, D. Phytochemicals: plant against cancer. Nutr Action Health Lett 1994;21 (3): 1, 9-11.

Schlosser, E. Fast Food Nation: The Dark Side of the All-American Meal. New York: HarperCollins, 2002.

Schlundt, D. Randomized evaluation of a low-fat diet for weight reduction. Int J Obesity, 1993; 17: 623-629.

Schmidt, EB, Dyerberg J. Omega-3 fatty acids: Current status in cardiovascular medicine. Drugs 47: 405-24. 1994.

Sears, Barry. Enter the Zone. New York: HarperCollins, 1995.

Self-hypnosis may cut stress, boost immune system: http://www. reventdisease.com/news/article/hypnosis. See also Journal of consulting and clinical psychology 2001; 69.

Sena, Kathy. Avoid energy drainers: *Let's Live Magazine,* Aug. 1995

Sergio, AR et al.: B-carotene and other carotenoids as antioxidants. J Amer Coll Nutr. 1999; 18:426-433.

Serraino, M, Thompson, LU. The effect of flaxseed supplementation on early risk markers for mammary carcinogenesis. Cancer Lett 1991;60:135-42.

Shils, M, Olson JA. et al. Modern Nutrition in Health and Disease: Baltimore: Williams and Wilkins, 1999.

Simopoulos, AP. "Omega-3 fatty acids in health and disease and in growth and development." Am. J. Clin Nutr, 1991; 54-438-463.

Simopoulos, AP, Kifer RR, Barlow SM, Eds. Health effects of Omega-3 polyunsaturated fatty acids in seafoods. World Review of Nutrition and Diabetics, ed. Simopoulos AP. Vol.66.1991, Karger: Basal, p. 591.

Simopoulos, AP, Robinson J. The Omega Diet: The Lifelong Nutritional Program Based on the Diet of the Island of Crete. New York: Harper Collins, 1999

Sorisky, A, Robbins DC. Fish oil and diabetes. The net effect. Diabetes Care. 1989 Apr; 12(4): 302-4.

Stevens, LJ, et al. Omega-3 fatty acids in boys with behavior, learning and health problems. Physiology and behavior, 1996; 59(4/5): 915-20

Steward, Leighton H., Morrison C. et al. Sugar Busters! Cut Sugar to Trim Fat. New York: Ballantine 1999.

Steinmetz, K, Potter J. Vegetables, fruit and cancer. I. Epidemiology. Cancer Causes Control. 1991;2(Suppl):325-357.

Stitt, P. Factors in flaxseed that help prevent cancer: 52nd Annual Flax Institute of the United States, 40-42, 1988.

Stubbs, J. et al. Energy density of foods: effects on energy intake. Crit Rev Foods Sci Nutr. 2000;40:481-515.

Subway Nutritional Fact. http:// www.subway.com.

"Tea…can it save your life?" Health Smart Today. Winter 2002-03 p 26

The Complete Book of Minerals of Health. Prevention Magazine Staff. Emmaus, Pa: Rodale Press, 1981.

The New American Plate. The American Institute for Cancer Research. http://www.aicr.org/NAPbook.htm

The Oprah Winfrey Show. http://www.Oprah.com

Theriault, A, Chao J, et al. Tocotrienol: A Review of Its Therapeutic Potential. Clin Biochem, 1999; 32 (5): 309-319

Thompson, LU, Rickard SE, Seidl MM. Flaxseed and its lignan and oil components reduce mammary tumor growth at a late stage of carcinogenesis. Carcinogenesis, 1996; 17(6): 1373-1376.

Tomatoes, Lycopene and Prostate Cancer. Proceedings of the Society for Experimental Biology and Medicine 218, 129-39, 1998.

Torjesen, PA. et al. Lifestyle changes may reverse development of the insulin resistance syndrome. Diabetes care, 1997; 30: 26-31.

Trichopoulou, A, Katsouyanni K, Stuvers S, et al. Consumption of olive oil and specific food groups in relations to breast cancer risk in Greece. J Natl Cancer Inst 1995;87:110-16.

Upritchard, JE, Sutherland WHF, Mann, JI. Effect of supplementation with tomato juice, vitamin E and vitamin C on LDL oxidation and products of inflammatory activity in type 2 diabetes." Diabetes Care (2000) 23:733-738.

Veggie nutrients dip in tests. New House News Service, Washington, *Omaha World-Herald,* 6, January 29, 2000.

Vickers, MH, Breier BH, McCarthy D, Gluckman PD. Sedentary Behavior During Postnatal Life is Determined by the Prenatal Environment and Exacerbated by Postnatal Hypercaloric Nutrition. The American Journal of Physiology-Regulatory, Integrative and Comparative Physiology. July 2003.

Walford, RL et al, "Biosphere Medicine" as Viewed from the 2-year First Closure of Biosphere 2. Aviation, Space and Environmental Medicine 67: 609-617, 1996.

Walford, RL et al. Physiologic changes in humans subjected to severe, selective calorie restriction for two years in Biosphere 2: Health, Agina and Toxicologic Perspectives. Toxicological Sciences 52:61-65, 1999.

Walford, RL, Liu RK et al.: Longterm Dietary Restriction and Immune Function in Mice: Response to Sheep Red Blood Cells and to Mitogenic Agents. Mech. Aging and Development 2: 447- 454, 1974.

Wansink, Brian (1996), Does Package Size Accelerate Usage Volume? Journal of Marketing, 60(1), 1-14 or www.foodpsychology.com

Weil, Andrew, MD. Eating well for Optimum Health: The Essential Guide to Food, Diet and Nutrition. New York: Alfred A. Knopf, 2000.

Weil, Andrew. Spontaneous Healing: How to Discover and Enhance Your body's Natural Ability to maintain and Heal Itself. New York: Alfred A. Knopf, 1995.

Weindruch, R, Walford RL et al. The Retardation of Aging in Mice by Dietary Restriction: Longevity, Cancer, Immunity and Lifetime Energy Intake. J. Nutrition 116: 641-654, 1986.

Weindruch, R, Walford RL. Dietary Restriction of Mice Beginning at 1 Year of Age: Effect on Life-Span and Spontaneous Cancer Incidence. Science 215: 1415-1418, 1982.

Weisburger, JH et al. Tea polyphenols as inhibitors of mutagenecity of major classes of carcinogens. Mutat Res. 1996; 371: 57-63.

Weisburger, JH. Nutritional approach to cancer prevention with emphasis on vitamins, antioxidants and carotenoids. Am J Clin Nutr. 1991;53(Suppl):226S-237S.

Wendy Nutritional Fact. http:// www.Wendys.com.

Westman, EC, Yancy WS, Edman JS, Tomlin KF, Perkins CE. Effect of 6-month adherence to a very low carbohydrate diet program. Am. J. Med. 2002; 113: 30-6.

Westman, EC. A review of very low carbohydrate diets. Journal of Clinical Outcome Management. 1998; 6: 36-40.

Willcox, BJ, Willcox DC, Suzuki M. The Okinawa Diet Plan: Get Leaner, Live Longer and Never Feel Hungry. Clarkson- Potter/ Publishers, 2004.

Also see: Willcox, B. Living to 100: ABC Sydney. http://www. abc.net.au/sydney/stories/s1329191.htm.

Willet, WC, Manson J, Liu S. Glycemic index, glycemic load and risk of type 2 diabetes. AJCN. 2002; 76(1): 274S-280S.

Willet, WC, Stamper MJ, Speizer FE. Relation of meat, fat and fiber intake to the risk of colon cancer in a prospective study among women. N Eng J Med. 1990.Dec.

Willett, WC. "Intake of trans fatty acids and risk of coronary heart disease among women. Lancet, 1993, 341, 581-585

Willett, WC. Eat, Drink and Be Healthy: The Harvard Medical School Guide to Healthy Eating. Simon and Schuster, NY. 2001.
Also see http://www. hsph.Harvard.edu/nutritionsource/pyramids.html.

Womersley, Tara. Three glasses of wine a day "a health risk". http:// www. news.scotsman.com/index.cfm?id=427712004.

World Cancer Research Fund. Food, nutrition and the prevention of cancer. A global perspective. Washington D.C. American Institute for Cancer Research. 1997.

Wu, D, et al. Effect of dietary supplementation with black currant seed oil on the immune response of healthy elderly subjects. American Journal of Clinical Nutrition 1999;70:536-543.

Yam, D, Eliraz A, Eliraz B, Elliot M. Diet and Disease – The Israeli Paradox: Possible dangers of a high Omega-6 polyunsaturated fatty acid diet. Isr J Med Sci; 1996; 32: 1134-1143.

Yehuda, S, Mostofsky DI, Eds. Essential Fatty Acid Biology: Biochemistry, Physiology and Behavioral Neurobiology. Human Press, Totowa, New Jersey, 1997

Yoon, S, et al. "The therapeutic effect of evening primrose oil in atropic dermatitis. Patients with dry scaly skin lesions are associated with the normalization of serum gamma-interferon levels." Skin pharmacol Apply skin Physiol, 2002; 15(1): 20-25

Zurier, RB, Rossetti RG, et al. Gamma-linolenic acid treatment of rheumatoid arthritis. A randomized, placebo-controlled study. Arthritis and Rheumatism, 1996; 11:1808-1817.

# Index

## #



## A



## B



## C



## D

## E



## F



## G



## H



## I



## J



## L



## M

## T



## U



## V



## W